Praise for
Hard to Bear

'In *Hard to Bear* Isabelle Oderberg manages to weave expert research into a personal narrative of grief, hope, and love. It is an important book that reveals the personal heartbreak of miscarriages and the way it fundamentally changes a life beyond the narrow clinical view of just a "cluster of cells". Yet, in all the grief, the heartbreak, and the feeling of being unseen and unheard, Isabelle's book is more. It is also about joy and grace. The joy of family, and friends, and all the tiny moments that call us away from grief. It is finally arriving at the grace of treating ourselves more kindly, knowing that the healing we desperately sought, the hope that there will be a time when the pain is all gone, shouldn't be the intention, even, when things are hard to bear.'

— **Nyadol Nyuon, lawyer and human rights activist**

'Told with love, sass and journalistic rigour, this courageous and compelling book will be a lifeline for so many families whose grief and loss has for too long been unspeakable.'

— **Jess Hill, author of *See What You Made Me Do***

'An unbeatable combination of compassion and courage, help and hope.'

— **Kaz Cooke, author of *Up the Duff* and *You're Doing it Wrong***

'In *Hard to Bear*, Isabelle Oderberg shines a light on the lamentable lack of care and attention paid to miscarriage – by medicine, governments and society at large. Her personal testimony keeps you gripped to the story while the science and wide-ranging interviews have you growling in shock and anger at the incredible lack of knowledge surrounding pregnancy loss – and the easy dismissal it sometimes receives from those who should know better. This incredible book should be another nail in the coffin to medical misogyny worldwide.'

— **Gabrielle Jackson, author of *Pain and Prejudice***

'This book runs loudly and proudly towards a topic we too easily ignore.'

– Gina Rushton, author of *The Most Important Job in the World*

'Funny, wise and forensically researched. *Hard to Bear* is brilliant.'

– Samantha Maiden

'With a journalist's passion for research, combined with the painful knowledge of lived experience, Isabelle Oderberg unpacks the silence, shame, and medical failures around the remarkably common experience of miscarriage. Fierce, frank and deeply compassionate, *Hard to Bear* is a long overdue reckoning with early pregnancy loss. This book will be a salve to thousands and propel a much-needed cultural conversation. Oderberg is the warrior we need to give miscarriage the attention it deserves.'

– Yves Rees, author of *All About Yves*

'Reading Isabelle Oderberg's remarkable *Hard to Bear*, I was struck by two words, shame and secrecy, and asked myself a question. How is it possible, when considering the loss of a new life through miscarriage that I would think so much about the raw emotions underpinning such loaded terms? Particularly when *Hard to Bear* is essentially a work dealing with love and grief. Isabelle Oderberg has managed to present us with a work of great care, while confronting us with the experiences of women who having suffered deeply, are sometimes punished further. We all need to read this book and shift the ways in which we value all life, old and new.'

– Tony Birch, author of *Dark as Last Night* and *The White Girl*

Hard to Bear

Investigating the science and
silence of miscarriage

Isabelle Oderberg

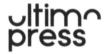

'I Celebrate Your Life, My Baby' quoted with permission: (Judith Durham/Rachel Stanfield-Porter/Simon Barnett), Musicoast © 1998. Words by Judith Durham, Rachel Stanfield-Porter & Simon Barnett. Music by Judith Durham.

'Brick House' Written by Lionel Richie, Milan Williams, Ronald LaPread, Thomas McClary, Walter Orange and William King © Brenda Richie Publishing / Jobete Music Co Inc. / Libren Music / Old Fashion Publishing / Cambrae Music / Macawrite Music / Walter Orange Music / Hanna Music. Licensed by EMI Music Publishing Australia Pty Limited International copyright secured. All rights reserved. Used by permission.

'failing' by j wallace skelton in *Interrogating Pregnancy Loss* quoted with permission from Demeter Press.

Gravidity and Parity by Eleanor Jackson quoted with permission from Vagabond Press.

Published in 2023 by Ultimo Press,
an imprint of Hardie Grant Publishing

Ultimo Press	Ultimo Press (London)
Gadigal Country	5th & 6th Floors
7, 45 Jones Street	52–54 Southwark Street
Ultimo, NSW 2007	London SE1 1UN
ultimopress.com.au	

   ultimopress

 A catalogue record for this book is available from the National Library of Australia

Hard to Bear
ISBN 978 1 76115 050 0 (paperback)

Cover design Alissa Dinallo
Cover artwork Amy Hiley
Text design Simon Paterson, Bookhouse
Typesetting Bookhouse, Sydney | 11.75/15.75 pt Bembo MT Pro
Copyeditor Deonie Fiford
Proofreader Rebecca Hamilton

10 9 8 7 6 5 4 3 2 1

Printed in Australia by Griffin Press, an Accredited ISO AS/NZS 14001 Environmental Management System printer.

 The paper this book is printed on is certified against the Forest Stewardship Council® Standards. Griffin Press holds chain of custody certification SCS-COC-001185. FSC® promotes environmentally responsible, socially beneficial and economically viable management of the world's forests.

Ultimo Press acknowledges the Traditional Owners of the Country on which we work, the Gadigal People of the Eora Nation and the Wurundjeri People of the Kulin Nation, and recognises their continuing connection to the land, waters and culture. We pay our respects to their Elders past and present.

Hard to Bear was written on Boonwurrung Country.

*For Jack, Royston, Roxie-Rose, Mum, Dad, Jules
and the seven magical angels who complete my circle.
I love each of you more than words could ever say.*

Hope deferred sickens the heart,
But desire realised is a tree of life.

תוחלת ממשכה מחלה־לב ועץ חיים
תאוה באה

PROVERBS 13:12

Contents

PREFACE

It's Only the Beginning

'Few subjects of such clinical importance as the factors associated with recurrent miscarriage are so bedevilled by inconsistency, imprecision and unwarranted assumption.'

G.M. Stirrat[1]

'If women were educated about miscarriage in school, then *this* wouldn't happen,' the doctor said, gesturing towards me. All of me. 'You'd know miscarriage was just a normal, natural thing that's supposed to happen and you wouldn't be crying about it.'

It was June 2018. I was in the middle of my sixth miscarriage, sitting in a chair, bleeding, cramping and sobbing into a tissue. I was in the office of one of Melbourne's most pre-eminent obstetricians. A Cervical Celebrity.

As I walked out of his office, paid my bill and dragged myself towards my car, keeping my head down because my eyes were as puffy as campfire marshmallows, I had a moment of clarity, through the grief and the hormones.

This obstetrician spoke as a clinician who views a miscarriage solely through a scientific lens; a loss like mine was simply a chromosomally challenged cluster of cells, not compatible with life and requiring expulsion or removal. This man had delivered hundreds, possibly thousands, of babies and he was one of the best in the state, possibly the country.

But I also knew he'd never felt a baby move inside him; he'd never felt that magical connection, then lost it.

A miscarriage is a full stop, when you want to keep reading.

There would be no happy ending with a perfect cherub in my arms, keeping me awake at night, giggling at me as I blow raspberries on her tummy, and peppering my life with the hilarity of projectile vomiting and explosive poonamis.

This was a feeling that the obstetrician would never understand and, despite decades working in obstetrics, it wasn't something he was trying very hard to understand. A doctor doesn't have to be female or have experienced pregnancy to show compassion or empathy and provide high-quality care, but all doctors have to listen. And there wasn't a lot of listening going on in that room.

Even though I have come to understand what he was trying to tell me, his gruff dismissal of my grief is only one example of how I felt unsupported in the midst of this loss. And it's a common experience.

I think many people, especially doctors, would be horrified if they truly understood some of the trauma they're causing their patients with their words, actions or inaction.

Patients and those close to them are routinely failed in myriad ways before, during and after miscarriage. They may be failed by medical specialists, a lack of medical knowledge or a lack of answers to better explain their situation. Or maybe it's a lack of understanding from partners, friends and family. The loss associated with miscarriage can be debilitating and affect all areas of a person's health: physical, psychological, emotional, spiritual and social.

In Australia, a conservative estimate is that each and every year at least 103,000 families experience miscarriage; the definition of miscarriage being the loss of a pregnancy before twenty weeks of gestation.

A vicious catch-22 applies to miscarriage and pregnancy loss. It is the most common 'complication' of pregnancy, and yet due to its prevalence there is a level of complacency and dismissiveness towards it, despite the trauma it can cause, both physically and mentally.

I found it absolutely fascinating when I read the autobiography of one of Australia's most renowned obstetricians, Professor Caroline De Costa. The book traversed her entire career across multiple continents and all the different cases she treated. Stillbirth? Yes. Fistulas? Yes. C-section versus vaginal birth? Yes. She opined extensively on her activism around abortion rights. But nothing about miscarriage.

In 2020, non-profit health service provider Jean Hailes for Women's Health added some questions about miscarriage to its national survey. It found that among almost 4500 respondents from around Australia who had been pregnant, more than a third had experienced miscarriage, with that number rising to over 40 per cent among those with a disability. Almost 60 per cent of respondents overall said they had not been given enough information about miscarriage (or stillbirth) to manage their loss.

We are failing people who experience pregnancy loss, whether they have that experience directly, or as a partner, a family member or as a part of an extended support network. We are failing them in almost every aspect of their care.

Early pregnancy loss can lead to severe depression, PTSD, anxiety or even suicide. A lack of cohesive and effective public health policy, and the related deficiencies in care, can compound the trauma and related fallout. It can even affect the way we parent subsequent children, if we are able to conceive successfully. It can be a potential marker for other adverse pregnancy outcomes such as preterm birth and increase a patient's likelihood of heart attack, thrombosis or stroke later in life.

But the good news is: we can fix this. There is a way forward. And that's what I aim to deliver with *Hard to Bear*.

This book is – as all investigation or analysis should be – underpinned by a broad and diverse range of lived experience. Not just mine, but the hundreds of people I have engaged with over the past eight years. Whether a person has experienced one loss or seven, there are commonalities in that experience that weave their way through almost all the stories I hear, in the grief, the loss and, far too often, the disappointment from failures in care. In order for people to share completely and honestly, many names have been changed to protect privacy or the privacy of family or treating doctors. I have also made a concerted effort to include as broad a range of experiences as possible; miscarriage affects all people, no matter their gender, sexual orientation, ethnicity, colour of their skin, class, religion, disability or any other aspect of their identity or reality.

While the Cervical Celebrity wounded me with his dismissal of my grief and my experience of loss, he also gave me a great gift: the desire to write this book and find a way to improve care in every way for all people affected by early pregnancy loss.

Between each chapter of journalistic reportage, you will find snippets of my own story. I felt it was important to understand that my all-encompassing drive to change the status quo around early pregnancy loss was fuelled by my own lived experience. These vignettes aim to offer a context and insight into what has propelled this quest: the ugly, the bad and, importantly, the good.

INTRODUCTION

Hello

Most people are aware of the culture of silence around miscarriage. People don't sit around over a coffee talking openly and at length about miscarriage, unless perhaps you're a counsellor, nurse or doctor. Yet, according to the most commonly accepted statistic, at least one in four of your friends who have been pregnant have experienced miscarriage, as well as others who weren't even aware they were pregnant.

Many of the people I talk to who have experienced miscarriage say they felt an overwhelming disbelief when told they were losing their pregnancy. We're taught from a young age that pregnancy equals a baby. We're never taught about the alternative scenarios and, even as adults, we rarely talk about it. The taboo persists. Often even the nuts and bolts of miscarriage – the different ways that loss materialises and the steps we take to medically treat it – are misunderstood, if known at all.

So this is what I like to call the nuts and bolts section. The building blocks of understanding. The tools you need for the journey.

Pregnancies are dated using the first day of the patient's last period. But life doesn't always go according to plan and sometimes it's difficult to know that date or what date a pregnancy may have been conceived. Not all conceptions are on an anniversary, a birthday or Valentine's Day, or if you've been together a while or already have kids, that one day a month you put aside for 'adult time'.

Today, early scans can assist with both dating and monitoring early pregnancy progression and fetal and placental growth. From six to ten weeks gestation, if you need or choose to have a scan, it will often be internal, and called a transvaginal ultrasound (later it's the more common ultrasound on the abdomen). This is conducted using a large probe inserted into the vagina. Often a condom and lubricant are placed over the probe.

I am proud to say there wasn't a single occasion when I was given a transvaginal scan that I didn't crack a joke to the ultrasonologist about buying me dinner first. That's true commitment to a gag – I had well over twenty internal scans through the course of my many, many pregnancies.

Unless there are any serious concerns, it's preferred that first pregnancy scans take place from six weeks gestation, because there isn't much to see before then, and by that stage you should, in theory but not always, be able to see a fetal heartbeat.

What even is a miscarriage?

Put quite simply, a miscarriage is when a pregnancy 'fails' before you hit twenty weeks gestation. It is usually marked by a lack of development or slow growth, either of the fetus or of a gestational sac.

Interestingly, not all countries have the same definition. For instance, in the UK pregnancy loss is defined as a miscarriage until twenty-four weeks, but a loss after twenty weeks in Australia is called a stillbirth. Where stillbirth is mentioned, I will reference it specifically, but in these pages when I write about pregnancy loss or miscarriage, I am referring to loss at or before twenty weeks of gestation.

Medically, a miscarriage is classified as a 'pregnancy complication', even though it actually means a pregnancy is ending, not that things are getting a little tricky. It is, in fact, the world's most common 'pregnancy complication', diagnostically speaking.

Sometimes there is bleeding. Sometimes not. Sometimes there is cramping, sometimes not. These can all be common signs that your pregnancy is coming to a premature end. But here's the rub: those symptoms can also be a normal part of pregnancy. The only way to confirm a miscarriage is by a scan, two blood tests a few days apart that confirm a drop in the pregnancy hormone hCG (human chorionic gonadotropin) or, to put it bluntly, expulsion of the fetus.

It's not an exact science (nothing ever is, apparently) but hCG – the hormone produced by the trophoblast cells which become the placenta in early pregnancy after implantation – should approximately double every two to three days in the first four weeks of a pregnancy. After six weeks it doubles every ninety-six hours, until twelve weeks, when it starts to tail off.

A single hCG test can confirm the presence of a pregnancy. But two blood tests a few days apart can establish whether the growth of the placenta is progressing at a healthy rate. If the numbers come up short, it can sometimes be the first indication that a pregnancy may end in loss.

Eight roads to grief

Broadly speaking, there are eight kinds of miscarriage:

- A *chemical pregnancy* ends before reaching five weeks of gestation.
- A *missed* or *delayed miscarriage* is when a pregnancy has stopped growing or an embryo has failed to develop and your body hasn't realised yet. The news they're having a miscarriage can often come as a complete surprise to the patient because often there's no reason to think anything is wrong.
- A *blighted ovum* is when a pregnancy has a gestational sac but no fetus. It can also be called an 'anembryonic pregnancy' because there's no embryo.
- A *threatened miscarriage* is another way for doctors to say they have a hunch you're having – or are going to have – a miscarriage, but they're not game to confirm it. Threatened miscarriages do not

always progress to miscarriage, they do sometimes resolve as viable pregnancies.

- A *complete miscarriage* means the entire pregnancy has left your body.
- An *ectopic pregnancy* occurs when an embryo implants outside of the uterus, often in the fallopian tube.
- A *molar pregnancy* (hydatidiform mole) is caused by a placenta that develops in an irregular way, with little sacs of fluid, a bit like a bunch of grapes. Molar pregnancies are surgically removed. In some cases the placenta can become malignant and develop into a rare form of cancer called choriocarcinoma.
- Finally, there is *recurrent miscarriage*, classified as either two or three consecutive miscarriages, depending on who you're asking.

There is a glossary at the back of this book, which goes into more detail around each type of miscarriage, as well as the inclusion of a host of other terms, should you lose track (like I did multiple times while writing this book).

So, what now?

Treatment options for miscarriage depend on a variety of factors, including what sort of miscarriage you are having, your medical history, your psychology, your personal preference and sometimes the preferences and beliefs of your treating doctor. Equally there's a persistent misconception that miscarriages happen quickly. Sometimes they do, but in some cases they can take weeks or longer to be complete.

When I had the absolute privilege of interviewing Professor Arri Coomarasamy, one of the world's leading miscarriage researchers and the director of Tommy's National Centre for Miscarriage Research, he told me the reason he decided to become a miscarriage specialist.

'It started when I was a junior doctor and I would work in a delivery suite and there would be a mother who might have sadly had a stillbirth and I would see the care that they would receive; tender, loving, very involved, totally compassionate, as it should be,' he said.

'And then you might be called away to the early pregnancy unit, you will see a woman who's had a miscarriage and it's the total opposite. The healthcare providers don't take the time. They don't seem to appreciate that the woman has gone through a major life event . . . it would be verging on a dismissive level of care really, and this would be the same clinician.'

Best-practice treatment for a miscarriage is to offer one of three options, with the patient making the decision about which route to take, with advice from their doctor. The first is to wait to pass the miscarriage naturally, as you would a period (expectant management). The second is to take medication to bring on the miscarriage (medical management). The final option is a surgical intervention to end the pregnancy (surgical management).

In the case of a missed miscarriage or a blighted ovum, sometimes the bleeding starts a few days or weeks after the patient is even aware of their loss or the bleeding may have already started. If not, you may choose or be required to take medication to bring it on. The medication used is called misoprostol, which causes the uterus to contract. There is debate as to whether it should be used with the progesterone-blocker mifepristone for miscarriage management – the two are often used together for medical abortions – but at the moment, Australian clinical guidelines only specify the use of misoprostol in miscarriage management.

Until twelve weeks gestation, the surgical procedure to end a pregnancy is a Dilation and Curettage (D&C). After twelve weeks the procedure is a Dilation and Evacuation (D&E). It is similar to a D&C, but the doctor may also use medical instruments like forceps to remove some tissue.

Late miscarriages are less common and take place in the second trimester (fourteen weeks onwards). In those cases, a parent may need to 'give birth' to their child or children. This can be incredibly traumatic for some, but it can also be welcomed by others if they want a chance to say goodbye.

Both surgical assistance and the prospect of passing the miscarriage at home (with or without medication) can be confronting.

There is no compelling evidence that one method of management is superior to another, but there is a minor risk with expectant management or medication-induced miscarriage that the process will be incomplete and you will still need a surgical intervention. According to a 2012 examination of risks around miscarriage management, the researchers concluded, 'Given the evidence, women's preferences should play a large role in management plans.'[2]

That doesn't stop some medical professionals – or the system itself – exerting a degree of undue influence over the choices people make when faced with these decisions during their time of grief. Family and friends can also exert pressure to choose a specific treatment. Ultimately, while the choice of treatment should be informed or advised by the treating doctor, the final decision should be the patient's alone.

I've chosen to have D&Cs and I've chosen to have miscarriages at home by myself. Each loss is different. Each has different circumstances and contexts. There is no one-size-fits-all strategy for dealing with pregnancy loss. A D&C or D&E are considered relatively minor procedures with low risk, but no matter how small, all surgical procedures come with risk. They are conducted under a general anaesthetic and although complications are rare they include bleeding, infection, uterine perforation or damage to surrounding pelvic organs.

•

I can't find any record indicating when pregnant women started comparing fetus sizes to edibles, though admittedly I got distracted and needed a snack. But it definitely seems de rigueur nowadays to compare your unborn baby to food. Probably because comparing it to something you handle every day can help give what sometimes feels like an unfathomable concept – another human growing inside you – some semblance of reality.

The first twelve weeks of a pregnancy sees rapid growth of a baby, which progresses from being a cluster of cells to a fully formed fetus by week twelve; at seven weeks the baby is the size of a blueberry and six weeks later the size of a lemon. (Our first living child was initially dubbed Oliver Prunus – we had downloaded an app that gave his size at the time as somewhere between an olive and a prune.)

Women constantly face pressure to do things 'naturally', including giving birth. This can sometimes translate to 'vigorous' encouragement that patients pass miscarriages naturally. But many patients are not warned about what's involved with this process. Essentially you go into labour and birth the fetus at home. If the embryo is the size of a poppy seed (four weeks) this may mean passing primarily the lining of the uterus and some clots, which can be quite large and alarming. If, however, the fetus is the size of a raspberry (eight weeks) or an olive (nine weeks) or even a plum (twelve weeks), there is a very good chance the fetus can be seen or, in some cases like mine, identified and held.

Part of the trauma can come from being unprepared for all that this entails. Some patients are simply told to go home and wait to miscarry, but not given any real insight into what that really means, what will happen and what they may see. 'I wasn't expecting the pain to be that strong,' Cassie told me. 'I didn't want to take Nurofen because I was still pregnant and you can't take Nurofen. So I only took Panadol. And yeah, I was screaming in pain, it felt like I was giving birth, that kind of contraction.'

Quite apart from the psychological effect of being totally unprepared to birth a fetus at home, there's also physical risk if people are sent home to 'ride out' a miscarriage naturally or wait for a D&C, without being properly informed of the risks or things to look out for. Some miscarriages can develop serious complications.

One of those potential complications is haemorrhaging. If you're passing a miscarriage, there's going to be bleeding. While every miscarriage is different, and each patient can experience different levels of bleeding, there is a point where you can bleed too much. If a patient bleeds through a pad in less than two hours, they need to see a doctor. If they bleed through a large pad in less than an hour they need emergency medical attention.

Another aspect of the bleeding that can be especially frightening is the clots. These can vary in size and are undeniably gruesome – especially when you're not expecting them. If the clots resemble the size of a golf ball, a patient should seek medical attention. But a clot the size of a marble? Well, that's not a problem. Not medically, anyway.

Getting down to the nitty gritty

Let's now turn our attention to the clinical definition of miscarriage and how it is formally diagnosed. Which – be warned – can be confronting.

For a pregnancy to be clinically recognised, it means that it has either been seen on an ultrasound or that the 'products of conception' have been identified. The products of conception are placental or fetal tissue. While 'products of conception' is the medically preferred term in Australia, I will be using the term used by Tommy's National Centre for Miscarriage Research, which is 'pregnancy tissue'.

This means the clinical definition does not include pregnancies that were confirmed at home with a home pregnancy test or with a urine test at the GP. It wouldn't include those who knew they were pregnant and then miscarried at home in private. Not all people have access to early ultrasounds. Or access to any ultrasounds at all. This particularly affects people of lower incomes or in regional or remote areas where services are thin on the ground.

While going from a positive pregnancy test to no detectable pregnancy may result in a doctor assessing that you 'probably' had a miscarriage, it's not enough, even with other context, to acknowledge clinically that a miscarriage has occurred.

False-positive pregnancy tests are rare. A test confirms the presence of hCG, which is only present when there is a pregnancy. Where false-positives do occur, they are usually because the body hasn't yet cleared the presence of hCG after a previous loss.

A much more likely incorrect reading is a false-negative, when someone tests too early in the cycle and a test comes up negative even though there is a pregnancy present, because the hCG is too low to get a positive reading.

We will return to the topic of how miscarriage is clinically diagnosed in chapter three, because it's an issue central to my questions around data collection, on which public health policy must be built.

What's in a name?

In assessing what a miscarriage is and how we define it, we need to briefly touch on the clinical name for early pregnancy loss, because it isn't miscarriage.

Back in 1985, a letter arrived at the offices of renowned medical journal *The Lancet* in London. The letter had been written by three doctors from the Department of Obstetrics and Gynaecology at St Mary's Hospital Medical School in London. The lead author was Professor R.W. Beard and the letter presented a request to the medical fraternity: 'It is curious that, in a language as descriptively rich as English, no clear distinction is made between a spontaneous and an induced expulsion of the contents of the uterus in early pregnancy, whereas the French have the words *fausse-couche* and *avortement*.'[3]

What he was referring to was the formal medical terminology for miscarriage, which was, and still is in Australia, a 'spontaneous abortion'. He continued: 'Doctors use the word "abortion" regardless of whether it was a spontaneous or induced event, yet our patients always speak of "miscarriages" unless they have had a termination of pregnancy.'

The letter spoke about the doctors' deep admiration for the pain women and their partners endure after miscarriage, especially recurrent miscarriage: 'It is remarkable how uncomplaining these women are, but one constant comment they make is how deeply offended they are by the use of the word abortion to describe their condition.'

It ended: 'We hope that your readers will agree that a change from "abortion" to "miscarriage" is not just a semantic quibble but is well-justified on humanitarian grounds.'

As late as 1998, thirteen years after Professor Beard's letter to *The Lancet*, the Royal College of Obstetricians and Gynaecologists in the UK was (again) advised to change the use of this term to 'miscarriage' or 'early pregnancy loss', which it did.[4] In Australia the phrase 'spontaneous abortion' is still used in research, as well as teaching, which is deeply concerning.

Some of the doctors I've spoken to in America have even stopped using the word 'miscarriage' reasoning that it implies wrongdoing and encourages self-blame. I did an informal poll in an Australian feminist doctors' group with the help of a friend and the overwhelming consensus was that the term 'miscarriage' should continue to be used, as some patients (and doctors) find the term 'early pregnancy loss' too clinical.

In my many interviews with doctors from all around Australia, they tell me they would never use 'spontaneous abortion' in front of patients.

But unfortunately, it's a case of best practice not translating into real life, because I have had this terminology used in my presence, as have many of my interviewees, and I've seen it used repeatedly when reading about pregnancy loss.

My concern around the use of this phrase is that it feeds into dangerous church-based cultural themes of blame and intent around women and pregnancy loss – a topic we will look at in more detail in chapter one.

For now, all we can do is acknowledge that the totally inappropriate terminology of 'spontaneous abortion' remains officially unchanged in Australia, which has never followed the precedent set by its peers in the UK and elsewhere. Until it shifts, the language will continue to slip into doctors' and nurses' interactions in front of or with patients and further compound the confusion and grief of loss.

Lady Sings the Blues

I was bleeding. Not a heavy bleed like a period, it was more like a watery bleed. How I imagined amniotic fluid to look. It was light pink and there was enough of it for my brain to register that I was unlikely to be getting good news today.

I had to go back to the front desk and ask for a pad, but hyperventilation kicked in midway through my sentence. I whispered that I 'needed a pad because I was . . . BLEEDING'. The last word exploded out of my mouth like a cannonball and the whole room fell silent. Every eye turned to me and I felt their pity soaking through my skin. I wanted to scream, but instead I focused on not passing out as panic set in and I struggled for a lungful of air.

The nurse blanched and ran out the back to grab a pad, came back, put her arm around me and steered me into a separate waiting room. The night before the appointment, my friend Melissa had told me she was coming with me. I insisted I was fine, but she wasn't asking for permission. Now I called her from the private room. She rushed to park and arrived as I was called in for my scan.

The doctor doing the scan was sympathetic and kind. She inserted the huge wand, covered in a condom and lubricant, and a bubble came up on screen. The gestational sac. She showed me gently where it was collapsing in on itself and explained that's why the bleeding had started. It looked like a used tissue, crumpled and tossed in a corner. A corner of my body. I'd been holding on to hope, swollen in my chest. And at that moment, reality set in and the balloon of hope burst. A miscarriage. I was having a miscarriage.

I remember howling. A noise I had never made before. Involuntary and completely uncontrollable. Despite my embarrassment, I couldn't stop. I remember Melissa crying and squeezing my shoulder. I remember the doctor's stricken, grey face and her repeating, 'I'm sorry, I'm so sorry,' as she moved the wand around, her eyes searching the screen for anything that would make her diagnosis wrong. There was nothing.

I was taken back to the private room while they called the locum who was covering for my doctor, Dr Stan, because he was on holiday on the Gold Coast. I remember calling my acting manager at the office. A staunch and no bullshit doyen of publishing, he doesn't appreciate things like 'tears' in the workplace. He was unflinchingly kind and told me not to come back to work until I was ready.

After a few minutes, the locum was put through to the phone in the room. It was a doctor I didn't know. A doctor I had never spoken to before. It was no one's fault, but it was less than ideal.

This was the first time I'd been pregnant. I'd spent my whole life trying not to get pregnant but now, happy and in love, I'd slipped up, though it was a happy slip-up as we'd planned to have kids later that year. The truth was, though, my decision to start a family had been made several years earlier.

||||||

The seed was first planted, as all the best seeds are, on a boozy night out. A close friend of mine, Geoff, a high-flying bachelor journalist I'd worked with in London, came to visit in 2009. He stayed a couple of weeks and took me to a fancy, ludicrously overpriced (if you weren't earning English pounds sterling) Japanese restaurant to say thank you. We drank all the sake and we ate all the fishy things and when we got home we danced around the living room with my one-eyed pug Bronson and talked about all the most important things that besties talk about.

'I just don't want to die and have my gravestone say "she was a great journalist",' I told him. 'I want it to say that I loved and I was loved.'

'Don't be ridiculous, Isy,' he scolded in his Pommy accent. 'There is nothing more important than being a journalist.'

Eight years later Geoff was stabbed in a terrorist attack at our old stomping ground in London Bridge. As he lay recovering in hospital, he messaged me because he couldn't talk. He'd changed his mind; journalism wasn't everything. There was more to life. But I'd already figured that out for myself.

|||||||

My own realisation that I wanted something more than a stellar career to cuddle at night was cast in stone in 2014, when I was thirty-four years old. I told my mum I was ready to have a family, with or without a partner. Well, I didn't so much 'tell her' as 'accidentally float the idea aloud' while visiting her in Hong Kong, where she lived with my dad and where I had grown up.

'Why don't you just go to a club and take a guy home and fuck them?' she shouted at me over the terrible pop music and racks of spandex miniskirts in an H&M store.

'Mum, I can't do that. What if the baby eventually wanted to meet their dad? What would I say? Plus, I want a baby, not an STD that makes my clitoris fall off.'

What I didn't expect was such an enthusiastic response. I really shouldn't have been surprised, my parents have never been what I would describe as conventional. But I was still proud that she wasn't fazed by my planned abandonment of the nuclear family option. Her excitement didn't make a difference to my decision-making, but it did help me understand how much she wanted me to be a mother and it helped me find comfort in my own parental aspirations.

By then I had spent close to two decades working as a journalist in London and Melbourne and a few other places in between. I had risen to the highest levels of where I wanted to go. I had broken stories, pioneered new methods of reporting, sat in a room with Rupert Murdoch to shoot the breeze and met more than my fair share of celebrities and politicians.

But after years of dating, or perhaps a better expression would be 'attempted dating', I had come to the conclusion that, while I'd had long-term relationships, everything I had achieved in my life

I had ultimately done on my own. I knew that I was what you might call 'a handful' and I was starting to wonder whether there was a man on Earth who wanted to be with a successful, independent, stubborn woman like me. I wasn't prepared to wait to find out.

As much as my mum and I fight like two wasps trapped in a jam jar, we are incredibly close and having her blessing to have a baby on my own helped the idea crystallise in my mind. Suddenly I was excited. And I don't mess around.

||||||

As part of the preparation for intrauterine insemination (IUI), I had to attend a mandatory counselling session. Mum came along and I asked her how it felt knowing I'd never partner after I had a child. She started cackling. 'Why on Earth would you think that?'

I shrugged. 'Well, no one's going to want to partner with a single mum.'

She laughed again. (All this laughter was starting to get a little irritating.) 'Darling, look at the divorce rate! If guys don't want to be with single mums, it's going to be slim pickings,' she reasoned.

I realised that any man I wanted to be with would be impressed I'd decided to have a baby on my own instead of waiting for a man to help me achieve my dream of having a family. For years my mum had told me she was tired of me dating boys and it was time to date men. Someone who could be, and was looking for, a true equal – a strong, independent woman with things to do and places to be.

So if I was going to be a single mum, I was going to do it my way. Several friends offered to donate sperm, but I politely declined. As the daughter of two lawyers, I wanted this experience to be completely kosher and not have a friend suddenly decide they wanted to co-parent with me. It's difficult enough to co-parent with someone you love.

In 2014 I went to Melbourne IVF. Three months after that I chose my donor, and eight weeks after that I was having IUI, the medical version of a turkey baster. As I sat in the doctor's office, my feet in the stirrups, I looked at my mum, who was holding my hand. Her eyes started to well up.

'Mum. Stop. Just stop. There doesn't need to be emotion or love in this room for there to be a successful conception,' I snapped.

The doctor laughed. 'Actually, that's true of any conception.'

After the procedure, I started the two-week wait to see if it had taken, though it felt like a year.

My brain was a swirling mess of hypotheticals, plans and phantom babies that all had my eyes.

Maybe back in that room, laughing with the doctor, I should have let my mum's love flow. I'll never know. But the blood test was negative. It didn't work.

||||||

Three months later on a freezing day in July, while preparing for my second round of IUI, I walked into a room of journalism Masters students at the University of Melbourne to give a guest lecture.

The first person I laid eyes on was the now-prominent Aboriginal journalist and activist Jack Latimore. Or as I call him these days: husbo.

There was an intermission of a fortnight between him asking me out and our first date, during which we texted like teenagers and spoke almost every night on the phone.

'Seriously, you're lovely, but you don't want to date me,' I told him on one of those calls.

'I'm pretty sure I do. But tell me why you think I don't,' he said in his laid-back Blackfulla-style.

'Well, I want to have a baby but I don't need a man to do it, so I decided to do it with donor sperm and I'm just waiting to start my second round . . .' and I continued to blather on.

'Well, now I'm just impressed,' was his comment.

Of course he was.

Two months after that, we realised we were very much in love and, in a joint decision, I put my second attempt at IUI on hold.

We moved in together quickly and agreed that once his Masters was finished we would try for a baby, somewhere in the middle of the following year.

In late February 2015, I realised I was pregnant. I'd never been pregnant before. Jack wasn't happy. The timeline wasn't right. He hadn't graduated yet, he had more to do. I knew there was no going back and, once we got past the shock and relationship reverberations, I started to get excited. Because the pregnancy was unplanned, we went for a scan to figure out how far along I was and find out the baby's due date. The earliest that can take place is six weeks and two days. The baby was small, indicating I was earlier along than I had suspected. This is not uncommon, and I was told to come back in a week or two for a follow-up scan.

That next time, the news wasn't good. There was no visible fetus, no heartbeat and growth was slow. Too slow. The ultrasonologist warned us that none of these things was a good sign. Miscarriages are marked by slow growth. She wasn't ready to call it, but she strongly suggested that a miscarriage was a likely outcome and that we should prepare ourselves. Reading back over my medical records from that period, she wrote 'threatened miscarriage'. Such an interesting phrase. One I would hear a lot over the next five years.

We had already planned a trip to the Easter music festival Bluesfest, held just outside Byron Bay, where I would be reviewing acts for a local music publication. Of course, I wasn't going to cancel. I don't cancel things. So off we went.

I wandered around the festival grounds like a zombie for five days, crying, wearing a preposterous neon yellow rain jacket my dad had bought me when I was nineteen. It was still too big and I felt very small. People stared at me as I cried through Nikki Hill. I sobbed through Pokey LaFarge. I blubbered through Trombone Shorty.

I went to the massage tent and poured my heart out to a total stranger while he tried to get the knots out of my neck. He looked bewildered and uncomfortable, asking polite, if reserved, questions, and when I left I saw him visibly relax. Every night and every morning

I prayed. I prayed harder than I had ever prayed in my life. To whom I'm not quite sure.

I talked to my baby. I told the baby that I wanted them. That they just had to be strong and focus on growing. Everything would be all right. Jack said it would. And anyway, bad things didn't happen to me. This was just a hiccup. 'Come on, baby, don't let me down,' I whispered into my belly.

When I got back to Melbourne, it was time for my follow-up scan. We had my step-daughter for the week and I didn't want her to know what was going on. I wanted to protect her. I told husbo I would go to the scan on my own, that I had made my peace with the situation and would be fine. I explained it was better for his daughter, who so desperately wanted a sibling, not to know.

I walked into the ultrasonologist's office where the waiting room was full to the brim of glowing, heavily pregnant women. I checked in at the desk and then redirected myself to the toilet. I pulled down my pants. My head started pounding in time with my heart, which felt like it was rising up through my chest and into my throat. It was choking me and I couldn't breathe.

||||||

After the scan the locum doctor on the phone asked me whether I wanted to have a dilation and curettage (D&C), a day procedure with a general anaesthetic where the cervix is dilated and any remaining fetal tissue is scraped or suctioned from your uterus. It means you don't have to pass it naturally as you would a period. I adored my doctor, Dr Stan, and said I wanted to talk to him before I made any decisions.

Dr Stan called me that night, despite being on holiday. He said he wouldn't be back for another week and that he wanted the locum to do the D&C – it had been a drawn-out process and he wanted it to be over for me. 'You've been through enough,' he said.

Two days later, on 9 April 2015, I had my first D&C. My brother took me to the hospital so Jack could stay with his daughter at home, which was what I wanted. I arrived at the hospital at 6 am. I felt empty and didn't know if it was the fasting or the grief. I woke up in recovery and my friend Dani, a doctor, was standing over my bed, visiting before I was discharged. It took me a minute to realise where I was, who was looking at me and why I was in a hospital. And then I panicked.

I put my hands on my abdomen. It was empty. I was empty. Really empty. This little person I'd spoken to, I'd pictured, I'd implored to keep growing – they were gone.

'I'm not pregnant anymore,' I gasped and I felt like I was hyperventilating.

'I know, Isy, but you're going to be okay,' she said calmly, using her most soothing doctor voice. She stayed with me, her hand on my hand, until I stopped sobbing.

I found my brother outside. He sat with me while a nurse prepared me to be discharged. When they talked about vaginal bleeding he almost turned inside out. But mostly he was a mensch.

The nurse showed me the rundown of the procedure: I was put under at 8.06 am and it was completed at 8.12 am. Six minutes. It took six minutes to take my baby away.

One of the benefits of a D&C is that it's easier to retain fetal tissue for sampling. Mine showed a triploid molecular karyotype, which means that instead of two sets of chromosomes, there were three. Dr Stan said humans have forty-six chromosomes and yet mine had sixty-nine.

While there was some solace in this knowledge, the feeling was conflicted.

My baby was and always will be perfect to me.

But was she even human?

||||||||||||||||||||||||||||||||||||||||||||||||||||||||||||||||||||||||||||||||||||||||||||||||||||||||||||||||||||||||

1

Don't Speak

The silence around miscarriage is commonly accepted, but where does it come from and does it exist in all cultures?

There is one word that is always unavoidable in any discussion of miscarriage: silence. In my observations of support groups, and hundreds of interviews and conversations about pregnancy loss, there is a consistent narrative that always presents itself: 'I just didn't realise how many people go through this until it happened to me.' And that's because while the culture around miscarriage is shifting slowly – some might say impossibly slowly – it remains a topic not raised in polite conversation. Despite that, the history of miscarriage, its interpretation and its place in public discussion have not been stagnant. The way it is viewed, interpreted and discussed has changed markedly over the years.

When I started my miscarriage journey, I observed pretty quickly how frequently the silence was acknowledged (ad nauseam) and how often it was the subject of column inches, celebrity interviews and news stories about people looking to 'break the silence and start a conversation'. Yet there wasn't a huge amount of time or energy given to unpacking the why and the how this silence came to be. And it seemed to me that if we want to dismantle the conversational vacuum, we can't do that if we don't understand where it comes from.

But before we launch in, we need to ask ourselves why it is important to break down the silence. Why does it matter? Is the silence damaging? How?

In 2015, 1000 people across America were surveyed about miscarriage and the results were staggering.[5] Of the participants who had experienced a miscarriage or whose partners had experienced miscarriage, 47 per cent said they felt guilty, 41 per cent felt they had done something wrong and 28 per cent felt ashamed. While miscarriage rates fall somewhere between 15 per cent and 30 per cent of pregnancies, 55 per cent of respondents believed miscarriage occurred in 5 per cent of pregnancies . . . or less. Silence propagates misinformation and reiterates that there's guilt to be felt. And that guilt makes us feel isolated and lonely, a feeling expressed by a heartbreaking 41 per cent of respondents in the survey.

Going back to the start

Miscarriage makes two appearances in the bible. The first is in the book of *Exodus*, when the Jews are promised that 'none will miscarry or be barren in your land. I will give you a full life span', if they follow the laws of Moses.[6] Conversely, when the Israelites are being naughty, they're told in the book of *Hosea*, 'Give them, O Lord—what will you give? Give them a miscarrying womb and dry breasts.'[7] Right, so reward is no miscarriage, punishment is miscarriage. Got it.

But what constituted a miscarriage back before we had the 'pleasure' of transvaginal ultrasound? Lara Freidenfelds explains beautifully in her book *The Myth of the Perfect Pregnancy: A History of Miscarriage in America* that, historically, when pregnancy tissue could be examined after miscarriage or early pregnancy loss, it generally didn't look like a baby. She notes that 'in evidence from court records, medieval and early modern lay people described early pregnancy metaphorically in terms of the coagulation of milk or the curdling of cheese'.[8] Sometimes these losses were described as 'tumours' rather than as babies.

Indeed, pregnancies were only thought of as 'babies' after the mother had felt the 'quickening', which is the baby's first movement. This is when the baby was considered 'ensouled'.

For this reason, in Western culture, there was not thought to be any difference between drinking a concoction to 'bring down the menses' (kinda like ye olde timey version of a late morning after pill) as there was in a pregnancy ending before the quickening, which usually takes place around sixteen weeks into a pregnancy. They were thought to be the same and, therefore, the word 'abortion' was applicable to either circumstance, unlike the loss of a child after the quickening, which could see a mother charged with murder.

A large contributor to this was the total lack of knowledge around what a pregnancy was if there was no discernible baby and what could possibly cause the loss. With an information deficit like that, we should opt for the default and blame the mother, right? Right.

A letter written in Latin in the first century by Pliny the Younger to Calpurnius Fabatus, the grandfather of Pliny's wife Calpurnia, explains that Calpurnia had a miscarriage, caused by not taking 'precautions', because she didn't know she was pregnant.

'But she has paid a very severe penalty for her mistake, for her life was in the greatest danger,' Pliny writes. 'Consequently, though you will be very grieved to hear in your old age that you have been cheated, so to speak, of a great-grandchild which was on its way to you, yet you must be thankful to the gods that, though they have refused you the child for the present, they have preserved your granddaughter's life and will repair the loss later on.'[9]

While Pliny doesn't name the imprudent things his wife allegedly did, his contemporary, the physician Soranus, claimed that the seed could be 'evacuated' by fright, sorrow, sudden joy, and any severe mental upset, vigorous exercise, holding your breath, coughing, sneezing, blows and falls (especially on the hips), lifting heavy weights, leaping, sitting on hard sedan chairs, administration of drugs (unspecified), the application of pungent substances like garlic or onions (or leeks, preserved meat or fish), or anything that causes sneezing, want, indigestion, drunkenness, vomiting or diarrhoea; by nosebleeds, other bleeds (haemorrhoids, for example), relaxation due to a heating agent, like a hot bath, or by marked fevers, rigours, or cramps.[10] So pretty much, like, being alive.

From the first century, the blame game has been strong. Throughout history, it has traversed geographies, crossing cultural, anthropological, religious and ethnic boundaries, usually travelling hand in hand with its good friend and bedfellow, guilt. And when something has been a cultural, societal, psychological or indeed medical phenomenon for this long, you'd better believe its roots run pretty deep. Without an adequate, provable explanation for loss or a fix that actually worked, women became an easy scapegoat for their inability to carry a baby.

This blame permeates everything, even the stories we tell our children. Social worker and counsellor Margaret Leroy's 1988 self-help book *Miscarriage*[11] discusses the theme of the 'loss of child as punishment for wrong-doing', which occurs in number of fairy tales and legends, indicating this is 'a persistent part of human thinking about reproduction'. She gives three examples,[12] the first of which is *Rapunzel*, where a man steals a lettuce for his pregnant wife from a witch's garden. His punishment is that he must give her the child when it is born. The second is *The Legend Of King Arthur*, in which Ygraine commits adultery with Uther, magically disguised as her husband, and the result of their union (Arthur) is taken by Merlin immediately after his birth. The final example is The Brothers Grimm's *Rumpelstiltskin*, where the miller's daughter cannot pay for the gold spun out of straw by the manikin and instead promises to him her first-born child, punishment for the lie told to the king that she could spin straw into gold.

Some semblance of control

Throughout history, until science developed reliable contraception, no one with a uterus had control over their reproductive future. Until fairly recently in historic terms, childbirth was a dangerous business and the risk factors were higher if you had a baby nine months after each time you had sex. Having a baby each year of your reproductive life is not something many women would aspire to, even with maternal and child mortality rates nowadays much lower than anything physicians practising before the start of the twentieth century could realistically hope to achieve. Back then, miscarriage often came as a relief, because it was seen as nature's way of spacing out the babies. Natural family planning.

In her book *Lost: Miscarriage in Nineteenth-Century America*, Shannon Withycombe writes, 'In nineteenth-century America, when women's primary role was the bearing and rearing of children, I initially assumed that miscarriage would be considered a failure or a shameful event. Instead, I found individual women who described the experience openly, without reference to shame or failure, and some even expressed outright joy at the event.'[13] She quotes a letter from June 1879, from Mary Cheney to her husband about the loss of her tenth pregnancy after near constant reproduction for sixteen years. 'O Bliss, O Rapture unforeseen!'[14]

According to Freidenfelds, women in eighteenth-century America rarely recorded their miscarriages, but when they did it was matter-of-fact, with early pregnancy loss relied on as an important component of fertility control.

'Women could not become emotionally invested in early pregnancies they rationally hoped would fail. And women did not typically express guilt or grief when pregnancies failed, even into the second trimester. In an era when it was challenging enough to keep themselves and their already-born children safe and healthy, they had not yet taken on miscarriage prevention as an aspect of maternal responsibility.'[15]

By late in the nineteenth century, there was a shift towards over-medicalisation of miscarriage, despite physicians and doctors being at a loss to explain how and why miscarriage occurred. Withycombe argues that the medicalisation was grounded in a desire to secure pregnancy tissue so it could be studied.

'Some of the impetus for doctors to rush to the bedsides of pregnant and birthing women was that they might have a chance to obtain these tiny specimens – objects portable enough to put in one's pocket and yet magnificent beings that could expose a wealth of information about human biology.'[16]

Medicalisation with no real answers meant more blame. By the mid-1800s, as doctors sought to increase their involvement in patients' lives and increase their business and income, they were publishing health manuals and guides containing long lists of things women should and shouldn't do to prevent infertility and pregnancy loss with no scientific or medical proof. Lord spare us the expert male, operating on assumption.

'By the 1840s and 1850s medical writings on miscarriage causation expanded to include long lists of social pursuits, environmental aspects and anatomical conditions,' writes Withycombe.[17] The blame game was ramping up to new and wondrous heights.

The key players in the blame game

Given the Judeo-Christian propensity to misogyny, and what we've seen in the biblical references to pregnancy, it should come as little surprise that the Church had a substantial role to play in encouraging this blame and shame. Because if women are causing their miscarriages, ultimately they're giving themselves elective abortions. This confusion between elective abortions and miscarriage, culturally and religiously, has contributed to the taboo now surrounding miscarriage, a taboo that neither miscarriage nor abortion deserve.

Dr Rebecca Cox notes in her paper 'The ancient taboo of miscarriage'[18] that a 1915 paper found poverty and a lack of rest were the most likely culprits of miscarriage – a contention that was surprisingly on the money, given what we now know about how poverty can of course affect health and overall well-being. In 1950, a prominent UK-based surgeon claimed that 90 per cent of pregnancy loss was likely caused by induced abortion, in what hindsight tells us is clearly a ridiculous claim. But if you didn't have the knowledge to understand which pregnancies were ending spontaneously and which ones were induced, why not lump them all into the same category? Why not indeed.

Before I go any further, I will state for the record that I am fiercely pro-choice. Militantly so. But I also believe that the fight for pro-choice freedoms has restricted a movement to have miscarriage more widely acknowledged and better treated (medically and societally), an issue I will explore further in chapter ten. This intertwining of two very different issues continues today, driven primarily by Christian lobbyists.

Historian Daniela Blei wrote in 2018 that 'in the Age of Trump, a miscarriage will get you punitive policies. As governor of Indiana, Mike Pence signed a law requiring hospitals to bury or cremate every miscarriage, regardless of gestation stage.'[19] Perhaps if certain powerbrokers within feminism had taken note of these incremental yet very deliberate moves (and accompanying warnings) to criminalise miscarriage and police the contents of uteri, they would have put in a more concerted effort to head off the overturning of Roe vs Wade in 2022; we'll never know.

Even the word miscarriage indicates wrongdoing. You mis-carried it. You carried it incorrectly. You made a mistake. What about 'pregnancy loss'; well, who lost it? The mother of course. Seems a very irresponsible thing to do. Lose a pregnancy like that. This is a complaint I hear over and over in support groups and in my interviews with parents.

In the West, blame for miscarriage has been placed on a wide and ridiculous range of factors including the female body, diet, infidelity, sneezing, blasphemy, heavy lifting, prior sexual activity, abortions or, seemingly, anything else anyone could think of.

But while the blame game may look or feel different in other countries, it plays out nevertheless. One of the seminal comparative studies of pregnancy loss across cultures is *The Anthropology of Pregnancy Loss*, edited by Rosanne Cecil, published in 1996.[20] In each chapter, an anthropologist walks us through a different culture and their approach to pregnancy loss.

In her wide-ranging introduction, Cecil points out that in the field of psychology, there has been much work put into pregnancy loss in recent years (well, back in the '90s when this book was written), unlike in anthropology. She points to many studies that show there is much to unpack in the way other cultures view loss. One such study is Edwin Ardener's study of the Bakweri people of Cameroon in 1962, which found that a distinction was not always maintained between miscarriage and stillbirth and 'the subject of pregnancy loss was clearly painful for the women'.[21]

Anthropologist Olayinka M. Njikam Savage built on Ardener's work with her research in 1991–93, and in chapter five of the book writes that, 'In Cameroon, religious views and cosmic views are closely intertwined with health beliefs'. She explains that pregnancy loss at any gestation is viewed as an indication of disharmony between the living and dead, though it can also be caused by practical factors like workload, physical abuse, a woman's sexual impropriety (sex during pregnancy is okay with your spouse, but no one else, apparently) and diet.

Interestingly, Savage notes, the Bamileke people, like the Bakweri, 'believe that crying over a miscarriage or stillbirth angers God, as a result of which he might not send another child or might send one after a long intervention'. This appears to be a mechanism through which women can be supported and encouraged to move on and get pregnant again as quickly as possible. If a woman does not act quickly to re-impregnate herself, this can be interpreted as an overt admission of guilt 'of having sold or pledged her babies (even before conception) to supernatural forces in return for longevity, wealth and success'.

In chapter four of Cecil's book, J.A.R. Wembah-Rashid explains that in the matrilineal societies of south-east Tanzania, efforts are made to prevent miscarriage ('the pregnancy fell down'), but little mourning takes place if the pregnancy is malformed or too early to be considered human. The four reasons for pregnancy loss are: meeting with an unclean person, if the mother has a dispute with someone, ancestor spirits are not kept happy, or illness.

Patricia Jeffery and Roger Jeffery also discuss 'falling babies' in rural north India, where this sort of loss is blamed on 'excessive heat'. Also, there is a particular threat posed by attacks with evil spirits, which can happen when pregnant women venture too far from human habitation or the domestic space. For that reason, it's much safer to stay home. How convenient. If, however, a pregnancy is deemed to be lost due to evil spiritual possession or a curse, subsequent pregnancies can be protected with amulets.

In rural Jamaica, Elisa Janine Sobo found that, in a perspective similar to historic Western tradition, a pregnancy is not seen as containing a fetus or a baby until the quickening (first movement). But unlike in Western societies, 'ancestral ghosts or duppies are frequently implicated in bringing on the horrible and perilous condition of "false belly"'.[22] False belly is a concept Sobo says is used to 'make sense of the emotionally and often physically painful occurrence of miscarriage or the birth of a monstrously malformed baby'.

I find this last example fascinating, because I read it as a deliberate strategy to blame miscarriage or pregnancy loss on something out of the woman's control. While I know this doesn't improve understanding of why miscarriage can happen or alleviate it, it makes for a refreshing change.

It's a similar story for the Abelam people of Papua New Guinea, as described by Anna Winkvist in chapter three of Cecil's book, based on research conducted in 1986. 'When miscarriages and stillbirth occur, Abelam explanations are related to social and spiritual rather than physical causes, for example, conflicts within the family or spirits who have been offended.' Other causes can be failing to pay the *nianmi* (healer) or angering the *wala* (spirits) which assist in reproduction, but can be dangerous if annoyed. Interestingly, however, if a woman works through her entire pregnancy, the baby will be strong and healthy. How very convenient indeed.

In more recent research, Dr Susie Kilshaw, the Wellcome Trust Principal Research Fellow at University College London's Department of Anthropology, has been working to compare the experiences of miscarriage with women in the UK and Qatar, where Kilshaw herself experienced miscarriage. She found that Qatari women's strong faith means that they are able to embrace the 'kismet' view of pregnancy loss that can irk so many women in the West, who are frustrated at hearing the old adage 'Oh well, it was meant to be,' when they're seeking out support.

In an article in the anthropology magazine *Sapiens*, Kilshaw writes about how Qatari women view their miscarriages as part of God's will and plan. She quotes one woman, Kholoud: 'You don't know what your child will grow up to be: He may grow up to be disabled or a corrupted person or disobedient, or he may kill his parents. So Allah didn't want him to be born because he wants the best for you. We believe in this, and this is why we stay strong when we have such experiences.'[23]

While this seeming abdication of medical or personal responsibility for early pregnancy loss may be a relief, faith in divine intervention could delay patients from seeking medical analysis of the loss, and where there is an underlying cause, they may suffer more losses than they need to.

The World Health Organization (WHO) ran a campaign called 'Why We Need to Talk About Losing a Baby' and several women shared testimonials about the cultural interpretations of loss in their communities. Larai, a 44-year-old pharmacist from Nigeria, described how beliefs around losing a baby due to witchcraft or a curse persist.

'Child loss is surrounded by stigma because some people believe there is something wrong with a woman who has had recurrent losses, that she may have been promiscuous, and so the loss is seen as a punishment from God,' she explains. 'In most traditional African cultures, these feelings are exacerbated because the worth of a woman is often determined by the children she carries to term.'[24]

Sitting in our discomfort

As a society, we are not good at discussing or processing grief. We're not good at sitting with our own or supporting others as they sit with theirs. The grief of miscarriage is one of the reasons that the silence persists, but there's another factor that elevates our discomfort to even greater heights: menstruation.

'Menstrual blood is seen as unclean, dangerous and polluting in many cultures,' writes Leroy in *Miscarriage*. 'It is one of the oldest and most widespread taboos, in fact the very word taboo is said to originate from the Polynesian word for menstruation, "tupua".' This is something I have seen referenced many times in Western literature, though I couldn't find any evidence that 'tupua' meant menstruation in any Polynesian language (though there are many). Certainly in many cultures and religions – including Islam, Hinduism and Judaism – there exists some form of belief that menstruation is 'unclean', and in some cases you are forbidden from visiting sacred sites until menstruation is complete for that month.

In their book *About Bloody Time*, Karen Pickering and Jane Bennett argue that the menstrual taboo is a device of the patriarchy. 'It reifies male strength and power at the same time as holding women back by making them anxious about their bodies and causing them to struggle with bodily confidence from the time they begin menstruating.'[25]

They go on to add, 'Patriarchal systems not only create an environment in which the menstrual taboo thrives, but they reinforce and strengthen it; and everyone plays a role, including other women and girls who are more likely to pass on their internalised shame, to become a tormentor, to judge the way people manage their periods, to project their feelings about menstruation onto other's experience of it.' Possum Portraits, the only charity in the world to provide free memento mori–style artwork created from photos of babies born sleeping to grieving parents, is based in Melbourne. I wrote an article about them in 2022, when one of the only advertising options they had for fundraising – with their local radio station – stopped them from placing ads. The short, tasteful, advertisement had prompted several complaints from female station members, because it had made them 'uncomfortable'.[26]

The silence around miscarriage occurs at the intersection of two of society's most uncomfortable topics: vaginal bleeding and death. And the discomfort it imbues is in no way limited to men. In a column for *The Age* and *Sydney Morning Herald* ironically entitled, 'The "ugly" side of pregnancy loss is the part we most need to see',[27] I tried to describe the true face of miscarriage, but the word 'clot' was edited out.

By a female editor.

Dos and don'ts

Feelings of blame around pregnancy loss stretch back almost to the dawn of time. They are ingrained and stubborn. That doesn't mean we can't shift these feelings, but it does mean we need to really understand them and examine the provenance before we can move forward. Simply acknowledging their existence isn't enough.

People who experience pregnancy loss must be told that losses are not their fault, and we need to stop the constant barrage of dos and don'ts to pregnant people so they aren't manipulated, even subliminally, into thinking something they did caused their loss. Having that latte on the way to work is not the reason you had a miscarriage. These are issues we will discuss in chapter thirteen.

We also have to distance ourselves from this constant trope of 'pregnancy loss as punishment' for wrongdoing. If this means abandoning the stories we've told for generations, so be it. This damaging blame leads to loneliness, isolation and guilt. It compounds the grief and ensures we continue, as a society, to not understand the extent of the problem.

Two Princes

'I fucking told you!' I screamed at husbo, pointing an accusatory finger in his face. 'I fucking told you, didn't I? I fucking did! I fucking told you!'

The adrenaline had apparently kicked in. And so too had my English accent, which resurfaces whenever I'm drunk, emotional or angry.

The ultrasonologist was twisting in her seat uncomfortably, ironic given that she wasn't the one on the bed, legs akimbo with a giant, white, condom-covered wand in her vagina.

My husband was staring at the screen, completely still. Staring at two little flickers.

Flick, flick. Flick, flick.

'I fucking told you it was twins,' I shouted triumphantly. He turned to me. His face shifted slowly into a half-strength, slightly strained smile.

'Yes, you did,' he forced out.

Underneath his big, bushy beard, he looked pale.

||||||

After the loss of my first pregnancy, Dr Stan told me I couldn't try again for two cycles, meaning until after I'd had two periods. There's not usually a reason to wait with a 'natural' miscarriage but lots of doctors prefer you wait after a D&C to make sure you don't pick up an infection. While there's no 'requirement' to wait, medically speaking, and it comes down to personal preference, there may be another reason to hold off. It gives you time to process the loss and deal with your grief – and to gird your loins psychologically – before you head into another pregnancy.

But having to wait to try again, when every single hormone coursing through your body is telling you how badly you need to be pregnant, is agonising.

It's the closest I can imagine to how a heroin addict feels when they need another hit.

Every single cell in your body craving. Aching. Screaming.

I started on the task of convincing Jack to throw caution to the wind.

I tried to convince him with a nod and a wink. He said no.

I tried some good old-fashioned Jewish guilt, which slid off him like butter on a cob of corn.

I tried to seduce him with promises of sexual activities I'd only read about in books and magazines. He said yes . . . But slipped on a condom.

I gave up and waited. Eight long weeks I waited.

Then it was time. But just a few short weeks after the deed was done, he set off overseas to China and I was filled with a good old-fashioned, black-and-white style melancholy.

It was the first time we'd been apart for more than a night since we'd moved in together. And his first trip overseas was to a place I was indelibly connected to. I was a committed Sinophile. I grew up in Hong Kong, studied Chinese history and politics as well as Mandarin and had backpacked around China several times.

That he was undertaking this landmark journey without me, to a place I so desperately wanted to show him, left me feeling sad.

||||||

I walked in the door from dropping Jack at the airport and I threw up. I knew I was pregnant before I did the test. Lo and behold, up came the line on the stick. I did one more test, just to be sure. I knew false-positive pregnancy tests were all but impossible, but I had to see the line come up twice before I could believe it.

I started messaging Jack the pictures of the positive readings, but he was already on the plane, phone off. He saw them when he landed in Shanghai. He was happy, but his reaction seemed muted. Though maybe that perception was just my instinct telling me not to get my own hopes up too high.

|||||||

During my first pregnancy, I had shocking nausea and sickness. The first clue I might be pregnant had come when I arrived at a friend's house for dinner. She had made fish. Kristen is an excellent cook and her food is always a treat, but I found myself having to force it down. Before we left I had returned the entire dinner to her toilet bowl.

The nausea that set in almost straight away with this second pregnancy was fast, fierce and full of fury. And it was unrelenting. Before I ate, after I ate, sometimes I even had to excuse myself in the middle of a meal.

I bloated up and looked visibly pregnant, even though I was only four or five weeks in. I couldn't keep my eyes open and even felt nervous driving. Sometimes I would need to sleep when I got home from work, then I would eat dinner and go straight back to bed.

When Jack got home from overseas, we lay in bed, chatting as you do, and I whispered, 'I think it's twins.' He laughed.

I told my mum I thought it was twins; she laughed too.

|||||||

When we first walked into the ultrasonologist's office I was shaking and teary. I was so scared. During my first pregnancy, I had known exactly how far along I was, what the scan should show and the necessity of there being a healthy fetal heartbeat.

The wait to conceive again had been interminable. The wait to get to this first scan an eternity. In reality it was about two weeks, but it was enough time to tease my fears and anxieties into a state of absolute frenzy.

The female ultrasonologist and obstetrician was short, snappy and aggressive. I explained as soon as she walked into the room that my previous pregnancy had ended in loss and that I was incredibly nervous about the scan she was about to give me.

I might as well have told her I was wearing green shoes, because nothing changed in her manner, her face or her approach. If anything, her demeanour hardened.

When she inserted the wand, I finally lost control of the nervousness building in my chest and spat out the trembling questions I'd been trying so hard to contain.

'What can you see? Is there a heartbeat? What size is it? How many millimetres? Please tell me there's a heartbeat. Please?'

She was not impressed.

'If you stop talking and asking me questions, I'll be able to concentrate and see and then I'll be able to tell you,' she barked, her words slapping me across the face.

I went utterly silent. I didn't breathe for what felt like twenty minutes. It was probably less than a minute. And then we saw them.

Flick, flick. Flick, flick.

Pregnancy 1. Pregnancy 2.

It was the first and last time that ultrasonologist scanned me.

I called the clinic that afternoon and made a complaint. They put it down to a language barrier. Except she was a Chinese-speaker and I grew up in Hong Kong. I'm used to a language barrier and cultural nuances. Her English was completely perfect. She'd done two degrees in Australia. Two. They just couldn't accept I had been treated poorly or that my situation warranted any sensitivity.

In a strange twist of fate, I googled her years later and found her profile on the website for the ultrasound clinic.

'When Sarah is not at work, she is a dedicated mum to active twin toddlers.'

Pregnancy 1 was a good, healthy size and had a beautiful heartbeat flick, flicking away at 118 beats per minute. Pregnancy 2 had a heartbeat of just ninety and was half the size of their sibling.

The ultrasonologist told me, completely devoid of emotion or empathy, that Pregnancy 2 was very small and 'might not be viable' and to come back in a week. But I had seen a heartbeat! And Dr Google reliably informed me that once you see a heartbeat, your risk of miscarriage falls significantly.

Dr Stan called that afternoon and his enthusiasm was, shall we say, contained.

He told me gently that it wasn't unusual for a twin pregnancy to become a single pregnancy. And Pregnancy 2 was very small.

But they both had heartbeats!

He agreed with me that we could choose to be optimistic.

I called my mum, my dad, my brother.

'How was the scan?'

'It was great! They both had heartbeats!'

'Um . . . they both?'

I called my friend Alice, a mother of twins, and she exploded with happiness. 'I always knew this would happen to one of my friends eventually!' she shouted down the phone, so excited at the prospect of supporting a friend through twins. I wrote down all the details she gave me for multiple-birth support groups on Facebook and sent them all join requests.

I googled twin cots. I googled twin prams. I googled matching clothes. I googled breastfeeding twins. I fell well and truly down the twin vortex. I could see my babies in my mind's eye. And both of them were perfect.

I told myself it didn't really look like blood. It was more pink than red. I told myself bleeding is very common in the early stages of pregnancy, which it is.

Exactly one week later another doctor did my follow-up scan. She was kind and patient and moved slowly.

Up came the image on the huge screen in front of us.

Flick, flick.

Just one heart, just one beat. One sac. One baby.

And nothing else.

No second baby. No second empty sac. No collapsing sack. No nothing.

Was it a figment of my imagination? Had Pregnancy 2 ever existed?

Dr Stan called me. He sounded sad. Vanishing twin syndrome.

My smaller baby hadn't made it and had been absorbed by my remaining baby and my body.

And then, there was one.

||||||

I was very confused. Was this result good or bad? My feelings vacillated wildly.

One minute I was relieved. It meant a pregnancy with far fewer complications, much more likely to result in a healthy birth.

The next moment I was filled with sadness. I had lost one of my babies. They wouldn't have twin cots and matching onesies. Would my remaining child always have a piece of their soul missing?

But with time, the excitement of my remaining baby's development took over. Strong and healthy and perfect on all their scans.

We started to make jokes to try to ease the bad days. I would put on a Russian accent and don my fake fur ushanka hat and proclaim, 'Our baby strong like ox, eat twin sibling!'

But it was always to cover the anxiety and fear. Relaxing into the pregnancy, enjoying the sensation of life growing inside me was challenging. There were dark shadows in the periphery of my forward vision and I wondered when they would materialise into something more sinister than just a distant, obscure threat.

Loss had robbed me of the beauty of a naive pregnancy filled only with promise. It left behind scar tissue, although everyone promised me it would heal with the arrival of my new baby.

When I was diagnosed with gestational diabetes, a reasonably common and manageable condition, I cried for days. I couldn't even get out of bed. My body had again let me down and my baby was at risk. At risk of diabetes, at risk of weight gain. At risk of premature arrival.

I started on a strictly controlled diet, and later insulin, but it felt like the shadows had become slightly darker and more menacing.

||||||

One warm summer's day, I was heavily pregnant and we were walking down Acland Street in St Kilda, past the European cake shops, the most famous of which my grandmother ran in the 1960s. We popped into a new Aboriginal art gallery to have a stickybeak.

A Central Australian fulla wearing an Akubra appeared. He smiled at us, gave a pointed nod to husbo and, without asking, put his hand on my belly.

'Strong boy you got there.' He smiled.

It further cemented Jack's totally unshakeable belief that we were having a boy. He wouldn't even entertain a discussion of girls' names.

'What's the point? It's a waste of time.' He'd shrug.

I wanted the sex to be a surprise, but fear of Jack's disappointment in the delivery room if it was a girl made me want to be sure.

The ultrasonologist was a gentle, kind, older gent. I was incredibly nervous, as I was during all scans, but the twenty-week scan is important and can reveal anomalies not yet identified.

'Do you want to know?'

I had been able to claim victory in our first scan, but this time it was Jack's turn.

||||||

We had been arguing over names for months. I was adamant that I wanted our son's name to start with R, to match his older sister, but we simply couldn't find one we both liked. Rolo. Roland. Remington. None were the right fit.

One night, I was on the couch and Jack was sipping on a whiskey as I looked on jealously.

We were listening to song after song of our favourite country music. As we listened, he told me a story about when Roy Orbison had come to his father in a dream.

As he came to the end of the story, Roy singing 'I Drove All Night', husbo paused.

'What about Roy?'

||||||

Royston Albert Lewis Latimore was born in March 2016.

|||||||||||||||||||||||||||||||||||||||||||||||||||||||||||||||||||||||||||||||||||||||||||||||||||||||||||||

2

The Fame

*(Mis)representations of miscarriage across popular
culture contribute greatly to misunderstandings across all
facets of the experience.*

Despite being a voracious consumer of popular media, when I turned
my attention to depictions of miscarriage in music, film, TV and literature, I found myself coming up with very few examples off the top
of my head. So when I began to research this issue in earnest, I did it
the twenty-first century way: I crowdsourced it on Twitter.

As I waded through the hundreds of responses and suggestions,
the first thing that hit me was the range of examples. Deleting the
double-ups, in just a few hours, I was pointed to fifty-five instances
on TV, eighteen instances in movies, twenty in books and sixteen in
music, and a handful in comics, graphic novels and poetry. Not bad
for one tweet. Though admittedly, when you consider how many
thousands (millions?) of depictions you see of pregnancy, it's still very
light on, and certainly not reflective of the rate of loss in the population.

Another interesting factor was how many of those examples were
actually not of miscarriage but of elective abortion (again, zero criti-
cism of depiction of that issue or indeed that choice). But what it does
indicate is a confusion and lack of nuance in popular culture of what
I would describe as miscarriage or pregnancy loss.

Something else I noticed was how many of these movies and TV shows I'd watched, how many songs I'd listened to and books I'd read, and yet I didn't recall most of the examples. I have no doubt that the blame for that can, at least in part, be placed on many of those depictions being incidental, rather than central. A side dish, if you like, rather than the meat and bones of a storyline. The other source of blame is likely my memory, which can be patchy at the best of times. But nevertheless, many of my responses were along the lines of, 'Really?' 'Seriously?' 'What episode?' It was unnerving to say the least.

That old chestnut

There are a lot of tropes in popular culture, especially TV and film, that rely on or involve miscarriage. A common one is the 'good girls don't have abortions' trope. This is when a character discovers an unwanted pregnancy and instead of them doing something awful like, say, taking control of their own body and fertility and making good decisions for their future (i.e. having an abortion), writers wrap the storyline up nicely with a big red bow and, you guessed it, a miscarriage. Examples of this trope are: Neve Campbell's Julia Salinger in *Party of Five*[28], Jennie Garth's Kelly Taylor in *Beverly Hills 90210*[29] and Jemima Kirke's Jessa Johansson in *Girls*.[30]

Another common theme is miscarriage through violence or extreme trauma, like car accidents or domestic violence. In reality, the majority of people who experience miscarriage never establish a cause for the loss. But it would be terrible to burden viewers with that sort of ambiguity, right? Best to give them an additional violent, dramatic twist on which to blame loss. After all, we know miscarriage goes hand in hand with blame, so it makes perfect sense. Examples of this trope are A.J. Cook's JJ in *Criminal Minds*[31] (car crash), Marina Squerciati's Kim Burgess in *Chicago PD*[32] (beaten up) or Victoria Principal's Pam Ewing in *Dallas*[33] (falls off a hayloft). Or Vivien Leigh's Scarlett O'Hara in *Gone With The Wind* (falls down a flight of stairs). Or Mimi in the Britney Spears movie *Crossroads* (also falls down a flight of stairs). You get my drift.

The irony is that, for a mental health issue that gets little societal or medical support, a miscarriage is relied on regularly to create 'insane' female characters. In *The Hand That Rocks the Cradle*, Rebecca De Mornay's lead character is sent mad by a miscarriage she blames on Annabella Sciorra. In a *Private Practice* story arc, which unfolds over several episodes, character Katie Kent, who had been diagnosed with schizophrenia and is portrayed by Amanda Foreman, is sent so far into psychosis by her miscarriage that she engages in the horrendous crime of fetal abduction.[34]

Interestingly, *Private Practice* was a spin-off of *Grey's Anatomy*, which featured four miscarriages in its nineteen-season run. Two became among the most impressive, iconic depictions of early pregnancy loss I can name. In one, Dr Bailey – a senior, accomplished and talented doctor played by Chandra Wilson – laments her inability to help her unborn daughter even as she helps so many patients in the hospital.[35] This sense of powerlessness is something that affects so many people who experience miscarriage, especially in the post-boomer feminist fight for women to have total control over their fertility. The second storyline involved titular character Meredith Grey, played by Ellen Pompeo, whose miscarriage takes place as she's in the operating theatre. She continues to treat the patient even as blood is spreading across her thighs.[36] This idea of working through miscarriage is something many of us know all too well and figures prominently in the reality of loss.

Thank you for the music

Music isn't short on examples of pregnancy loss being used as inspiration for song. One of the best known of these is the heartbreaking Beyoncé song 'Heartbeat' or her husband Jay-Z's song 'Glory'. Lily Allen, who experienced both miscarriage and stillbirth, wrote the song 'Something's Not Right'.

But the poetic nature of music means a lot of the songs thought to be about miscarriage are actually either ambiguous or in some cases not about miscarriage at all. Examples include the goddess Dolly Parton's song 'Dover', a tale of abandonment over an extra-marital pregnancy and subsequent stillbirth. Another example is Ben Folds Five's song 'Brick', which is about lead singer Ben Folds' high school girlfriend getting an abortion.[37] And then there's folk singer's Joanna Newsom's 'Baby Birch', which, despite being heralded within the loss community as a song that resonates, is in fact deliberately ambiguous.

There is nothing wrong with people who have experienced miscarriage finding solace in music or art that doesn't necessarily portray it. Interpretation is of course personal and subjective. Interestingly, in the case of Newsom, she has repeatedly refused to be drawn on the song's meaning and maybe that is her intent – to allow people who see their story in the words to enjoy that comfort.

There are also artists who've witnessed the pain of early pregnancy loss in people close to them and been inspired to create. Ed Sheeran wrote about his friend's grief after miscarriage in his song 'Little Bump'.

International music legend Judith Durham – who passed away just months after I spoke with her representatives for this chapter – had not experienced child loss herself, but she was unexpectedly deeply moved to co-compose and record the hauntingly beautiful 'I Celebrate Your Life, My Baby' after a friend showed her a compilation of poetry and stories written by parents who had lost a baby. In the opening verse of the resulting song, she sings:

Where do I start? How do I feel?
Sad and empty, cheated and lonely
You were my life, you were my babe
I was so excited, I longed for you only
Did I do wrong? Why did I lose you?
You lived here inside me, tears I still cry
Friends couldn't know how much
I was grieving
Just you and Mummy were saying goodbye
© 1998

The recording was released in 2011 on her *Epiphany* album and subsequently on her compilation album *Colours of My Life*.[38] With music by Judith and words inspired by Simon Barnett and Rachel Stanfield Porter, it remains direct and heartbreakingly resonant.

Life imitating art imitating life

Surely the most famous depiction of miscarriage in art is by the phenomenal Frida Kahlo. I travelled to Sydney in 2016 to see her exhibition at the National Gallery of NSW with a very teeny tiny five-month old Roy. Among her many depictions of miscarriage (Kahlo had three pregnancy losses) is a 1932 lithograph (her only lithograph in fact) called *The Miscarriage*[39], which featured in the exhibition.

It shows Kahlo, naked, blood running down her leg and into the earth, nurturing the soil and the plants. She has a fetus inside her and a larger fetus outside her body, both connected to her, with a large branch and leaf growing out of her shoulder. She had an abortion, because carrying a pregnancy was not considered safe, but after that she also had a miscarriage and she wrote the following to her doctor.

'*Doctorcito querido* [dear doctor]: I have wanted to write to you for a long time than you can imagine. I had so looked forward to having a little Dieguito [a small Diego, after Diego Rivera, her partner] that I cried a lot, but it's over, there is nothing else that can be done except to bear it.'[40] She had seemingly resigned herself to a future without a baby.

Author Kylie Maslen wrote about Kahlo's depictions of miscarriage in her book *Show Me Where It Hurts*, where she discusses Kahlo's painting *Henry Ford Hospital* (1932), which depicts Kahlo lying in a pool of blood, with a fetus still connected to her.

'In Kahlo's case, by viewing her work simply as that of a tragic woman who was denied her maternal right to children, audiences appease the patriarchal structures that continue to impede access to healthcare,' Maslen writes in her book of essays, which traverses topics relating to the author's life with chronic pain.[41]

I would build on Maslen's writing with my own interpretation of Kahlo's work; both the lithograph and the painting feel sterile and very lonely. In the lithograph, she presents herself in the style of scientific specimen drawings. To me, it's a commentary on the dehumanisation of women by a patriarchal medical system.

In the painting, she lies on a bed, just a white sheet and her blood. 'Civilisation' (buildings and high rises) is very far off in the distance, giving the painting a sharp sense of isolation. I see it as a commentary on medicine's failure to understand loss and treat patients holistically. There is significant patriarchy and politics in the way women are treated by the medical system (outlined beautifully in both Maslen's book and also in Gabrielle Jackson's *Pain and Prejudice*). This is an issue we will explore more deeply in chapter four.

Fame

This is the part of the book where I wanted to talk to you about celebrities being open and honest about their miscarriages. More and more frequently celebrities seem to be using their social media presences to acknowledge a loss, either recent or historic.

I wanted to explain how celebrities are using their platforms and fame to break down some of the stigma and how this has the potential to support other people and shift the culture of silence. But I ran into a roadblock.

To start with, I made a list. A tremendously long list of anyone in the public eye who had experienced a miscarriage, and who had been open about it and discussed it. The list included a vast array of celebrities across many continents, including Australia, from the A, B, C and even D-grade levels. They were singers, actors, writers. Not all of them had experienced miscarriage, some had portrayed it on TV or in a movie. But they all had one thing in common.

Not a single person would talk to me. Not one agreed to be interviewed. I placed requests through friends or contacts mostly, but even then, with people willing to recommend me as a journalist, each one declined. Where I lodged an inquiry with a publicist, they would reply within minutes (clearly they had no intention of running it past their client) to decline.

I have worked as a journalist since I was sixteen. Never in my working life have I encountered an issue that literally no one would talk to me about. One prominent celeb I spoke to told me they didn't want to be interviewed because they feared possible backlash in the media, which they'd felt on previous occasions when they'd openly discussed their losses or challenges with fertility.

Clearly I don't have a right to anyone's story and I would never pressure anyone into sharing it. Having said that, the fact that not one single celebrity would talk to me is perplexing to say the least. I suspect that at least partly it is about control, image and sharing only on their own terms. So many of the glimpses we see into the celebrity world are stage-managed, despite attempts to make them look authentic on platforms like Instagram.

I also wonder whether it's in part because their grief drove them to share something intensely personal at the time, and having moved beyond it, they don't wish to revisit?

Anything, just anything at all

Should we be grateful for any representation of miscarriage? Or should we hope for more than just its existence in popular culture? Should we hope for realistic portrayals that help educate people on a topic that will touch all of us in some way?

The popular TV show *The Bold Type* – which tells the story of three young millennial women who meet working at a magazine – featured a central storyline of a miscarriage for a principal character, Sutton, played by Meghann Fahy, back in 2020.[42] I was alerted to this by a close friend who called me excitedly to tell me and suggested I watch it and write a column on it, which I did for *Guardian Australia*.[43] Watching the episode, bursting at the seams with anticipation, knowing that this show's predominantly young female audience could benefit from this potential for education about loss, my excitement melted away as the storyline unfolded. Hence the headline on the column I then wrote, 'From undercooked statistics to over-simplification: what *The Bold Type* got wrong about pregnancy loss'.

'Twenty-seven seconds. That's how long it took for a doctor on the American comedy-drama *The Bold Type* to give lead character Sutton a scan and then tell her she was having a miscarriage,' was the op-ed's opening line. It was in this scene that the doctor tells Sutton that 10 per cent of pregnancies end in miscarriage. Say what? A very conservative estimate is one in five or 20 per cent. The doctor then says Sutton will start to bleed in up to forty-eight hours. There's no way of knowing if or when someone will start to bleed after a missed miscarriage. It could be a day, it could be a week, it could be more. Sutton is never offered a follow-up appointment. She's not offered counselling. 'Should women expect that perhaps in 2020 such a potentially devastating event should be depicted with some semblance of accuracy?' I asked at the time.

I think we all know the answer to that question. I added, 'It's not popular culture's responsibility to educate the public, but we can and should aim to do better than homogenised, sanitised, and misleading depictions of the reality that millions of women worldwide experience, along with their partners, friends and families.'

For an example of a much more ambitious and successful depiction of miscarriage, we have to travel back to what is arguably one of the best shows ever made, *Six Feet Under*. In the opening episode of season five of the show, which revolves around a family who run a funeral home, central character Brenda has a miscarriage the day before her wedding to Nate.

She wakes up to find she is bleeding. She and Nate go to the doctor. After a scan, the doctor confirms she is miscarrying and says she needs a D&C. Their wedding is the next day, so Brenda chooses to delay the D&C until the start of the following week. 'This is so not the vision I had of the night before my wedding. Where's the stripper?' Brenda says as she takes a Vicodin for the pain. Her mother realises what's going on when Brenda declines a thong to wear under her wedding dress, instead opting for 'granny panties', presumably to hold a large pad to catch the bleeding. The mother tries to tell Brenda how common it is, throwing out the best line I've ever heard about the prevalence of miscarriage, 'More women have miscarried than have masturbated with a dildo, they just don't talk about it.'

This depiction has it all. It has Brenda blaming herself and Nate for telling people too early, wondering if it's something she did that caused it ('all that anonymous cock', as summarised by a vision Brenda has of Nate's dead ex-wife) and hoping that it's as common as everyone tells her it is ('it fucking better be'). A stellar performance by Aussie actress Rachel Griffiths pulls it all together and makes it educational, poignant, realistic, central and everything else a miscarriage depiction should be.

The fact that you see the grief of those around her – her mother lamenting that there's nothing she can do to help and Nate crying in the doctor's office quietly and in secret after she's taken away for her D&C – rounds out an absolutely beautiful story that should be recognised as the way this can and should be done.

Two of the other depictions that resonate strongly within the loss community happen to appear in children's cartoons. The first is the Pixar/Disney film *Up*. Its depiction of ambiguous infertility grief on behalf of both partners – and the isolation felt by the female partner – is particularly effective and poignant. Many patients or couples who have experienced early pregnancy loss tell me this scene is the cinematic depiction they feel falls closest to reality. Interesting that it should be an animation that achieves this result. Importantly, both this and the next example provide parents with an age-appropriate opening to discuss loss or infertility with younger kids.

Children's TV juggernaut *Bluey* might seem footloose and fancy-free, but it's actually got a really excellent track record of addressing some of the 'stickier' issues kids need to learn about. In the episode 'The Show'[44], there's a blink-and-you'll-miss-it moment when Bluey and her little sister Bingo put on a show for their parents Chilli and

Bandit. Bingo sticks an inflated balloon up her top to play a pregnant Chilli and the balloon bursts. Chilli grimaces and Bandit grabs her hand. After this split-second moment, Bingo runs off devastated, thinking that she's ruined the show. Chilli follows her and explains how to pick yourself up and carry on. Many viewers interpreted this as representative that Chilli had experienced a miscarriage.

There seemed to be some heated debate online as to whether it is indeed a reference to miscarriage, so I reached out to the makers of the show and asked them. This was the response from *Bluey* writer Joe Brumm.

'"The Show" indeed does point at Chilli having a miscarriage. In fact, this is what the episode is about essentially, Chilli is passing down her method of coping to Bingo,' he wrote. 'I can't say too much about who it is based on as the person involved wouldn't want me to. But the key aspect of the experience relevant to this episode was the fact that her other children still needed taking care of, so there really was no choice for her but to pick herself up and keep going. Which I always admired.'

When a Man Loves a Woman

I walked up the laneway beside my house. My mother was holding one elbow, my dad was holding the other. We walked up together, Mum and I both sobbing, and turned right into the easement behind my house. Together, we walked through the backyard, Mum and Dad either side of me as I tried not to trip over, thanks to my tear-filled eyes. The crowd parted and through them we walked, past almost everyone of importance in my life. I walked onto the deck that adjoins our house and stepped under the chuppah.

Over the preceding four weeks I had sewed the chuppah myself. I created it from lacy curtain fabric, the kind I picture in an old house in a town with 500 residents, absolute maximum. I sewed an Aboriginal flag out of sheer chiffon in black, red and orange and then stitched little embroidered Stars of David around it. I took my place next to Jack and in front of my cousin Emilie, our celebrant. My brother stood next to us, holding our son. My bridal processional was 'Brick House' by the Commodores and I was giggling and grooving as I sang along with Walter Orange, 'She's mighty mighty, just lettin' it all hang out'.

Though we had never wanted to get married, here we were. We were deeply in love with each other and with our baby, a crazy red-haired eccentric who made us laugh more than we'd ever laughed in our lives. Everything was going to plan.

We wrote our own wedding vows. We didn't promise to love each other forever. We promised to be friends forever. To support each other. To respect each other. To always be a family. When Jack's foot came down on the glass, crushing it to the cheers of our friends, family and our son, I had no idea how much our commitment to each other – and the life we had planned together – would be tested.

There's something special about the doctor who delivers your children. Especially when you've navigated loss and they've shown you compassion and care like Dr Stan. I'll never forget his words to me before he lifted my son out of my body. 'Are you ready for life to never be the same again?' I laugh when I think that he probably said that before delivering each and every one of the bajillion babies he must have helped into the world.

But he wouldn't be saying that to me, or anyone else, again. Dr Stan was dead. My doctor had been felled by a heart attack in his sleep. He was fifty-nine.

||||||

I finished maternity leave and started a new job. The 'Didgerijew', as we'd come to call baby Roy, was a year old and my desire for a second child was starting to grow; understandably given how perfect my prodigal son was turning out to be. It was time to find a new doctor.

Of course I wanted a doctor who was good at their job, smart and professional. I also really wanted someone I liked. Someone who shared my sense of humour. Even then I had a sense that it was going to be incredibly important that I shared a connection with my doctor. I think somewhere deep in my heart, in my intuitive mind, I knew it was going to be a long journey to living baby number two.

I had spent many years wondering why I had a propensity to choose male doctors and, deciding to confront that bias head-on, I had already promised myself that my new obstetrician would be a woman. A few weeks later I walked into Dr Lovely's office. I told her I was interviewing for new obstetricians given that my old one was dead and I would like to invite her to interview for the position.

She was short. Busy. Blonde. Self-assured. I couldn't pronounce her surname (and still can't). But I could tell she was listening to me and taking in what I said. She heard me. She understood. She didn't laugh at me when I asked to do some preconception genetic screening, despite having a living child. In fact, she thought it was a good idea.

But the clincher was her reaction to me inviting her to interview for the new role of 'my obstetrician'. She laughed. And when she laughed, she snorted. A big, full-bodied nasal snort, right out of both nostrils.

The deal was sealed. Dr Lovely was mine. And in a way, she always would be.

||||||||||||||||||||||||||||||||||||||||||||||||||||||||||||||||||||||||||||||||||||||||||||||||||||||||||||||||||||||||||||||||||||||||||||||||||||||

3

Count on Me

How many patients experience miscarriage each year?
Your guess is as good as mine.

To the vast majority of people, no matter their sexuality, data isn't sexy. Most lovers aren't whispering sweet data nothings into each other's ears or planning candlelit dinners to mull over new pivot tables and modelling. That doesn't mean it's not important.

When I started writing this book and hunting for some definitive numbers for losses under twenty weeks in Australia, one statistic kept popping up everywhere, touting that 103,000 families are affected by pregnancy loss in Australia each year. This number is attributed to miscarriage support charity Sands Australia, which in 2020 merged with Red Nose, another charity that provides support in the wake of miscarriage, stillbirth or newborn death. Researching the figure before their merger, I found it on the Sands website.

But where did it come from? It's used extensively in media coverage, on health websites, charity websites and so on, but no sources or citations are ever given beyond Sands. I approached Sands before the merger back in June 2020, emailing a request for the source of the data. A reply bounced into my email inbox simply stating that the one in four number is the 'widely accepted worldwide figure' and 'acknowledged worldwide to be likely at the lower end of the scale as not all miscarriages are known or recorded'. The 103,000 figure is 'based on our current birth rate in Australia and then applying the 1 in 4 principle'.

So really they couldn't actually tell me the source of this figure, because there wasn't one; it was a guesstimate.

Well, that's okay, I thought. I'll just go and source some data myself. I love a good quest. Off I went to all the usual suspects to find the hard facts so I could get going on the fun bit: the analysis.

Except that The Australian Institute of Health and Welfare (AIHW) doesn't track miscarriage rates. Neither does the Australian Bureau of Statistics (ABS) or the state or federal Department of Health. It transpires that Australia doesn't collect or collate data on its most common 'pregnancy complication'. It just . . . doesn't. This, to put it mildly, is staggering.

Without this data we have no clear picture of early pregnancy loss in this country. We don't know who it's affecting, why, where or when. We don't know if it's rising, falling or going sideways. We're flying blind. Without this information, an effective public health policy is nigh on impossible to develop or implement effectively, let alone fund.

In May 2021, *The Lancet* published a series on miscarriage, which included an extremely strong editorial and three papers authored by some of the most important and highly regarded researchers in this space.

A key recommendation of the first paper, entitled 'Miscarriage matters: the epidemiological, physical, psychological, and economic costs of early pregnancy loss' – which had twenty-five authors comprised of the world's leading doctors and researchers in the pregnancy loss space, including Mary Stephenson, Raj Rai, Lesley Regan, Siobhan Quenby and Arri Coomarasamy – was that data needed to be central going forward.

'We recommend that miscarriage data are gathered and reported to facilitate comparison of rates among countries, to accelerate research, and to improve patient care and policy development,'[45] the paper read.

At this point, we need to do two things, friends. First, we need to unpack why it's so important that we have this data and what it can help us achieve as part of our roadmap to better care.

And then we need to establish what we know, what we don't know, what we need to know, and how to fill those gaps most effectively.

Counting the cost

The World Health Organization (WHO) defines 'health policy' as 'decisions, plans and actions that are undertaken to achieve specific healthcare goals within a society'. You only need to talk to a range of people who've experienced early pregnancy loss in this country to know that public health policy on this issue is failing. The data is the underlying structure on which the entire policy needs to be pinned. In the words of the WHO's Deputy Director-General, Zsuzsanna Jakab, the 'backbone' of public health and strong decision-making is high-quality health information.[46]

Research released in 2021 put the cost of miscarriage to the UK economy at £471 million. No research exists around the Australian cost of miscarriage, but the UK population is around 2.6 times the size of our population. I approached several organisations to see if someone could help me calculate the cost of miscarriage to the Australian economy but was told it would take millions of dollars that I unfortunately don't have. Apparently, I can't just divide £471 million by 2.6 and then use the current exchange rate to give me a figure of $340 million, because that would be simplistic and utterly ridiculous. Small point of order: the tally has been funded and executed for Australian stillbirths – we do have stillbirth data – showing a five-year cost of $682 million for the period from 2016 to 2020, with an assumed stillbirth rate of 2700 per year by 2020.[47]

Australia's birth rate is in decline and has been for some time. As reported in 2022, in 2020 the rate of women giving birth dropped to its lowest level in a decade to 56 per 1000. In fact, Australia's birth rate is now below replacement level, so the only reason the population is growing is thanks to overseas migration. This has been influenced by a number of factors, including more reliable contraception, climate change, housing affordability, job insecurity, increasing average maternal age and improving gender equality in the workplace.

Demographer Dr Liz Allen explains that with these changes, childbirth is being pushed out to a later and later stage. 'We're seeing now a constraint on the birth rates as a function of the way that we live our lives.'

There is another reason miscarriage data is incredibly important. Patients who experience miscarriage are more likely to experience a range of health complications, including adverse outcomes in subsequent pregnancy, thrombosis and heart attack. Dame Lesley Regan is Professor of Obstetrics and Gynaecology at Imperial College's St Mary's Hospital Campus and an Honorary Consultant in Gynaecology at the Imperial College NHS Trust. She is also principal investigator of the Recurrent Miscarriage Tissue Bank. In 2022 she was appointed the UK's inaugural National Ambassador for Women's Health.

'We should be using pregnancy, or a woman's physiological response to pregnancy, to predict what she needs in the future,' she explained to me. 'I would argue – from the feminist point of view – that if that was the case for men, we would have done it a long time ago.'

Money, money, money

Money might not be able to buy you love, but you know what it can buy? A fuck-tonne of medical research and resources for comprehensive medical treatment. And this is where the numbers game comes into play.

Medical research is funded in a number of ways, including private companies looking to make a profit (big pharma), philanthropy or government. It's incredibly difficult to make a case for funding if you don't know exactly how many patients an issue affects.

'It's very important to understand and quantify the weight of the health burden . . . meaning the number of people that it's impacting and the extent or type of impact it has on their lives,' explains Professor Sarah Robertson, an Adelaide-based specialist researcher in the area of reproductive immunology.

'Actually, being able to quantify that is really important in the case of miscarriage, because it is quite likely it is one of the reasons that research into miscarriage is perhaps under-funded; we don't fully appreciate the weight or extent of the health burden.'

Australia punches above its weight in medical research, ranked in the top ten of countries by per capita spend, adjusted for population size, but in this area we are falling behind.

'Compared to other areas of reproduction and pregnancy, we are underdoing it when it comes to miscarriage research,' says Professor Robertson. 'It isn't because we don't have the capability, we definitely do. But what it does require is quite a lot of dedicated infrastructure, especially in regard to bio-banking.' A bio-bank, or bio-repository, is used to store biological samples, like tissue, for use in research.

What is the rate of miscarriage?

The human body is not very efficient when it comes to fertility.[48] Unlike men, who are constantly either producing sperm, or thinking about it, women are born with all the eggs they will ever have.

According to the Cleveland Clinic,[49] during fetal life, a woman may have up to seven million eggs. By the time she is born, this has reduced to one million eggs and this reduces even further. Only 300 to 400 eggs will be released during a woman's reproductive window. An extremely high number of fertilised eggs are thought to miscarry before implantation takes place. That number could be as high as 75 per cent.[50] So that time you had unprotected sex and didn't get pregnant? Maybe you did. Of a sort, anyway.

When researching the rate of miscarriage, there are two principal ways studies are conducted. The first is to get a group of people together and monitor them before everyone starts trying to conceive, the second is to do it retrospectively. There are benefits and drawbacks to both.

If you start monitoring people with blood tests before they get pregnant, you may end up catching miscarriages that would have otherwise been put down to a heavy flow or a late period. If you end up doing it retrospectively, you're working with self-reporting or memory recall, which isn't always as accurate as we might like.

The results of studies around pregnancy loss vary widely. Some show miscarriage rates are as low as one in five preganancies[51] and there are studies that show it could be as high as one in three.[52] It's important to note here that researchers do acknowledge that recruitment for many miscarriage surveys or research is disproportionately skewed away from marginalised groups such as those in low-income brackets, people of colour and the LGBTIQ+ community.

In a paper for *The Lancet* Professor Siobhan Quenby stated that a review of nine studies that collectively tracked about 4.6 million pregnancies found the pooled risk of miscarriage was 15.3 per cent.[53] This is lower than the commonly recognised one in four number, mostly because it is based only on clinically recognised miscarriage.

Arri Coomarasamy, director of the world's leading miscarriage research organisation, Tommy's, told me that he estimates that the number is much likely closer to 25 per cent, but acknowledges it could be higher. We just don't know.

In 2009, 5806 women aged between thirty-one and thirty-six years old were interviewed for the Australian Longitudinal Study on Women's Health[54] to obtain a full reproductive history. The conclusion drawn from this study was that the rate was one miscarriage for every four live births. Researchers noted there was a 'huge variation in the calculable rates, which would be higher again if the groups with no live births were included'.

Professor Hugh Taylor, the Chair of Obstetrics, Gynaecology and Reproductive Sciences at Yale, told me he believes the rate is 'much higher than commonly recognised'. Professor Regan agrees with

Professor Taylor. 'I personally think that the miscarriage rate is about 50 per cent . . . I think about 50 per cent of human conceptions are lost. And I think there's quite good data to support that. But if you raise expectations like that, what are you going to do in terms of how you are going to manage people and look after them?'

There are indeed several studies that bear out what Professors Regan and Taylor are saying. We begin that part of our journey in the days of the highest hair and most padded of shoulders. The Wilcox study[55] – which Taylor described to me as 'an old classic' – was published in the highly respected *New England Journal of Medicine* in 1988. The study recruited 221 healthy women from before their baby's conception. It conducted regular urinary analysis to detect hCG and found that one third of the positive results didn't proceed to delivery (meaning they resulted in pregnancy loss), though only one third of those were 'clinically recognised'.

'It could be higher than 30 per cent,' says Professor Taylor. 'In a normal, healthy, young woman, almost every month you'll ovulate, if the sperm is there, it will fertilise, you'll make a blastocyst and it'll start to try to attach to the uterus. So it depends on what you define as a pregnancy loss. There are a lot of losses that are in that first day or two.'

In America the Longitudinal Investigation of Fertility and the Environment (LIFE) Study[56] recruited 501 couples between 2005 and 2009. Participants completed blood and urine tests and also used a Clearblue Fertility Monitor to track intercourse relative to ovulation. The study was primarily aimed at tracking environmental factors affecting fertility, which we will discuss in chapter fourteen, but found the rate of pregnancy loss was 28 per cent.

Obviously much has changed in the years since the Wilcox study, and I'm not just talking about how some of us (but not others) moved on from super-strength hairspray and electric blue eyeshadow. There has been progress since the mid-2000s of the LIFE Study too. Parents have a better understanding of fertility cycles, conception, and greater access to super-sensitive at-home testing options and better medical care. Without seeing a doctor, you can know within days of implantation whether you're pregnant. A higher proportion of people experiencing loss know what is happening. Simultaneously, maternal age has continued to climb and we know that miscarriage rates mirror at least some of this increase.

When Jean Hailes for Women's Health added questions about miscarriage to its national survey, 34.3 per cent of the 4347 respondents said they had experienced miscarriage. 'I was really surprised by the percentage of people who said they'd experienced one, it was much higher than I was expecting,' says chief executive Janet Hailes Michelmore. 'It indicates to me that the official statistics are massively undercooked.'

Can you feel it in your waters?

When I spoke to early pregnancy loss researchers, obstetricians and scientists, I always asked them, based on their gut feeling – especially those working on the frontlines of health – whether they thought miscarriage rates were going up. Every single person said yes. Paused. And then qualified the statement.

As the veil lifts, it's difficult to say whether rates are on the rise or whether we just have more visibility over them. Other issues similar to this which have been cocooned in silence might be rape or domestic violence. In addition to the slow erosion of the taboo, other factors contributing to increasing visibility of miscarriage include better technology, like transvaginal ultrasounds, and high-sensitivity home pregnancy tests. Increasing maternal age is another factor, as is, possibly, increasing paternal age, but almost certainly sperm quality.[57]

'My gut is I believe it's going up, but I don't know because we can assess early pregnancy better than ever before, so are we just recognising more early pregnancy losses? I haven't seen a big jump in the later losses,' says Professor Taylor.

What little research we have indicates that miscarriage rates are rising. A key study from the US analysed self-reported pregnancy loss from 1990 to 2011 and found that, excluding abortion, the risk of pregnancy loss rose 2 per cent each year during the reporting period, after adjustment for maternal characteristics such as age.[58]

Back in the 1950s, a sociologist by the name of Joseph W. Eaton and a psychiatrist, Robert J. Weil, did a large study into Hutterite communities in America. Like Amish and Mennonite communities, they trace their origins to the Radical Reformation movement of the 1500s. These days they live in communities across western Canada and America. One aspect of the study looked at natural fertility and was long used to provide insight into how fertility declines in mothers over the age of thirty-five. But recently, more current data points to a general decline in fertility. Part of this is attributed to increased maternal ages, but looking at comparative ages from current data next to the original study shows that fertility is on a downward trend.[59] There are other indicators too. The annual number of rounds of IVF initiated each year in Australia had been rising by around 2 to 3 per cent annually, though it seems to be accelerating. From 2015–19, there was an 11 per cent jump. Between 2018 and 2019, the jump was over 6 per cent.[60]

What's going on down under?

While we don't have the full picture of data we want or we need, let's see if we can make a likely estimate of miscarriage numbers.

Hospitals log the reasons people are treated and the number of discharges (which they call – romantically or perhaps heartbreakingly – 'separations'). So, as a first step, what we can do is look at how many hospital discharges there were for miscarriage-related treatment, using data collated by the AIHW. In 2018–19, hospitals in Australia treated 85,383 cases of 'pregnancy with abortive outcome' and 'spontaneous abortion'[61], which combined cover what amounts to miscarriage, give or take. The terminology, and therefore data, is (some believe deliberately) obfuscated, which we will get to.

We don't know what number of repeat patients this number would include, but we do know that recurrent miscarriage only affects 1 per cent[62] of parents, so the number of repeat patients being treated for miscarriage is unlikely to be high. Even if we err on the side of caution and take out 1 per cent of miscarriages for repeat or recurrent patients (853), that still leaves 84,530 patients total.

We also know that an extremely large number of miscarriages never reach hospital. They are managed by GPs or obstetricians. Or at home. Or not at all, if the person who is pregnant doesn't even know it has happened. Studies from Finland and Denmark suggest that one in five miscarriages are not treated with a hospital admission.[63] This number would represent an additional 21,133 miscarriages, meaning our number is now at 105,663, an increase of around 2663 miscarriages annually from the commonly referenced Sands number.

We're starting to see that even with conservative estimates, the '103,000 families' figure may be planted on the very cautious side of the white picket fence. The real number could be higher. But how much higher?

According to Jacqueline Rek, AIHW's Manager of the National Perinatal Mortality Data Collection and the National Maternal Mortality Data Collection, another way to calculate the number of miscarriages in Australia per year would be to look at how many pregnancies get to twenty weeks. This, incidentally, is how Sands reached its 103,000 number.

If the miscarriage rate in Australia is one in four, then around 100,000 losses would be close to the right number, though not included in this increasingly frustrating equation is how many pregnancies we don't know about because they occur 'outside the system'.

But what happens when we apply miscarriage rates at the higher end of the scale to the Australian live birth rates, which Rek told us were around 300,000 per year, and this time assume that there's a 32 per cent rate of loss? All of a sudden we're looking at around 140,000 losses a year.

Are you as dissatisfied with this data deduction as I am? We're left with so many possibilities and no clear answer. The statistics we do have are so varied that it's clear we need to be collecting and collating this data properly so we can better inform policy and start resourcing medical professionals to best support patients and their families. There could well be a much larger cohort of people requiring care, and improvements in care, than we initially thought.

Where to now?

Miscarriage care has so many touchpoints. Patients can be under the care of a GP, an obstetrician, a midwife, or not under the care of any medical professional and miscarry at home. Professor Coomarasamy believes there are three layers of data that need to be collected, from hospitals, GPs and community.

Starting with hospitals, that information could be collected via an expansion of the Medicare codes to include codes that reflect miscarriage. Right now, data is rolled up, in part to obfuscate abortion data, with deliberately opaque Medicare coding. This coding needs to be clear and the lines delineated, with miscarriages that occur while in the care of a hospital (irrespective of department, for instance an early pregnancy assessment centre or emergency department) centralised.

GP management or oversight of miscarriage can also feed into the same central repository, whether by reporting or coding. However, there is some concern that GPs, already under huge time constraints and pressure, would refuse any additional reporting into a central repository despite the benefits better visibility would bring. When GPs are being pressured to cut minutes from their already fleeting appointment times, what seems to you and to me like a simple additional task amounts to a heavy burden.

For miscarriages that happen at home, away from medical professionals, or that are not clinically recognised, a self-reporting mechanism by the patient could be one way to bridge this gap. This would require broad advertising and promotion of the reporting framework through informal and formal support networks and healthcare professionals.

While self-reporting is flawed in some respects, together with GP reporting it would go a long way to including many of the forgotten miscarriages because they don't meet the definition of 'clinically recognised', a narrow view of what makes a miscarriage. It is also my view that the requirements for a miscarriage to be clinically recognised are locking out the groups most at risk of experiencing one. That includes people who have little to no contact with medical systems or contact that starts very late in pregnancy: people of colour, those on a low income, those who live with disability, people for whom English is a second language, members of the LGBTIQ+ community, or people who represent more than one of those groups.

Waiting on the World to Change

'What do you mean you can't do a scan? I came to a women's hospital so you could do a scan.' It was a Friday night in March 2018. Husbo was having drinks in the city. Being a basement bar, his phone had no signal. I was six weeks pregnant and had started bleeding. So much blood. Huge clots. I was terrified. I'd avoided passing my previous two miscarriages 'naturally', but my doctor didn't want me to have another D&C unless absolutely necessary, which I understood, while simultaneously being petrified. How much blood was too much? How big a clot was too big? Also the pain. This low, deep thud of pain. Like a fist clenching and squeezing. Clenching and squeezing. Clenching and squeezing. I was giving birth.

In a panic and with my toddler asleep in his bed, I had called my brother and my parents. My parents came to sit in the house with the Didgerijew. My brother tore over in an Uber (he had imbibed a few and didn't feel safe to drive) and off we went into the chilly Melbourne night.

||||||

My brother was trying not to giggle. No poker face, that guy.

'Hey, Dad, can you grab the cheese?'

'The cheese?'

'Yep it's just on the top shelf of the fridge, wrapped in foil.'

Dad grabbed the foil-covered package.

'Roy wants some, can you just unwrap it?'

Dad unwrapped layer after layer of foil as we all went raspberry red trying not to laugh. He was left holding several balls of foil and a positive pregnancy test.

I'll never forget the look of joy on my parents' faces. My mum cried, of course.

That night, before a dinner of takeaway with the whole family around my cramped kitchen table, was the last time in my life I celebrated a positive pregnancy test. Well, one of my own, anyway.

|||||||

'So what's going on?' asked the Uber driver curiously in a heavy Eastern European accent.

'I'm having a miscarriage,' I said, confident that it would shut him up.

'Oh, how do you know?' he asked.

'I'm bleeding heavily and I'm cramping and I'm six weeks pregnant.'

The topic of vaginal bleeding usually shuts people up. But not always, apparently. Pretty much everyone in my family has a dark funny bone, so my brother was trying to stifle his giggles as the Uber driver launched into a list of all the women he knew who'd experienced miscarriages. His sister, his mother, his sister-in-law . . .

I nodded and smiled, but inside I was praying for him to just shut the fuck up.

Shut up.

SHUT. UP.

|||||||

The triage nurse in the emergency department was sympathetic until I told her I'd had a dating scan at six weeks and two days, because with that she knew the pregnancy wasn't ectopic and was measuring a week behind.

After that, the staff lost interest and time seemed to grind to a snail's pace. They apparently decided it was likely a miscarriage and I didn't need treatment. Or care, empathy, sympathy or, indeed, dignity. The hospital was quiet. I was the only patient in the waiting room. I was the only patient behind the curtains. In the whole time I was there I didn't see or hear a single other patient. It was quiet. Too quiet. All I could hear was me. My own panicked voice, my sobs and my grunts as the squeezing came and went.

'We're not calling in an ultrasonologist because it's not life threatening. Just come back on Monday.'

Don't worry about whether or not your baby is dead for three days. Just put it aside and come back on Monday.

And that's how I ended up standing over my toilet bowl at home, after two hours of contractions, holding my tiny little baby, the size of a blueberry. No one had explained how to retain the tissue for testing. No one had prepared me for this moment. For what I might see. For how it might feel.

I was in shock. I was confused and I was totally and utterly alone, in every sense of the word. So, in a complete state of panic, I did something for which I will never forgive myself.

I flushed her down the toilet.

|||||||||||||||||||||||||||||||||||||||||||||||||||||||||||||||||||||||||||||||||||||||||||||||||||||||||||||||||||||||||

4

Bad Medicine

It's impossible to understate how many horror stories there are about miscarriage care in this country; they simply shouldn't be this easy to find. How and why is the system letting patients down?

Something that struck me, or perhaps floored me, when I started to investigate early pregnancy loss in Australia, is just how easy it is to find horror stories about the care patients receive . . . or indeed the total lack of care on offer. Whenever I made a public callout, even for highly defined experiences within a specific geographic location or complication type, I would get so many responses. I would have to set aside hours of time so I could respond to every single person who messaged me. It really shouldn't be this easy to find real-life case studies that demonstrate such serious gaps in our medical system.

As you might imagine, there are a multitude of issues that converge, as well as services that overlap, to create the sort of systemic and cultural problems that lead to these gaps in care.

In addition to the deficits in physical care, there are also cultural issues in medicine that affect how patients are treated when they seek care. This is why *The Lancet*, in its miscarriage series, was very clear in stating that 'the era of telling women to "just try again" is over'. It's a cultural distinction that doesn't fit with what we do know about miscarriage, medically speaking. It is nevertheless persistent, despite a wealth of information to back up the potential physical and psychological consequences. This could be related to long lapses in time between research and applying the results to clinical environments. The delay between the publication of research and the application of that work in medical practice can be as high as seventeen years.[64]

That in itself a huge issue that needs to be addressed by the medical fraternity.

There is one additional contextual overlay to bear in mind. We hear a lot about how the Australian hospital system is under-funded. And while sometimes this is used as an excuse for sloppy care or medical judgement found wanting, there are real consequences for every Australian patient seeking care. But what does that really mean? What does it look like? And how does it affect early pregnancy loss care?

That depends in part on who you ask, because we're not all equal in the eyes of the health system, a fact amplified during the Covid-19 pandemic. If English is your second language, if you are queer, genderqueer, have a disability, are not white, are a woman, have mental health issues, have a lower income, are Aboriginal or Torres Strait Islander – or if you identify as any combination of the above – these are all components that can affect the quality, cultural safety or suitability of the care you receive.

In addition, the Australian health system is stretched far beyond capacity, let down by successive state and federal governments failing to give the funding needed to deliver the world-class care that we as a nation could absolutely afford, should we make that choice. Years of relative funding cuts have taken their toll. Healthcare workers have been stretched beyond what is reasonable and at some levels (for example, nursing and midwifery) are paid far below their worth. And that was before the advent of a once-in-a-lifetime global health pandemic. Winter isn't coming for healthcare. It's here. And it's fucking freezing.

In 2019, the AIHW confirmed that the public hospital elective surgery waitlist had swelled to 890,000 patients for 2018–19. Only

760,000 patients were admitted to surgery during that time period, showing the capacity gap. This isn't botox for your worry lines. Elective surgery is any surgery that can be scheduled in advance and is therefore not classified an emergency: joint replacements to give someone back mobility, cataract surgery so people can see, tonsillectomies for sick kids or even hernia corrections. The average annual growth in elective surgery waiting lists is around 2.5 per cent[65], so each year the list widens out just a little bit more.

Meanwhile emergency department data for the same period of 2018–19 showed that of the 8.4 million presentations each year in Australian public hospitals – 23,000 a day – only 71 per cent of patients were seen on time for their urgency category, down from 74 per cent in 2014–15. The overall number of presentations was a 4.2 per cent increase on 2017–18.

Why am I telling you this? Because before we launch into all the ways the system fails patients who experience early pregnancy loss, we have to understand that the system is failing more generally due to a lack of critical resources.

Two final notes. This chapter seeks to identify and address gaps in care. That means the ways we go wrong. We can never forget that there are a lot of doctors working hard, doing their best, who genuinely care about the people they treat. We should never forget that they exist and that not every patient has experienced the gaps I will outline, though an unacceptable number do. Also, when I refer in this chapter to medical care, I am excluding psychological treatment, which is of course of equal importance, and will be addressed in chapter eight.

Long and winding road

So. You think you're pregnant. Maybe your boobs are on fire. Maybe you did a wee on a stick. Did you look in your diary and realise you're a couple of weeks late? Chances are you'll be heading to your GP.

When a patient attends a GP clinic to confirm a pregnancy, the first step is usually a urine test, a blood test for hCG levels or perhaps an ultrasound if the patient is unsure of their dates. Once a pregnancy is confirmed, the next step is a specialist referral. If you're a public patient this would be to your local public hospital, which you would visit for the first time somewhere around twelve to eighteen weeks. If you're planning to go private, the referral would be for a private obstetrician, and they generally see patients from around nine weeks, though this can happen earlier.

GPs primarily come into contact with miscarriage or pregnancy loss when the loss is before the patient is in the care of an obstetrician or midwife. It would be best practice in the case of a suspected miscarriage to order an hCG test, or indeed two to establish whether it is rising and at what rate, and/or an ultrasound. When a miscarriage is confirmed, the three options for management must be given and explained (medical, surgical or expectant, aka 'natural'). If the patient opts for surgical or medical management, they are usually referred to hospital (an early pregnancy assessment service if available or emergency department) or in some cases a private clinic like the not-for-profit Marie Stopes Australia, now known as MSI Australia. It is the only national family planning organisation in Australia and offers the full breadth of family planning services from contraception to abortion and everything in between.

Kate's miscarriage was confirmed by her GP with blood tests. She was referred to her local hospital's early pregnancy assessment service to arrange a D&C, but they never called her back. Luckily Kate could afford to get a D&C privately. 'I called Marie Stopes and booked in with them and they were really good; they were really, really lovely and understanding and handled it really well.' But when she turned up on the day, it was a challenging process. 'It was just kind of miserable because you're there, and this is nothing on Marie Stopes, but it's an abortion clinic. You're surrounded by people who don't want their pregnancy. It's just a different vibe.' The cost of a D&C at Marie Stopes starts at $620 for those with Medicare.

Frontline fatigue

The Royal Australian College of General Practitioners' (RACGP) *General Practice: Health of the Nation* report for 2019 showed a growing number of GPs had seen workload growth in the previous two years and 29 per cent of GPs disagreed or strongly disagreed that their work–life balance had improved over the past five years. 'Job satisfaction and positive perception of work–life balance have deteriorated since 2013, which will compound the current slow growth in GP numbers across the country and increase the difficulties in recruiting and retaining GPs in the future.'[66]

GPs are specialist generalist medicine practitioners and identify or treat 10,000 medical conditions. They are truly at the coalface of community medical care and they see it all. 'I remember the Dean of Medicine at Monash University sitting us down in first year medicine way back when saying, "You will be lifelong learners",' explains Royal Australian College of General Practitioners President Dr Karen Price. 'And that's what we are, and most of us actually enjoy it, as long as you've got the time, space and, frankly, sometimes the money to afford to be able to do it.'

The reality is that GPs are under-funded, under-resourced and face huge pressure within a system that often doesn't let them do their jobs in the way they would like. 'Medicare is being made so cumbersome; it's based on activity, it's based increasingly on [item numbers] and it's dividing healthcare down into ever smaller parts,' says Dr Price. 'And that's not good for general practice, it doesn't work; it's not the philosophy of care, or training that we have. So we really are pitted against the system. And I understand that the health insurer wants to try to audit what we do, but all the evidence points to generalism being the best way to run your health system.'

Many GPs provide phenomenal supportive care to patients experiencing miscarriage. Some do not. Where care is lacking, it's usually due to time pressures or subscribing to the outdated cultural protocols like 'just try again'. 'When we have systems of care that really focus on volume and activity, and disease, instead of focusing on quality and person-centred care, you need time to be able to do that, and you need the hospital or general practice or whatever service staff to have enough time to actually really see the person in front of them. If they're rushed, stressed, hurried, and have millions of people to see, it's going to be very hard for any health service to deliver that patient the care that's needed,' says Dr Price.

Dr Price also acknowledges the role played by the lag in the time it takes for research to become integrated into practice. 'Evidence takes a long time to trickle through, and not only that, but evidence does have to be tested. There is always the early adopters and then there's the people who watch and wait and see what happens, because you don't want to be the first and you don't want to be the last to adopt a new change in treatment. There's often a bit of what we call "clinical variation" and, in practice, that's reasonable.' She adds with a laugh, 'It doesn't move along in a nice linear fashion, that would be lovely, but that's not the real world.'

I should also take a moment to point out that GP care can operate differently in regional and rural areas, where many take part in shared care with public hospitals. These doctors do additional training in obstetrics so they can do much of the routine maternity monitoring, when patients can't regularly travel the long distances required to access their nearest hospital. Many of those GPs are able to dispense drugs for medical management of miscarriage and some may even be able to perform a D&C. However, some GPs have told me that regional hospitals are making shared care arrangements more difficult and it is becoming less common.

What use is a vagina?

American radio and TV host Art Linkletter once said, 'Sometimes I'm asked by kids why I condemn marijuana when I haven't tried it. The greatest obstetricians in the world have never been pregnant.'

Obstetrics is the field of study for pregnancy, childbirth and the post-partum period. But like all areas of medicine, it falls prey to the same misogynistic and patriarchal views on which modern medicine (and you could say society more broadly) is built. These translate into the cultural, medical and practical ways in which patients who do not identify as male are disbelieved, misunderstood and treated with less care.

Obstetrician and gynaecologist Dr Kara Thompson says there are clear gender biases in Medicare item rebates that can't be explained by differences in difficulty or time required for services. She points out that the Medicare benefit payable on a woman's pelvic ultrasound is $102.20. To scan a scrotum, the rebate is $113.95.

'This makes no sense for a number of reasons,' she explains. 'Firstly, female pelvic scans look at more organs and structures than a scrotum scan and the range of pathology can be more varied and subtle, endometriosis for example. Secondly, the type of scanning equipment is different. Scrotum is all external and requires one type of probe. A pelvic scan on a woman is usually both transabdominal and transvaginal. This requires two different probes, and special cleaning and sterilisation procedures for the internal scan. Thirdly, the time difference is significant. Pelvic scans take longer, as there are more organs and more details to be assessed. In addition, the time required to use two probes, and this often requiring a woman to go to the toilet between scans to empty her bladder and the sonographer stepping out to give the woman privacy to undress. If the sonographer is a male, a chaperone is required for an internal scan, which is a significant extra personnel cost.'

This creates a disincentive for hospitals to provide out-of-hours ultrasound services, which are expensive. 'It goes some way to explaining why you can get an X-ray or CT any time day or night in hospital, but it is very difficult to get a pelvic ultrasound,' says Thompson.

Interesting that of the pelvic ultrasounds conducted in this country, the overwhelmingly vast majority are done on women.

'It does feel like this is such an egregious example of gender bias in medicine that we should be able to get it rectified if we made enough noise.'

Australian journalist and author Gabrielle Jackson covers this topic in her incredibly important book *Pain and Prejudice*,[67] which addresses this topic broadly within the context of chronic pain. Jackson argues that, historically, women's pain was dismissed with theories of hysteria and 'the widespread idea that a woman is inherently irrational and brimming with uncontrollable emotions and bodily functions'.

While the medical concept of hysteria has been debunked, the cultural implications endure and have led to a raft of well-documented adverse health outcomes for women that persist today; women are less likely to be diagnosed with heart issues, medicine knows less about every aspect of women's biology than men's, women are less likely to be included in medical trials, and almost half of women diagnosed with auto-immune diseases will be told they are hypochondriacs or 'too concerned with their health'.

'There's a palpable anger towards conventional medicine, and doctors in particular, that needs to be confronted,' Jackson writes.[68] Writing in Croakey Health Media, senior public health registrar Dr Lea Merone explains, 'Studies have demonstrated that owing to gender biases, the pain of female patients is often taken less seriously than that of males; with women on average waiting significantly longer for diagnosis and pain relief.'[69]

In its series on miscarriage, *The Lancet* alluded to this double-standard, comparing the idea of non-interventional treatment in miscarriage as similar to treatments of other 'women's issues', such as menstrual pain and menopause. Women's pain and trauma cannot and should not be dismissed or ignored. One obstetrician described the dismissal of miscarriage and the failure to treat patients holistically to me as the 'obstetric equivalent of a teenager being told for five years that their painful periods were normal'.

The first council of the Royal Australian College of Obstetricians and Gynaecologists was appointed in 1978 and was an all-male affair, which reflected the fact that 95 per cent of obstetricians at the time were men.[70] But thankfully, change is afoot. By 2012, 80 per cent of the training cohort were female and predictions were being made that in the next two to three decades 'obstetrics and gynaecology will have a predominantly female workforce'.[71] The gap has continued to narrow, and by 2016 men made up 55.4 per cent of obstetric clinicians.[72] But there is still a glass ceiling.

Men continue to occupy the majority of the obstetric and gynaecology department head roles at many of Australia's biggest hospitals. Since the 1998 amalgamation of the Royal Australian College of Obstetricians and Gynaecologists (RACOG) and the Royal New Zealand College of Obstetricians and Gynaecologists (RNZCOG) to create the Royal Australian and New Zealand College of Obstetricians and Gynaecologists (RANZCOG), just one of its eleven presidents has been a woman.

One.

In a speciality that treats vaginas.

The waiting game

Though it is slowly showing signs of abating, there is a pervasive and dangerous idea that persists in the early pregnancy loss space around miscarriage being 'natural' and 'necessary' and therefore requiring no active care or management. It is true that more than half of miscarriages are both natural and necessary. Chromosomal abnormalities are thought to account for anywhere from 50 to 70 per cent of miscarriages. Ultimately, these pregnancies simply aren't viable, so the body expels them in a biologically imperative form of quality control. Some miscarriages will occur and complete 'naturally' and not need intervention. But just because something is natural, it doesn't mean it doesn't present physical risks. Miscarriage can be life-threatening or come with life-threatening complications, including sepsis, rupture or even cancer.

Equally, just because something is 'natural' or 'necessary', it doesn't mean it can't cause significant trauma. Irrespective of whether it presents physical or even life-threatening risk to the patient, miscarriage has been linked to post-traumatic stress disorder (PTSD), depression, anxiety[73] and even suicide.[74]

Research shows those mental health issues can persist for years, even after the birth of a subsequent living child.[75] It can result in anxiety and depression that moves far beyond subsequent pregnancies and influences parent–child attachment if a successful live birth is achieved, and even influences the way those subsequent children are parented, with higher incidences of what's known as 'helicopter parenting'.

With statistics showing that most miscarriages are a single anomaly event, many obstetricians encourage their patients to 'just try again' on the basis that a subsequent, successful pregnancy will 'fix it'.

The 'just try again' idea is not a strategy, it's a harmful dismissal. Indeed, *The Lancet* states that the 'insidious implication' that miscarriage 'should be managed with minimal medical intervention is ideological, not evidence based'.[76]

People who have experienced miscarriage are also at higher risk of preterm birth, fetal growth restriction, placental abruption, stillbirth in future pregnancies and other non-obstetric health issues like cardiovascular disease and venous thromboembolism.[77] This is another factor that seems to be roundly ignored in many obstetric and broader medical circles.

And then there are the miscarriages that aren't 'necessary', meaning they could be prevented. The miscarriages that are caused by underlying health conditions such as auto-immune diseases, an incompetent cervix, genetic disorders and so on. When we dismiss all pregnancy loss as being 'normal' and 'natural', the ones that are neither fall between the cracks.

This is why there is a push among advocates to test pregnancy tissue wherever possible in order to identify the miscarriages that have occurred without chromosomal abnormalities, indicating there might be something else at play, rather than the current standard, which is waiting until the patient has had three losses and been classified as experiencing 'recurrent miscarriage'.

In the 2021 editorial on miscarriage in *The Lancet*, the world's leading doctors and researchers in the field also pushed for a new graded model of care that would see patients screened for risk factors and offered online preconceptual advice after one miscarriage. After a second they would be referred to a nurse or midwifery-led service offering continuity of care, some investigations and regular ultrasounds during subsequent pregnancy for management of anxiety. A third miscarriage would qualify the patient for a full panel of investigation and intervention for recurrent miscarriage.[78]

Kate had seventeen miscarriages before, during and after her two living children. It wasn't until she finally got into the medical obstetric department at a Sydney hospital, after being on a long waiting list, and was then referred to a recurrent miscarriage clinic that she started to get some answers. Those answers included a blood-clotting disorder, similarities to polycystic ovary syndrome, fibroids and more. Does she believe at least some of her losses could have been avoided, and potentially she could have had more children, had those issues been identified earlier? 'I do. The thyroid would have been dealt with, the clotting issue would have been dealt with,' she says sadly. 'It chews up so much time, waiting for appointments, getting in the queue, getting on the treadmill, see this person, see that person, get these bloods. Months turn into years, turn into a decade. It is so long and it is so exhausting.'

Holistic, you say?

The medical system is highly aspirational. There are benchmarks, standards and key performance indicators. The Australian system just isn't geared to achieve them, primarily due to a lack of resources, but culture also plays a part. Two persistent sexy catchphrases bandied about are 'holistic care' and 'patient-centred care'. Holistic care represents the treatment of all aspects of a patient's well-being.

Patient- (or person)-centred care means placing the person receiving healthcare and their family at the centre of all decision-making about their health and treating them with care and respect.[79] The inability of many medical specialists to apply these theories in practice is the third factor contributing to sub-standard care.

In a 2018 study,[80] key barriers to patient- and family-centred care were staffing constraints and reduced levels of staff experience, high staff workloads and time pressures, lack of physical resources, environmental constraints and unsupportive staff attitudes. The same study identified key enablers of patient- and family-centred care as leadership focus, staff satisfaction and positive staff relations, formal structures or processes to support the care itself, staff cultural diversity and health professional values or role expectations. These findings were established through interviews at a 215-bed metropolitan acute care public hospital in Sydney, but the issues raised were consistent across other studies of a similar nature, including in Europe[81] and the US.[82]

Recasting the lens to encompass the whole view of the patient, moving beyond just their reproductive organs and biology, apparently proves challenging for some medical professionals. For a host of reasons, as detailed above, including time pressure or lack of insight or empathy, some clinicians simply don't have an interest in or ability to treat the patient holistically. This might include looking at how stress levels affect the patient's ability to conceive or carry a baby to term, or referring them for psychological support or giving advice on healthy conception. Or doing a full physical examination to ensure a pregnancy loss is complete and the patient isn't at risk of further complications. Or ensuring the patient is provided with whatever follow-up they need post-loss.

When it comes to emergency medicine, holistic care is more complicated. Emergency medicine is life or death: heart attacks, gunshot wounds, car accidents, severed limbs and burns. Triage – categorising presentations so that the most urgent cases are seen first – is key to saving lives. But it means that patients who present with cases that emergency department (ED) staff don't see as urgent are sometimes ignored, disrespected or given no information about where to find care. Unfortunately, this is what often happens when patients experiencing miscarriage attend hospital. Often they are bleeding, passing clots, experiencing contractions and, in some cases, absolutely terrified. Sometimes, in addition to being scared for the life of their baby, they're fearful they're going to die too.

Miscarriages or threatened miscarriages are seemingly always, no matter the length of the ED queue, at the bottom or close to the bottom of the list. There are two reasons for that. The first is this assumption that miscarriage is natural, not dangerous and not life-threatening, with the exclusion of ectopic pregnancies. The second is that there is a perception that early pregnancy loss happens 'for a reason', the pregnancy can't be saved and therefore intervention or care is pointless.

Queensland-based emergency physician Dr Kim Hansen would expect a miscarriage to be categorised as a category three in the five-category triage system, unless ectopic. Usually a category three would be seen within around thirty minutes to an hour, but these times are blowing out due to resource constraints and she says category three patients can now regrettably wait for three or four hours, or even longer.

'I don't think it's reasonable for anyone – it doesn't matter if it's trivial or not – to spend that much time in an emergency department,' she explains, 'and it just shows that the health system is not coping with the current demand.'

There are other factors for the extended wait too. If the examination needs to take place in a bed, not a chair, the patient is likely to wait much, much longer; beds are one of the most valuable emergency department commodities and there simply aren't enough of them.

And then there are the cultural issues.

There have been several instances of pregnant patients presenting in general emergency departments but failing to be treated because the attending doctor wanted the patient transferred to an obstetric department. In one case, a woman in Melbourne died because a doctor failed to identify sepsis that could have been treated with a broad-spectrum antibiotic. Transferring obstetric patients immediately out of EDs because no one wants to deal with them also means that sometimes ED staff are unable to provide really basic care in the case of an emergency.

'I remember someone coming in, in cervical shock during a complicated miscarriage with products stuck in the cervix,' one ED doctor told me. 'Removing them is a very simple procedure that involves a speculum exam, but no one who has trained there knew how to do it because pregnant women get funnelled elsewhere.'

Dr Hansen explains, 'I still think there is a view among some healthcare workers, though hopefully it's diminishing, that this is very complex, that it's "women's problems".' While the number of trainees coming through medical schools are now evenly split between men and women, she also says certain biases can be persistent. 'Studies show women's pain isn't taken as seriously as men's pain and, of course, that bias can come from female practitioners as well. The more we try to break down those biases and normalise that this is a mainstream part of medical care, the better. It's not just a single speciality that deals with women's health.' Interestingly, a 2016 American study found that nurses in emergency departments reported the least amount of confidence and knowledge to provide women and families with support in cases of presentation with miscarriage.[83]

Dr Simon Judkins has worked in both urban and regional emergency rooms and says that clinicians rarely get to spend the amount of time with patients that they would like and often they are 'very, very rushed'. He explains ED staff are often looking to move that patient to somewhere they can get the best possible speciality care, which is frequently not readily available. Communication in those circumstances can be very challenging and often falls short of what a patient needs.

'There is time pressure to see the next patient or the resuscitation patient or the palliative care patient who's dying and I think whenever you have a system that's working at capacity or over capacity, those extra bits, those very important parts of the doctor–patient relationship, get missed,' he says sadly.

But there's another factor he raises that must be acknowledged.

'Some of it is also probably related to individual clinicians' own level of stress and well-being. Working in an environment which is often very stretched and stressed, conversations with distressed people can be very challenging for the medical staff; they have never met the patient, and they are delivering terrible, terrible news the patient doesn't want to hear.'

Reproductive psychologists Martha and David Diamond write, 'This work is not for the faint of heart. As any clinician who has listened to the physical details of miscarriages, or has borne witness to the "baby pictures" brought in by parents who have just experienced a stillbirth can attest, this kind of work requires not just specialised knowledge and training but courage.'[84]

Communication (or a lack thereof) with patients so they understand wait times, reasons for delays and so on is also a source of frustration for patients. 'Back when I went to medical school,' Dr Hansen explains, 'there really was very little education around communication, and in particular, the "soft skills", the empathy, compassion. It's getting better now, but I still don't think it's emphasised as a key skill along with clinical knowledge or procedural skills.'

Equally, time is required to explain management options in cases where action needs to be taken. When Estelle was diagnosed with an incomplete miscarriage in a Melbourne ED, she was pushed to make a decision on how it would be managed. 'Everything was falling down around me and I was having to make a decision on the spot, but I also felt like we were really on the clock. A doctor would come in and say, "Have you made a decision yet?" There needs to be some kind of broader understanding of those management processes . . . so you don't end up being put on the spot when you're not actually in any mental state to deal with it.'

When dealing with patients whose first language isn't English, these issues are even more acute. Most of the printed material on offer (and there isn't much) isn't translated for varying language groups. If you fall outside a white, high–income bracket your ED experience is likely worse. An American study that looked at the effects of race and socio-economic factors in the way patients were treated in ED featured some extremely worrying findings. We already know that people of colour and those on low incomes are more likely to experience miscarriage. But when they turn up at an emergency department for miscarriage or threatened miscarriage treatment, they're more likely to be admitted to hospital when compared with white, privately insured women, more likely to have surgery (including surgical sterilisation instead of contraception) and higher rates of complications, and are less likely to receive pain medication.[85] Basically, they're more likely to be paternalised and interfered with by the system, but not have their pain taken seriously.

In 1998, Leah went to hospital in Queensland. She had already had a fallopian tube removed due to an ectopic pregnancy. She was pregnant again but had started throwing up and was in tremendous pain, which was radiating up into her shoulder. A nurse told her off for lying on her stomach and accused her of only being there to seek pain medication. 'You're lying to us,' she told Leah. Despite Leah's incredibly high pain threshold, the pain in her shoulder was unbearable. Shoulder pain is common in ectopic pregnancy and is caused by abdominal bleeding. A doctor finally came to see her and within minutes she was being wheeled into surgery. She saw the nurse's 'look of absolute horror as I was wheeled past her. I hope it stayed with her for the rest of her life.'

All the best with your book

In 2007, at fourteen weeks pregnant, Jana Horska miscarried in the waiting room toilet at Royal North Shore Hospital's ED in Sydney. It was leaked to the press and sparked a firestorm of outrage over her treatment, or lack thereof. The furore sparked a Parliamentary Royal Commission and, as a result, several recommendations were made around miscarriage care, including the establishment and monitoring of early pregnancy assessment services (EPAS) in public hospitals across New South Wales. While progress reports were made in NSW Health's annual reports in the couple of years following the inquiry, these quickly dissipated. As did any mention of early pregnancy care.

I first started investigating EPAS clinics in New South Wales when a well-placed source told me off-the-record that many EPAS clinics, especially in regional areas, were operating in name only and weren't being adequately staffed or resourced. I approached NSW Health asking a number of questions about EPAS clinics in the state, for instance who had oversight, how they were funded and so on. I waited six months for a response. When it finally came, the response read, 'This information is not available,' and then added the passive aggressive afterthought, 'All the best with your book.' One of the queries was simply, 'How many EPAS clinics are there in New South Wales?' And another was, 'How many public hospitals are there in New South Wales?' None of this information was apparently being held by NSW Health. If NSW Health doesn't know how many hospitals there are in New South Wales, who in the name of Saint Dolly Parton does exactly?

EPAS clinics can provide some of the best care available to patients who are miscarrying. But unfortunately, they are understaffed, under-resourced and unable to always provide the care that they should. After further investigation, I wrote a news feature for *Guardian Australia*[86] on the unreliable, or in some cases non-existent, care being provided in EPAS clinics around the state. Just before the story went to print, I offered NSW Health one more opportunity to comment. They finally provided me with an actual statement to the effect of management, oversight and budgets are all the responsibility of local health districts. So they passed the buck and declared it not their problem. Big surprise. Not.

I spoke to Jana Horska about her experience that night in the Royal North Shore Hospital ED and she, like so many of the patients I interviewed, was generous and forthcoming about what was one of the worst experiences of her life. She told me what it felt like to squat on the floor of the ED waiting area as she suffered contractions, the lack of information or care given by staff and the eventual arrival of her baby boy on the floor of a toilet cubicle. She talked about her fear as she birthed her baby and screamed for her husband. How he burst in to the cubicle thinking she was dying.

Even now, she struggles with how much information to give her living children about their sibling and the circumstances of his passing. She expressed anger that women are still treated with such a lack of care when presenting in hospital emergency rooms with threatened miscarriage.

In that same article, I also told the story of Hannah, who went to an emergency department in 2021, after the hospital's EPAS clinic failed to return a multitude of calls. She was given painkillers and told, again, to call the EPAS. When the clinic finally called her back, Hannah explained that she suffers from a kidney disorder and is used to high levels of pain, but she was really struggling. She was also losing a lot of blood and concerned about being left alone. 'And she [the nurse] said to me, "Darling, it's just a miscarriage".'

This is not a problem in any way limited to New South Wales. I later extended this investigation into other states where there were clear examples of sub-standard care.[87] At eight weeks pregnant in 2021, Marie started passing large clots and went to hospital in Canberra. She was told she couldn't have a scan, not even at the fetal monitoring unit (FMU) which doesn't see patients until after twelve weeks. There was nowhere else to go. 'I feel like a problem for the system,' says Marie. 'I feel like I'm inconveniencing people. The advocacy you have to go through for yourself isn't fair.'

By fourteen weeks Marie was aware that something was very wrong, but made the mistake of calling and asking the FMU for a scan on a Friday afternoon. 'We're public servants, we only work nine to five,' the nurse told her. Two weeks later she found out her baby had stopped growing.

When Elsa started to miscarry at twelve weeks in Queensland in 2019, she attended an emergency department. She waited for several hours, watching people with minor injuries being sent through for care. She was then told it would be another three to four hours before someone would be able to see her, so she left. No one tried to give her any information or communicate with her. She miscarried her daughter Lucy at home in the shower that evening. In a panic, totally unsure what to do, she put her daughter in a container and put the container in the freezer. She contacted a private specialist the next day and was told to come in immediately. He examined her and found that the placenta was lodged in her cervix. Had Elsa not pursued medical care, this would have led to serious complications.

So while we can see the need for a wholesale shift in the way ED staff care for and treat patients experiencing miscarriage, if they're going to be referring those patients to EPAS clinics, work must be done there too. Clinic staff need to be provided with specialist training, referral pathways for psychosocial support and specialist obstetric staff to back up the staff midwives and nurses. Some EPAS clinics in this country do have all of those things, but they are few and far between. This must be prioritised nationally as a matter of urgency.

We don't talk anymore

Beyond the gaps in care, there are also deficits created when the systems don't talk to each other. These systemic issues are broadly applicable across medicine but can compound emotional and physical trauma when it comes to miscarriage care.

Stella was told in the fourteenth week of her pregnancy that her daughter Frankie had Down syndrome. The Melbourne hospital's genetic counselling service treated her with compassion and kindness. But before she could decide whether she wanted to proceed with the pregnancy or not, a scan at sixteen weeks confirmed the baby had died in utero.

It was then, in her distraught state, that Stella was told she would have to exit the hospital system and re-enter via the emergency department, essentially starting her hospital journey from scratch. She waited for hours in ED with no communication, surrounded by pregnant women and newborns, only to be told upon admission that she would have to wait another week for a D&C to end the pregnancy. Eventually, she had the procedure, but three weeks later, at twenty weeks, she was sent a text message reminder that she was due for her twenty-week scan.

'There were just all these ways that the system didn't link up, they really let the whole experience down, which is a real shame,' she explains.

This is a common issue among people who experience early pregnancy loss. There is no flag system to notify the various health touchpoints that they are at risk of miscarriage or indeed no longer pregnant. So they're often subjected to reminders and notifications because there's no way to extract their information. The systems don't talk to each other.

When Alice found out she was pregnant with her second child, she attended her GP clinic and was referred to the local private hospital. But before she got the letter from the hospital confirming her first appointment, she started to bleed. She knew something was wrong. Her GP referred her for an ultrasound, but being too early for a definitive diagnosis, she was asked to come back in two weeks. The bleeding increased and her follow-up ultrasound confirmed a complete miscarriage. It was while she was grieving that she received a letter from the hospital to attend her first appointment for a pregnancy that no longer existed.

'It was just one of the most surreal things, because I was calling to cancel the appointment and the lady was like, "Do you want to make a different day?" and I was like, "No, no", but I wasn't ready to even say I wasn't pregnant.'

When Anne attended an EPAS clinic with a threatened miscarriage, she had to sit in waiting rooms full of pregnant women, then describe why she was there over and over. No one had time to read her medical notes, and continuity of care wasn't a priority. These issues could be remedied by previous clinicians taking the time to update her notes, those notes being made available to all future clinics and then being read before or during appointments.

'The fact that you have to go back and forth to a thousand appointments, there's not just one person who can do it. You can't just go see a doctor that you trust, and they do the scan and they confirm it to you. It's also really difficult when you're in the middle of that to share that experience with so many strangers.'

In some hospitals overseas, medical notes of people who have experienced loss are indicated with a sticker on their file. This is particularly important for pregnancies after loss so medical professionals are aware they may be dealing with a patient who is experiencing PTSD or elevated anxiety. I'm not aware of any hospitals in Australia at the time of writing who use this simple and almost zero-cost technique.

Another systemic issue that compounds trauma for miscarriage patients is the location of the services they attend. I've been active in online miscarriage support groups for over eight years. I hear one complaint repeatedly: when dealing with a threatened or confirmed miscarriage, the last thing you want is to be seated in a room with heavily pregnant patients. It's been described to me as a form of 'mental torture'.

According to NSW government guidelines, EPAS clinics are supposed to have a discrete waiting area, but many are located within maternity wards. Rose had a loss confirmed via ultrasound in regional New South Wales and was then referred to the local hospital's EPAS. They took three days to call her back. When she finally went in for her appointment, she was surrounded by pregnant women.

I was buoyed in 2022 when the head of a recurrent miscarriage clinic at a large Melbourne hospital approached me after a discussion panel to tell me they were moving the clinic to the same location as EPAS, away from maternity. I congratulated him and his team for their ability to see the need and make the change happen. After all, even where there is desire on the part of the medical professionals – and there often is – they are still unable to tweak the system to make change possible.

After a pregnancy loss, I had a follow-up with the lead obstetrician/ultrasonologist at the ultrasound clinic where I had almost all of my pregnancy scans. At the end of the consultation I asked the doctor (who I knew well) whether I could provide some feedback and he said, 'Of course.' I suggested that when a patient attend for an urgent ultrasound for threatened miscarriage, they be seated in a separate area on the other side of the floor rather than in the main waiting area. Or they could even be offered to stay in the changing rooms until they were summoned for their scan. He looked at me, his face totally blank. 'Why?'

I explained that one of the most traumatic aspects of miscarriage is being seated in waiting areas next to heavily pregnant women talking about gender, names, and rubbing their bellies while you wonder to yourself, 'Why not me?', as your dreams of having a baby slip away. I said it was the complaint made more than any other in the numerous support groups I frequented.

'Huh,' he said. 'I'd never thought about it.' He expressed his gratitude for the feedback and off I went. Three years later, as I was writing this book, I checked in at the clinic to see whether any changes had been made when patients attend with threatened miscarriage.

Reader, they had not.

Four Horsemen

My fourth miscarriage was in March 2018. The same month we had tickets to see one of my favourite American rockers, Benjamin Booker. A girlfriend and husbo conspired not to let me stay home. I didn't take much convincing. I knew it would be good for me to get out of the house and Booker was my favourite.

A friend had slipped us a small amount of MDMA and recommended that we have a little bump to help us find some light in the darkness. So off we went, the three musketeers. We sang and danced until 4 am, sweaty and smiling, pretending we didn't have a single care in the world. For a short time, I felt alive. Something I hadn't felt for weeks.

But when my pregnancy test turned positive the following month, my insides calcified on the spot.

||||||

'When was the last time you had sex?' came Dr Lovely's voice over the phone.

'I'm pregnant, I knew it.'

'Isy, how did you do that?'

My body hadn't even had a period after my last loss and, again, here I was. But this time I had an awkward question to ask. The embarrassment crept up over me like a rosy glow and warmed up to the point where I felt like I might spontaneously combust.

'Hey, um, I didn't think I'd get pregnant so fast. And I, well, um, I went to a club and I had the tiniest little bit of MDMA. Does that matter?'

Dr Lovely laughed. 'No, not one bit. It's far too early for that to have affected the pregnancy.'

I miscarried a few short weeks later and the guilt was like a tourniquet around my neck. But I didn't have time for grief. I ripped off the tourniquet and ran in the other direction, turning my attention to getting pregnant again.

||||||

My friend Carmen's new baby was in the back seat as we drove around running errands. We snuck into McDonald's drive-through while the baby slept and giggled while we stuffed ours faces full of junk and chatted away. 'Mum's gone Mickey D wild!' I shouted as Carmen laughed and took another nugget.

I had met Carmen in my mother's group when Roy was born. We took a while to warm to each other but she'd become one of my closest friends and one of the only people I talked to openly about my losses. She and almost all the other mums in the group had welcomed their second babies. Despite being the first in the group to say I wanted to try again, I was the one whose dreams of a second child were becoming less and less likely to materialise.

On the drive home we chatted about her son Tommy's birth. And I recalled the day Roy came into the world and feeling my heart truly being full for the first time in my life. I turned to Carmen. 'What if I don't have that again?'

I pulled over and I cried. Not the way I'd cried before. This time they were huge, heaving sobs from right inside my chest, as I watched the thing I wanted more than anything else moving further and further away into the distance. It was the first time my faith in my happy ending truly wavered, but it wouldn't be the last.

|||||||||||||||||||||||||||||||||||||||||||||||||||||||||||||||||||||||||||||||||||||||||||||||||||||||||

5

Fast Car

There are some stark differences between the experiences of patients in the public system and those in the private system, and the pros and cons fall on both sides of the divide.

At the end of chapter twenty-eight of Mark Twain's *Adventures of Huckleberry Finn*, he makes use of a mid-nineteenth century proverb: 'You pays your money and you takes your choice'. While we live in a capitalist society where money buys you choice, nowhere is this more true than in the healthcare system.

Australia's healthcare system is world-leading for acute and emergency care, which often costs nothing for Australian taxpayers. But when it comes to some 'elective' surgery (anything that can be scheduled, like for instance a D&C) or treatments for issues considered not life-threatening, in many circumstances, whether or not you have private health membership is going to dictate what choices and options you have and the speed with which you are treated.

But the number of Australians with private health insurance is in decline, in large part due to climbing premiums. The biggest shrinking demographic in terms of cover is young people, aged 25–34.[88] At June 2021, 44.5 per cent of the Australian population had private hospital cover, a decline from 47.4 per cent in June 2015,[89] despite a slight uptick during 2020–21, thought to be driven by the Covid pandemic.

As a consequence, more patients are giving birth in the public system. Reassuringly for a lover of medical science like me, 96 per cent of all births in Australia in 2020 took place in hospitals, in conventional labour wards. Of those, a whopping 75 per cent were in public hospitals in 2019, leaving 25 per cent of those in the private system.[90] This marks a period of steady growth since 2010, when it was 70 per cent in public, and 2015 when it was 73 per cent.[91]

Private 'gap' fees (the amount a patient is out of pocket due to private insurance not covering all costs of care) can be staggering in obstetrics. While the cost of giving birth in the public system is often nothing, the cost of giving birth in the private system can be anything from a couple of hundred dollars to pay the insurance excess up to tens of thousands of dollars, depending on the services and specialists you choose to use and the hospital, even with top tier coverage.

If you're being treated in the private system, once you have a referral for your chosen obstetrician, you can have your first appointment pretty much whenever you choose. All things being equal, you will see that obstetrician consistently for all your appointments until you give birth, and that obstetrician is likely to be the person who delivers your baby. Many private clinicians now have an ultrasound machine in their rooms and you can take a peek at your baby each time you visit. This is particularly useful for high-anxiety pregnancies, such as those after loss.

If you are navigating the public system, you will be seen by whichever obstetrician is on duty, meaning there is no continuity of care, unless you are a high-risk patient. Interestingly, of the 1786 accredited obstetrician-gynaecologists working in clinical settings in 2016, only 36 per cent worked in the public sector,[92] which is a stark juxtaposition to the data showing 75 per cent of babies are being born publicly.

Having said that, many hospitals are shifting to midwife team-driven care models, and some patients, if low risk, with no complications, may not see an obstetrician at all. Currently Midwifery Group Practices are being trialled at a number of hospitals, but they're only able to take on a small amount of patients, and this is being dominated by educated, middle-class patients, rather than high-risk patients who could most benefit from the service. One obstetrician, who is extremely supportive of the service, says, 'It's great, but it's who you know rather than who needs the service most, like Aboriginal patients or patients who can't speak English. The patients who have higher levels of education and can advocate for themselves know it exists and ask for it immediately upon learning they're pregnant. They're dominating the places and it has to be managed better.' This is despite research from Melbourne showing that continuity of care for Aboriginal patients using the Midwifery Group Practices can drastically improve health outcomes for both mother and baby.

Another obstetrician who works in both the public and private systems told me there aren't enough jobs made available for obstetricians and gynaecologists in the public system, because there simply isn't the funding. It should be noted that moving to nurse/midwife-driven care also has significant cost benefits. The average taxable income for a midwife in 2018–19 was $68,231 (just as an aside, the average for women was $68,029 compared to $83,079 for men, who represent around 1 per cent of the workforce). The average taxable income for female obstetricians was $305,118, for men it was $426,128.[93]

Whether you see an obstetrician or not, if you are obtaining a referral for the public system, unless you're a high-risk or complex patient, you're going to have your first appointment somewhere between twelve and eighteen weeks. What this means is that if you do experience a miscarriage in your first trimester, the period in which you're statistically most likely to have one, you may not have even seen anyone other than a GP to confirm the pregnancy. This is why so many patients end up in emergency departments – they're not sure where else to go when they start to bleed and pass large clots, especially if it's their first pregnancy or first loss.

There are two other kinds of care worth mentioning. The first is a hybrid model where you give birth in the public system, but hire a midwife privately to attend all appointments, and the birth, with you, to give some consistency in your care. This can cost anywhere from $3500 to $6000. They are called 'midwives in private practice'. More common in regional areas is shared care, where a GP (who is registered with the nearest public hospital) shares your care with a public hospital for some of the routine check-ups, usually because the public hospital is some distance away, making it difficult to attend appointments. Most of those GPs have done an additional obstetrics qualification or certification.

20/20 vision

While you do pay for the privilege, if you're a private patient, you're much more likely to have had an early scan. Possibly even an extremely early dating scan. There are benefits to that, both physically and psychologically.

'Ideally you would like your patient, all patients, to be scanned before twelve weeks,' explains obstetrician Dr Marilla Druitt, who gives a number of reasons why, including more accurate dating, meaning fewer inductions and early intervention where necessary. 'If you only find out at twenty weeks that someone's having twins, you probably don't know what type they are unless they're boy and girl, in which case they've each got their own placenta.' In a highly ironic twist that feels like nature taking the piss, the older you are, the more likely you are to have a miscarriage . . . or twins. This is because the follicle-stimulating hormone ramps up as you age, in what seems like the body's last ditch effort to sew some oats. So as maternal ages rise, so too does the likelihood of twin conceptions. Another argument why scans should be offered earlier and more routinely in the public system.

When I mention to Dr Druitt that anecdotally I hear more examples of 'later' missed miscarriages in the public system than in the private, she puts that down to non-invasive prenatal testing (NIPT). The NIPT is a blood test conducted any time from ten weeks to identify aneuploidy, chromosomal issues like Down syndrome or Edwards syndrome, through the baby's DNA, which is in the mother's blood.

While the government announced in 2022 it would be funding preconception genetic screening, the NIPT is not funded at all and it's expensive at a cost of around $500. Because of that, Dr Druitt says 'most of the ultrasound places that offer NIPT won't do it without doing a scan just to check you've still got a live baby'.

Ultrasound screening is not as effective as NIPT; for instance twelve to fourteen week scans would only pick up around 70 per cent of cases of Down syndrome, whereas the NIPT has an efficacy rate of over 99 per cent.[94] Dr Druitt agrees the NIPT should be free for all patients. 'This is all just a gendered medicine problem. If blokes had this problem, they would have funded it 50,000 years ago. It's just that there are too many pregnant women that cost too much money,' she says.

Another benefit to earlier scans would be that you can establish a loss at an earlier gestation. Some argue that in this case there would have been less time to bond with the pregnancy and the trauma of the loss (where there is trauma) might not be magnified quite so much. Equally, some patients feel a huge loss when they have a miscarriage before they've been able to have a scan, meaning they never got a chance to see their baby or retain a keepsake marking their existence.

Is it really a choice if you can't choose?

As we know, but it bears repeating, best-practice miscarriage care management is that patients should be offered three options for management when a miscarriage is confirmed but not yet complete: expectant (natural), surgical (a D&C) and medical (medication). These options need to be fully explained to the patient, including the pros and cons of each option.

Unfortunately, these options are not always fairly or accurately presented to the patient, with influence coming from factors like cost or the clinician's personal biases. This can be further complicated by the power dynamic between patient and treating physician, one that can be heightened if the patient is in the midst of grief. This dynamic is also exacerbated if the patient is from a minority demographic more likely to be subjected to prejudice, racism or bigotry.

As American civil rights scholar Loretta Ross writes, 'Women of colour activists pointed out that the concept of choice masks the different economic, political and environmental contexts in which women live their reproductive lives. Choice, they argued, disguises the ways that laws, policies, and public officials differently punish or reward the childbearing of different groups of women, as well as the different degrees of access women have to healthcare and other resources necessary to manage sex, fertility, and maternity.'[95]

If the patient chooses the 'wait and see' route, they can sometimes be managed by the GP and assessed with a follow-up scan to ensure there is no retained pregnancy tissue. Some (mostly regional GPs) actually have additional obstetric qualifications so they can provide misoprostol or even, in some cases, perform a D&C. But in most cases, if a patient chooses the medical or surgical route, they are usually put back into the hospital system, either via emergency or through an EPAS.

There can be a delay of days to be seen and weeks to have a D&C, whereas in the private system you can be given a D&C within twenty-four to forty-eight hours, if the appropriate bookings can be made. Both of my D&Cs were done within forty-eight hours of the miscarriage being confirmed.

Rose negotiated the public system and wasn't as fortunate. She went to the GP, got a referral for a scan, the scan confirmed she had a missed miscarriage and she was then sent back to the GP but couldn't get in for a few days. It then took another few days for her to get into the EPAS and then not until the following week was she able to have a D&C. This meant that from diagnosis of a missed miscarriage to ending the pregnancy took ten days. For some patients, the wait can be an excruciating form of mental torture, something we'll discuss in chapter eight.

'I just wanted it done. I just wanted to escape that period of my life, the grieving,' Rose explains.

In both the public and the private system, choices for miscarriage management aren't given the way that they should be, but in the public system, there is resource and budgetary pressure that can result in patients being pushed in one direction or another, but usually away from surgery.

When Natasha found out she'd had a missed miscarriage at a nine-week scan, she started researching options herself before she attended her EPAS appointment. She walked in knowing she wanted a D&C. 'The cramping had stopped. I had morning sickness. I had sore breasts. Nothing was stopping. And nothing was going to stop any time soon,' she explained. Over the next three appointments, they tried aggressively to convince her not to have the D&C she wanted. Possibly because they didn't have capacity, possibly because many doctors see D&Cs as 'medically unnecessary', perhaps because they were conscientious objectors. Or a combination of one or more of these reasons. She stuck to her guns and eventually had the procedure.

One patient I spoke to was told they couldn't do her D&C at her local hospital for three weeks. She ended up at Marie Stopes. Another patient had misoprostol in the morning to prepare for her D&C, but when she arrived at the hospital she was pressured by three different clinicians to go home and wait to miscarry naturally. Another patient I met also ended up at Marie Stopes after a miscarriage because, in the wake of Covid, the hospital she went to made it clear to her that a D&C was simply not a priority for them.

One obstetrician who works in both public and private practice told me that, from their perspective, there are two primary differences between the way they work in each sector. The first is that she is able to spend more time with each patient in the private practice, where time pressures are not as severe. The second, interestingly, is how she can apply changes in research or best practice to the care she provides patients.

'I don't know if I could cope with just working in the public system the whole time.' She laughs. 'The bureaucracy just does my head in. I can change my practice the very next day, if a study comes out saying this is better than that. I don't need to go through seventeen committees and layers and layers of silliness. Private practice isn't subject to the same sort of regulation processes.'

Meanwhile, in private practice, doctors are accused of being more prone to over-medicalisation, with tests or procedures being ordered simply because a patient requests them or the doctor wants to appear to be actively managing a situation, when in reality there is little to be done. 'They [private and public] have both got their pros and cons,' the doctor explained.

Dr Druitt is based in Geelong and points out that Victoria is one of the safest places in the world to give birth. 'Perinatal outcomes are fantastic, particularly with preterm babies, so we're pretty good on the physical outcomes. Now we have to improve our psychological outcomes, which is all about shared decision-making,' she explains. 'The patient being at the centre of the story is not the doctor trying to convince the patient to do what the doctor thinks is the safest thing, or a midwife saying "birth is natural, intervention is bad". Those are the two extremes, most people are somewhere in the middle.'

But holistic and person-centred care gets very difficult when there's no continuity. 'For miscarriage management, in private you've got an obstetrician who can do the counselling and offer the medical and offer the surgical. Or you might have a fabulous GP who can sort everything out. But it's much trickier in the public setting, when you have people changing shifts and the possibility that you won't always be seeing the same healthcare worker.'

Maternity or not maternity, that is the question

When you get a positive pregnancy test, you are immediately classified as a maternity patient. But the minute you have a confirmed miscarriage, this classification seems to dissipate. Ironically, if you need any procedures relating to your miscarriage, they're likely to take place in a maternity ward. The question of whether or not people experiencing a miscarriage are maternity patients is an interesting one that was thrown into stark relief during the Covid-19 pandemic.

In New South Wales there was a concerted effort and campaign to allow support people to attend births during the pandemic. This was spear-headed by natural birth militant and Professor of Midwifery Hannah Dahlen. It was a success and NSW Health buckled and allowed one support person to attend with anyone giving birth. During the campaign, I asked whether they were also fighting for patients who were attending hospital either with a threatened miscarriage or for D&C. The answer from Professor Dahlen was, 'surely it would be allowed under compassionate grounds'. I'll take that as a non-committal no. In the UK, one father told of having to support his wife through a miscarriage by text message during the pandemic, something he described understandably as 'barbaric'.[96]

In Western Australia, June was taken to hospital with an ectopic pregnancy. It was the start of the Covid pandemic and, despite no cases being admitted at that point, the hospital had shut down an entire surgical ward to prepare for the possibility of an influx of infectious Covid patients. So, in addition to not having a support person attending, June was treated in the neonatal ward, the sound of babies crying all around her.

In Melbourne, when Trina attended the hospital for a D&C in the early days of the pandemic (it was later established that she had significant internal bleeding and the procedure became an emergency situation), she was told she would have to wait outside while they tried to find her Covid test results. She was not offered a chair.

Her support person had already left because she was told they wouldn't be able to attend.

'They sent me outside into the carpark. That's when I just broke down.'

People who experience miscarriage are consistently treated without the care or empathy afforded to other patients, compounding and magnifying their grief and creating additional layers of trauma.

The Letter

Dear Dr Lovely,

So I'm now over the worst of it (this was by far the most physically difficult one I've had just in terms of the duration of the heavy bleeding and the related fatigue), I thought I'd drop you a line. I've done a hell of a lot of thinking over the past few days and I know you're busy so I thought I'd just jot them down in an email so you can give it some thought and let me know what you think. I think it's also easier for me to just write this stuff down in the first instance. Of course, happy to come in for an appointment whenever, not trying to side-step coming down in ANY way, but I know you're busy and this is a form of self-care, I guess.

I would like to have a conversation with you about whether you want to continue to be my doctor (I hope you do!). I realise that I'm high mainten-ance. As much as I try to be calm, there's a limit to how much control I have. Pregnancy after miscarriage is supremely stressful, let alone when you've had five. I try to be as in control as I can, but ultimately I am always going to be pretty anxious. I feel like you've been frustrated with me. I know I am an extremely stubborn and frustrating person – wait until you meet Jack. He'll happily confirm that and offer you a shoulder to cry on.

I also wanted to explain to you the reason I wanted the early scan because I feel like maybe there's a bit of a misunderstanding. I know that there's nothing you can do if I am having an MC. I don't expect any early intervention for a five-to-six-week or even ten-week pregnancy. I know that if I'm miscarrying it's happening for a reason. The reason I want the early scan is that, for my own mental health, I want to know asap whether the pregnancy is likely to end. You said in your email to me that the scan the other day was 'inconclusive' and I know that's *medically* the case, but you and I both know that scan showed the growth was far too behind to have been a viable pregnancy. When I get that result, it's actually a relief. The unknown is the thing that scares me, especially when I'm bleeding. The scans are what allow me to 'cut my losses' in my head and start to grieve so I can prepare for the next cycle. At every early scan I've had (and I've had one in every single pregnancy) the ultrasonologist/

OB has been able to confirm the growth has been significantly slow enough to confirm a likely miscarriage. They've not once been wrong.

The other thing I wanted to discuss with you is whether there's any more testing we can do to figure out if there's something we've missed. Women in my support group are throwing all sorts of things at me that I should be tested for. Is there any more testing we need to do? Is there any point? This is where I feel totally lost.

Also a few friends have said 'you need to see a specialist'. But as far as I'm concerned you are a specialist. Is there such a thing as a recurrent MC specialist? I have googled my butt off and I don't think there is. Only OBs with a special interest but I already have an OB. (That's you, by the way, if the answer to my first question was yes.)

My final question is that, according to some of the reading I've done, the shape of the uterus or fibroids can have an impact on early MC. The ultrasonologist at the most recent scan said I had two fibroids. Is that an issue?

I hope you understand why I'm asking all these questions. I'm going to be thirty-nine in November. I feel like I'm running out of time and I just have this fear that something has been missed and I'm wasting time trying when it's not going to happen for me.

Isy x

||||||||||||||||||||||||||||||||||||||||||||||||||||||||||||||||||||||||||||||||||||||||||||||||||||||||||

6

Rolling in the Deep

Not all miscarriages are grieved. The differentiator between those who mourn their losses and those who don't view them as losses is all about perspective.

Mia was thirty-two. She'd been with her then partner for two months. 'When I found out I was pregnant, it was like a sign flashing in my head, like a visual sign saying: *no, no, no.* I was that adamant about not wanting to have children.' When Mia started to bleed she was sent for an ultrasound and was told that she had miscarried, because there was no fetus in her uterus. But that's because it was in her fallopian tube. Ectopic pregnancies can be incredibly dangerous or even fatal if not treated.

'I was at my boyfriend's birthday party and I started haemorrhaging really heavily and they had to drive me to the hospital. It was a bit spectacular and dramatic,' she says, rolling her eyes. 'And then I had to have emergency surgery. I thought that I'd had a miscarriage and I was super relieved about that, but then all of a sudden, being told, "No, you're actually still pregnant and not only are you still pregnant, but you're in an emergency situation." That was pretty traumatic.'

As Mia lay in her hospital bed in recovery, she considered the feeling of knowing she'd had one of her fallopian tubes removed. 'I didn't particularly mind. I did think, *This is terrible.* But then I did think that of all the people that this had to happen to, it's all right that it was me.'

Allsorts

In a letter to a medical journal, nurse and senior nursing academic Dr Sara Rich Wheeler wrote of the varying perceptions women who lose pregnancies before twenty weeks of gestation have, saying they range from no loss to loss of a pregnancy to loss of a baby. 'In other words, not all people feel like they lost a baby and consider themselves to be bereaved.' She finishes the letter by writing, 'It is just as bad to assume that everyone grieves and run the risk of making women feel bad for feelings they do not have, as it is to assume that no one grieves and allow women's needs to go unmet.'[97]

Equally, a small-scale, qualitative study with transmasculine and non-binary parents from Australia, the United States and the European Union found very similar responses to the general female-identifying population, in that the majority found pregnancy loss to be devastating.[98] Interestingly a small number saw a miscarriage as positive in that it confirmed they could conceive despite the use of hormone supplements.

Not all miscarriages lead to grief and mourning. Some people are relieved. Some are angry. Some are happy. Some are sad. There is no correct way to react. However, it is important to understand the variation in reaction, so parents can be offered support where needed following a loss, but also during any subsequent pregnancy, where they are clinically more likely to experience heightened levels of anxiety or other mental health instability.

Beyond the fact that we are all individuals with unique perspectives, there is another reason for this variability and it comes intertwined with the concept of fetal personhood. This is the interpretation of the fetus as a person, as opposed to a mass of cells. A baby, rather than a blastocyst, embryo or fetus. This is where we venture into psychology and interpretation, rather than biology or medicine. In Mia's case, she intentionally went looking for scientific terminology, in order to maintain her distance from a pregnancy that she didn't want. She never considered or called the pregnancy a 'baby'. 'I specifically looked up where it was at that point, and it was called a blastocyst, so I had it in my head it was a blastocyst.'

Dr Jessica Zucker, an American psychologist and founder of the #IHadAMiscarriage movement on Twitter, writes in her book about the moments after she miscarried her sixteen-week-old baby at home and the interaction she had with her husband during the frenzy of panic. '"Get a plastic bag," I shouted. "Put her in it so we can bring her to Dr Schneider's office." Anything but grounded, reeling from his own experience of this trauma, he shot back, "Why are you calling it 'her'?!" before descending the three flights down to our kitchen, where leftover grocery bags were stored.'[99]

Different people and cultures employ various thresholds for when pregnancies come to be seen as 'babies'. For many, historically, this threshold was the quickening, the first perception of a baby's movements. But for parents who have access to ultrasound technology and hyper-sensitive at-home pregnancy tests, this threshold has become progressively earlier. Take for instance social media announcements of pregnancy. It's not uncommon for parents to now pose for an announcement photo with a positive pregnancy test. The test represents a baby, not a blastocyst. Even if the pregnancy hasn't yet reached the threshold of viability, it's seen as a welcome addition to the family. It is a first step towards the creation of the concept of that baby as a person, from the moment the pregnancy hormones hit your bloodstream.

In a 2001 study, seventy-two women described their first or only pregnancy loss; 25 per cent described losing a pregnancy, 50 per cent said baby, 11 per cent said they lost a baby with a name often provided and 14 per cent felt they lost a child 'who would now be a certain age'.[100]

'For many women . . . the child begins when the decision is made to bear it,' wrote Shulamit Reinharz back in 1987. 'When a woman decides to become pregnant, her child, which hitherto had been only a potentially wanted thing, is transformed into an actually wanted thing. The child begins to exist.'[101] This occurs through the first imaginings of what that baby will look like, how it will change a family dynamic, their personality and so on. This is the start of a process of personification, the creation of a person within the mind.

Medical historian Shannon Withycombe writes of the scholarly contention that the 'cult of fetal personhood' began with imaging technology and reached a crescendo with Lennart Nilsson's iconic photographs of a fetus that graced the cover of *Life* magazine in 1965 (ironically, the iconic Nilsson photos were all, apart from one, taken of miscarried or terminated pregnancies[102]). But Withycombe also argues that what shifted for women was the idea of having more control over their medical fate.

'While women remained in a world where they had little and often no control over their fertility, they might be more apt to see their miscarriages as being subject to fortune and fate, and less interested in thinking of their pregnant bellies as holding another person. But once pregnancy became more controllable and its fate more predictable, women could begin to think of a person within,' she theorises.[103]

New and fascinating cultural norms, some of which persist today, actually sprang from moves to criminalise abortion in England in the early 1800s, before being taken up in America and Australia later in the nineteenth century. The difficulty at the time was that physicians couldn't differentiate between 'spontaneous abortion' (miscarriage) and induced abortion. Historian Lara Freidenfelds argues that doctors were then flying blind, as patients sought reasons for their miscarriages, fearful they might fall foul of the new laws around their reproductive health. This was the beginning of a new movement. 'Advice book authors told women in no uncertain terms that it was their responsibility to care for the developing babies in their wombs, not destroy them,' Freidenfelds writes.[104]

She points out that these laws resulted in another cultural development. 'In English legal tradition, women who gave birth to stillborn children in suspicious circumstances were often acquitted of infanticide if they could demonstrate that they had prepared child-bed linen.'[105] Whether it was for this reason or any other, there was a movement by department stores in the 1920s to create 'infant' departments. Catalogues started separating out baby products and marketing of this potential money-maker began in earnest.

Dr Linda Layne addressed commercialisation of pregnancy and childbearing in 2003, writing 'shopping is one of the strategies used by mothers and their social networks to transform an anonymous mass of cells into "our precious baby".'[106] But these days, it's not just linen, clothes or nursery items. Now it's also phone apps that track your journey, online forums for mums with the same due dates, baby product fairs, books about pregnancy and the early days of motherhood, parenting courses and the list goes on. For many, mothering begins at conception. And so does the shopping, often for clothes, what some would consider the ultimate tool of personification.

Another common social media announcement set-up is a chalkboard, letterboard or sign announcing the due date of the baby, with a pair of shoes or other item of clothing representing each parent and any existing siblings, plus a teeny tiny pair of shoes representing the baby. Because who doesn't love baby shoes, right? You can almost picture the little toes. The soft skin in the arch of the foot.

As a patient progresses through pregnancy, the phone apps, the baby book they're reading and updates from subscriptions to baby forums maintain a constant attachment to the little poppyseed growing within. A poppyseed that becomes an apple seed, that becomes a pea, that becomes a blueberry, that becomes a raspberry. You get the idea. As Freidenfelds writes, 'Smartphone pregnancy apps, introduced in the twenty-first century, are pregnancy websites on steroids. By pinging their users frequently, they aim to keep women engaged and thinking about their pregnancies all day, every day.'[107]

Interestingly, in the Jewish tradition, no baby gifts are given until after the birth. One might think that this is to encourage the delaying of connection, in order to protect against the grief of loss. But it appears that this is now primarily a function of superstition among the many Jewish families I spoke to. While the vast majority of them abided by the tradition of not giving or receiving gifts until after the safe arrival of the baby, connection was nevertheless formed through early imaging and pregnancy tests. Names were discussed extensively before birth among almost all the families I spoke to – though not revealed until a naming or at circumcision – and miscarriage was felt deeply as a loss by many, including myself.

In your mind's eye

Woody Woodburn is a columnist for the *Ventura County Star* in California. He wrote a column remembering the loss of his third child with his wife, in a missed miscarriage, on what would have been the child's eighteenth birthday. It's the last few paragraphs that really caught my attention, as he remembered his little Sienna.

'I visualised her this June at high school graduation ceremonies for the Class of 2021; imagined her last year schooling at home during the pandemic; saw her 13 years ago walking into a kindergarten class-room,' he writes. 'Too, I have imagined her getting her driver's license, learning to ride a bike, taking her first steps. Indeed, often when I see girls the same age she would have been, I imagine her in their place.'[108]

Nothing makes you plan for the future quite like a pregnancy. And there are curiosities that extend well into your child's yet to be realised life. Will they have my eyes? Will they be a writer like me? A lawyer like their grandparents? Will they have their own children for me to care for? And with these questions come images. Memories of events that haven't taken place. Memories of a person you've never met. Those who feel the most intense grief are those who are mourning their child, whether they were the size of a poppyseed or a cantaloupe.

In a 1994 German study that sought to differentiate the grief reactions between men and women after miscarriage, the researchers phrased it thusly, 'The major source of grief for both partners seems to have to do with relinquishing the hopes for, expectations of, and fantasies about the child.'[109]

When someone loses a friend, a partner or a parent, we all appreciate these are fully formed human beings. Others may have known that person, heard stories about them or made their own memories. A visualisation of that person can even be offered through photos or video. But when you lose a pregnancy, those closest to it hold the memories of a baby who doesn't yet exist, apart from in their mind's eye. As a consequence, it's much more difficult for those who haven't experienced the pain to understand, because it's a concept and vision that's almost entirely in someone else's head. In a paper on how to offer psychosocial support to people who have experienced miscarriage, Dr Sara Wheeler suggests that the practitioner listen for key words, 'Do they use the word baby repeatedly?' she asks.[110]

In addition to the lack of understanding surrounding fetal personhood and the related grief that compounds the feelings of loss, it can directly affect caregiving if these concepts are not understood by health professionals, especially those who work outside mental health fields. A 2016 study in *MCN: The American Journal of Maternal/Child Nursing* found that 'care is restricted by lack of understanding about the significance of miscarriage for the woman and family, minimisation of the loss, and uncertainty about whether this loss presents a longer lasting burden'.[111]

Just the first step

The fertility systems of humans are alarmingly inefficient. Scientists estimate that as many as 70 per cent of eggs are actually fertilised when released in conjunction with the arrival of sperm. The technology hasn't developed to the point where we know the data precisely, but it's thought that around 50 per cent of zygotes (fertilised eggs) don't progress into blastocysts that implant.[112] Of the pregnancies that do develop to the implantation stage, we know many fail before anyone is aware that the process has taken place, in what many would see as a late period or heavy flow. Whether we like it or not, miscarriage where there is a chromosomal abnormality is an essential part of the human reproductive process. It's a form of quality control to ensure that embryos with 'developmental errors' do not proceed to term.

I had the absolute delight of interviewing renowned science journalist Jon Cohen, the author of the 2005 book *Coming to Term: Uncovering the Truth About Miscarriage*. It is an exploration primarily of the science of miscarriage, a work which Cohen undertook after he and his wife suffered multiple miscarriages. He told me, 'If you don't have an identified problem, miscarrying in itself is not a problem. Miscarrying itself is a very positive thing that the body does. If humans brought to term 50 per cent of these embryos and fetuses that have chromosomal abnormalities that would be worse than miscarrying at five weeks, I will be brutally honest.'

When I spoke to Cohen, his daughter was four months pregnant, her previous pregnancy having ended in miscarriage, after which she turned to him for advice. I asked him whether he thought some of her pain could have been alleviated had she, and all of us, been better educated about the realities of miscarriage. He said there's no question that it's time for the taboo around miscarriage to end and education to begin.

'I want my daughter to know that if you get pregnant, it's just the first step. It doesn't mean you're going to end up with a baby in your arms . . . you have things that are in your control and not in your control.' He said he was astounded in researching his book how many things he learned about the biomedical aspects of the female anatomy. 'I could stop a dinner party cold by telling women there about their own bodies and that's wrong,' he says. 'Most women don't know how their bodies work, in terms of conceiving and carrying to term. And that should be learned at the same age as we tell young girls and young boys about the birds and the bees. It should be part of it then. And it isn't.'

Remember the Cervical Celebrity from the very first words of this book? Let me remind you. 'If women were educated about miscarriage in school, then *this* wouldn't happen,' the doctor said, gesturing towards me. All of me. As I cried into a tissue. 'You'd know miscarriage was just a normal, natural thing that's supposed to happen and you wouldn't be crying about it.'

These words have resonated in my head in the years since, as well as through subsequent pregnancies. Despite the brutal dismissal of my grief and pain, there is some truth in the Cervical Celebrity's words. Perhaps if all of us were educated about the reasons for miscarriage and the frequency of it, if we were less reliant on the myth that pregnancy equals baby, while I don't think it would totally alleviate the sadness and grief, it might go a long way to helping us all feel less alone, less isolated and less likely to engage in a raft of self-blame or even self-hatred. But surely Australian kids are being educated about the entire reproductive journey, which of course includes miscarriage. Surely.

Well, no.

The Australian national curriculum doesn't include any specific mention of miscarriage or pregnancy loss. A representative of the Australian Curriculum, Assessment and Reporting Authority went to great pains to explain to me that state curricula or schools can include it if they choose, but did acknowledge that other topics, like contraception and menstruation, are, in fact, included. So I did what any other obsessive, compulsive, researcher would do. I contacted every single state curriculum office and asked them if they include miscarriage or pregnancy loss in their curricula.

Out of all the states and territories, only New South Wales includes miscarriage or pregnancy loss specifically. Just the one state. How can we realistically be surprised that miscarriage is a taboo, never-to-be-mentioned topic, when we aren't even broadly teaching it as part of basic reproduction education to kids?

Don't tell me how to feel

The societal confusion over whether miscarriage constitutes loss and entitles the person who experiences it to grief or a period of mourning is another potential catalyst for suppression of those emotions, with people feeling they don't have a 'right' to feel sad, especially in an age where the vast majority of people are pro-choice (a tension that doesn't need to exist and one we will examine in chapter ten).

Eighteen years ago, Dani, a writer and journalist, experienced a vanishing twin pregnancy. At her eleven-week scan she saw two babies, but by the time of her next scan, there was only one. She was offered no support, no counselling, no information and, as a consequence, was made to feel like she couldn't pause to acknowledge the loss. It has taken some time, but she now looks back and is disappointed that she wasn't offered more support or care.

'It was definitely a traumatic loss. There are certainly losses that are more traumatic, but it was a loss,' she explains. Having not really experienced the desire to have children earlier in life, her hormones had well and truly kicked in by then and she desperately wanted a baby. She felt empowered as a woman to identify and embrace this desire and the loss ate into her confidence. 'I think it was also this vision of myself as powerful and the freedom. All the potential that's in your body. And then I felt like is that wrong? Did my body stuff up? Am I not this amazing tiger?'

Dani sees herself as strong, capable and intelligent, all things that she clearly is, both as a person and as a friend. Looking back on how little support she was given, she worries that someone else wouldn't have weathered the storm as well as she did. 'How bad that no one was nice to me about it. No one said anything. I was just waiting in a cubicle by myself. "Yeah, it's not there, oh well, get dressed." There wasn't even a pamphlet.'

It's okay to not be okay

A pregnancy also doesn't have to be planned for a parent to be sad when it's lost. With three kids, Sarah had considered her family complete and was using contraception when she got pregnant unexpectedly. She immediately started considering whether she wanted to proceed and have a fourth child or get an abortion. She saw her GP, expressed that she wasn't happy about the pregnancy and was considering her options. The GP ran a beta hCG test to see how far along the pregnancy was, but when the doctor called with the results, she told Sarah she was having a miscarriage. 'I sat on my floor and cried, pulled myself back together and carried on with the birthday party for my daughter.'

The pregnancy ended up being ectopic and required surgery. Because Sarah works in a medical field, her obstetrician asked her if she'd like to see the images of her surgery to remove the fetus. Sarah's voice cracks and she starts to cry. 'So I looked at it [the image] and I could see it and it was just this feeling of wanting to reach out and put it back,' she explains. 'I instantly regretted it. It made it so real. There was something there and it's not there now.'

Violence

Pip was twenty-five when she had her first child. When she'd found out she was pregnant, she knew she was going to have the baby, despite the pregnancy being a surprise. She never really considered any other course of action, despite being very much pro-choice. But when she became pregnant at thirty-eight, it was far more complicated.

By then, she had three children, but was separated from their father, with whom she had experienced a violent and abusive relationship. They had been separated for four years when she re-entered the dating pool with a 25-year-old lover. She was still very nervous about her ex, who was trying to maintain control over the family and create problems, but she was enjoying living her life again. The relationship (which she says is a generous way to describe it) with her younger lover was relaxed and based on mutual attraction.

'We were both on the same page.' She laughs. A mishap with a condom resulted in Pip's fourth pregnancy, but this time she wasn't twenty-five and wasn't interested in having another child. She called Marie Stopes and started looking into her options. When she had a miscarriage, she felt total relief, for multiple reasons including not having to make the decision to have an abortion, not having to procure one and not creating further issues with her former partner.

'Part of the relief was that, because I'm so inextricably tied up with my children's dad, who is extremely violent with me, across multiple platforms, now I didn't have to deal with all that. It would have just opened an even bigger can of worms, even though we've been separated since 2016.'

In fraught relationships and tense co-parenting, whether together or separated, frustration can often boil over and create toxic situations, or in the case of relationships where there is already violence or abuse, it can push an entire situation to breaking point. I spoke to many people who cited family violence as a reason they were relieved their pregnancy didn't progress.

But equally fascinating is research from Australia which shows that women who experience partner-based violence are more likely to experience miscarriages (as well as more frequent pregnancies and abortion). Therefore, when victims of partner-based violence are treated for maternal depression, a possibly troubled reproductive history may also be a contributing factor.[113] This is something we'll look at further in chapter fourteen.

Slipping Away

As I walked down the shopping strip in the winter sunshine, realising the rain had cleared, I searched the sky for a rainbow. I found myself looking for rainbows compulsively, convinced that perhaps if I saw one, it would herald the coming of just one more baby that would stick. The sticky baby. One that would stick around long enough to be born alive.

I walked into the beautician's shop, searching the shelves for something to buy. I had a gift certificate for a massage, but not wanting to reward my misbehaving body with kindness, I decided to spend it on products in the shop instead.

I grabbed a basket and started popping things in: hand cream, a candle or two, some lip balm. And then I saw it. A rack of crystal pendants on the counter near the cash register. My eyes wandered across the chart that listed each crystal with a photo of the colour and how they were supposed to heal you. Why do we even need modern medicine when we have crystals, right? If you believe that chart then aches, pains, depression, anxiety, whatever ails you, there's a crystal to fix it. And what about aromatherapy oils? If the crystals let you down, there's always those to try.

I felt like I was having an out-of-body experience. Hovering above myself, watching my body move, I picked each crystal up and let the weight of each sit in the palm of my hand. My eyes searched the text on the chart hungrily. Who was I, this stranger? I've always been a lover of science, a chaser of facts. But as I stood there, mourning yet another loss, I wondered, what if I was wrong? What if a crystal could help? What if it was the thing that was going to give me a baby? I suppressed all the voices screaming in my head to reject such stupidity. They were drowned out by my desperation.

Smokey quartz crystal. Helps you rise above, fight depression and bring balance. I unhooked it from the velvet stand. It had a little wrap of what looked like rose gold at the top, looping into a pendant.

I handed over my gift voucher. As I walked out of the shop, a bag of useless beauty paraphernalia in my hand, a hot flush of shame crept up my whole body from my toes to the top of my head until it felt like flames were fanning out above my head and lapping the top of the doorjamb. I rushed out into the street and my feet hit the pavement. I took off my necklace, reached into the bag for the small pouch holding the crystal, put the clasp through the loop, and put the necklace back around my neck. I tucked it safely under my jumper so I could feel it, cool against my skin.

As I set off back down the street, I rested my hand over my jumper and I could just feel it there. A hard lump on my sternum. I was the princess with a pea.

||||||

Each morning of each pregnancy I had a routine. Wake up, check my underwear for blood. Go to the toilet. Check the toilet paper for blood. Catch some urine, grab a cheap pregnancy test (you can order a hundred on Amazon for about $20), dip the stick. Take out the notepad. Use sticky tape to secure the stick to the paper, right below the others, note the date and time of the test and hop in the shower.

By the time I'd get out of the shower, the test would be complete. I'd look at the shade of the line. If the hCG in my body was increasing, so too would the darkness of the line. If the line was lighter than the day before it's an indicator that all might not be well.

This process involved a lot of squinting and significant lighting control. It was terrifically imprecise and unreliable. It was not recommended by any doctor. They would have been horrified if they'd known I was doing it. But any crumb of comfort, no matter how small, was one I wolfed down hungrily.

Every morning, the same ridiculous test, day after day, designed to ease the anxiety and help me survive one more morning, one more afternoon, one more evening, before I had to wake up and do it all again. Each day was a year. The crawl towards the seemingly all-important twelve-week mark continued at a pace so slow it felt like my life was barely inching forward. And as I limped into bed each night as darkness fell, I would congratulate myself on one more day without bleeding. One more day, closer to the twelve-week watershed moment. One day closer to meeting my second living child.

||||||

Loss number five came just six weeks after the fourth; I clearly didn't have a problem getting pregnant, everyone tried to reassure me. But all I remember was more scans, more disappointment, more blood, more clots, more cramps, more pain. More hushed meetings in my boss's office to explain why I needed to go home and why I wouldn't be in tomorrow. More of my son asking me why I was crying. More of my husband's loud sighs of frustration. More of my mum's sad eyes searching my face, looking for any indication that there was something she could do to help.

The whole period is a blur. But I remember with precision the growing awkwardness between me and every single person in my life. People ran out of words, ran out of comfort. In my mind they had run out of sympathy and patience. Of course no one wanted to be around me. No matter how upbeat I tried to be, I was the embodiment of grief and sadness. What do you say to someone whose life has become a constant cycle of death and loss?

||||||

I climbed the steps into the house. Alli and Carmen were already there. The latest miscarriage had been confirmed that morning. I walked into the room. I cracked jokes. Asked them how they were. But they wanted to know how I was.

And as I looked at them, in a rare show of weakness, I let my guard down. Just for a minute, but all the way down it came. Once the gate was open, it was a flood and I couldn't stop the grief from escaping me, just like I couldn't save the baby that was bleeding out of me. I remember repeating one line over and over as I tried to gulp down air and not choke on the tears streaming down my face.

'What am I going to do?'

I looked up. Carmen and Alli were looking at each other. They looked scared. More than scared. They looked utterly panic-stricken. They had no idea what to say to me or how to react. Who can blame them?

I took three deep breaths and with a strength inside me that I didn't know I had, I reigned in the tidal-wave of emotion I was surfing just moments before.

I wiped my eyes and I gave them a soggy smile.

'Sorry, no idea where that came from! I'm fine really.'

I loved these women like sisters and I am still blessed enough to call them my friends. But they had run out of words. And so had I.

7

We're All in This Together

The patient experiencing a miscarriage isn't the only person at risk of grief; partners, siblings, grandparents, friends and co-workers can also feel the sting from loss.

When Koen and his wife Abigail decided to start a family, they knew they might need a little bit of help. Abigail had polycystic ovary syndrome, so after two years of trying, she went onto some medication to help with ovulation and, finally, they got pregnant in 2019 and had their first scan in December. 'At the dating scan they found the first baby and then a couple of seconds later, she moved the equipment around and said, "Oh, and there's another one," and we were just shocked.' Koen laughs. 'We were so happy and never once stressed about having multiples. We were just so excited.'

By January 2020, they were due for a second scan. One of the babies was measuring slightly larger, though the risk of abnormalities was low. In February, Abigail noticed spotting. Doctors couldn't find anything wrong at the scan, but Abigail mentioned to a midwife that she had been experiencing Braxton Hicks contractions, which are also known as 'false labour' pains that can feel like an elastic band tightening around your belly. They're thought to be the body preparing for 'real' contractions and birth. Koen and Abigail were concerned. They had attended a twin information night at the hospital, where Braxton Hicks was described to prospective parents in detail, because twins do have a habit of arriving early. But the nurse didn't take their anxiety seriously. 'The nurse quickly dismissed us and said there was "no way that you're getting Braxton Hicks, it's too early".'

Later that month, Koen was out of town working and Abigail was at work. Between meetings, feeling noticeable contraction pains, she headed to the toilet to find she was bleeding heavily. Koen raced back on the train and when he arrived at the hospital he was told Abigail would be giving birth that day. He and Abigail were warned there was little chance for their babies, being born at nineteen weeks, so far off what is considered 'viable' at twenty-six weeks. Lily arrived first, 'absolutely beautiful, with the rosiest of cheeks and the cutest nose'. She was no bigger than Koen's palm. A short time later, her sister Ayla was born, 'slightly longer and with darker hair and cute eyelashes'. Both little girls were born sleeping. Koen and Abigail held their babies and mourned together for three nights in the hospital.

'They were just so perfect. Noses, eyebrows, they had their own characteristics. It was just really, really sad. But at the same time, I was just so happy that we were holding our children. It was surreal.' There was no solid reason given for the babies' premature arrival, other than a possible infection – Abigail had been treated for a urinary tract infection a few weeks before. 'I'm a scientist, and I think of most things logically and I couldn't find any logical reason as to why it happened,' Koen explains. He decided that he had to be strong and stoic to support Abigail. 'I had to be a man. I didn't want to show any sign of weakness.'

But then the dreams started. Nightmares during which Koen sobbed through the night. 'Once I was crying to the point where my throat was hurting the next morning. It was really strange. And again, this was not something that I was doing consciously, because I was sleeping. And then it went away.' His grief resurfaced around the holidays. 'We were watching a Christmas movie, it was November or December at that point, and of course, all Christmas movies have happy endings. That triggered me really badly, to the point where I was punching the couch and just crying bitterly. I think that was the most emotion I experienced consciously. The next day we were going to put up the Christmas tree and when we woke up I thought, "What's the point?"'

Koen told his boss about the loss of their baby girls and, with permission, his boss let his co-workers know. Of the forty people working in his lab, three immediately got in touch to say that they too had experienced loss and offered him their condolences. But he was shocked at how many people didn't acknowledge the loss at all, something he found extremely painful.

Another couple was particularly caring towards Koen and Abigail, filling their fridge with food and regularly checking in during their deepest grief. One of the highlights of Koen's year was taking their friend's very young daughter to the beach. He didn't realise at the time that she'd never been to a beach before. 'Her dad told me that he did that on purpose – even though he's a surfer and loves the water. He let me have that first experience because of our loss. He did that for me, which was amazing; allowing someone else to give his child their first experience of being in the water.'

Koen is still processing his grief and has started a blog. He's also in a Facebook group for partners who've experienced loss. When asked what advice he would give to partners who experience loss, he doesn't hesitate. 'You'll never be able to understand exactly what your partner is going through mentally and physically, the person who gave birth. But the important thing is to be flexible and reactive and talk about and share the grief with your friends and partner. Realise that you've both experienced the same loss. I think that's important to do as a male partner.'

•

Miscarriage doesn't just affect the people who are carrying the pregnancy, it affects partners, siblings, grandparents, workmates and friends.

In the words of proud Yolŋu woman Leila Gurruwiwi, who experienced several later-stage miscarriages before welcoming her gorgeous son Uzo, 'It wasn't just me that was waiting for this baby. It was a lot of other people that were waiting too.'

It has to be said, however, that in terms of family structure, we have moved far beyond the nuclear model. There is far more diversity that needs to be embraced. The support needed by a cisgender male partner is very different to what's needed by a queer female partner or someone who is trans or someone who is non-binary. There might be more than one partner in polyamorous families. The birth parent may be a surrogate. Care must be broad, non-gendered and tailored to the specific circumstance of the person in need. The grief and care needs of any person losing a pregnancy is valid, important and needs consideration.

Straight and narrow

When it comes to straight, cisgender couples, we know from a wealth of research that men and women grieve differently. Many of these differences are driven by gender binaries and societal expectations, rather than biology. I'm hopeful that as we shift away from gender normative structures, we will watch those differences dissipate somewhat, but this is the reality in which far too many of us live for the time being.

Toxic masculinity, both internal and external, mean that male partners in heterosexual relationships often don't talk about or openly express their grief when they are struggling. In a small qualitative study conducted in Australia, ten men whose partner had miscarried were interviewed about their response and feelings towards the loss. 'Most men described feeling significant grief following the miscarriage, with many describing their immediate emotional responses as sad, devastated or shocked. Men often described feeling the whole experience as being on a roller-coaster and they felt powerless or had no control over the outcome or their emotions at the time.'[114]

While men are less likely than women to seek medical care in general, the study identified that there was little support available for men experiencing the loss of a pregnancy, not only from professional services but also socially, thanks to the silence that seems to follow this particular kind of loss. Other studies also confirm that support is thin on the ground. A literature review by two of the authors of the paper I've cited above – the University of Melbourne's Professor Meredith Temple-Smith and Dr Jade Bilardi – states, 'perinatal loss can have negative implications for men's psychological and social well-being'. The paper recommends further research for 'enhancing support for men, and consequently their partners and families, who experience perinatal loss'.[115] Another study recommends that, in the case of recurrent miscarriage, healthcare professionals should be implementing screening for anxiety, depression and social support for both partners;[116] interesting given how few patients are screened, let alone their partners.

As we know, grief varies from person to person, and in each manifestation ways of processing can vary greatly. But let there be no question around whether the pain of miscarriage can be debilitating and crippling for men. Research undertaken in Melbourne back in 2011 showed that young men whose partners had had an abortion or miscarriage were twice as likely to develop depression than men whose partners had never been pregnant, 60 per cent more likely to have issues with alcohol, 80 per cent more likely to have issues with cannabis and 70 per cent more likely to have issues with harder drugs. While the findings are fascinating, the researchers emphasised they show correlation, not causation.[117]

Another study of 323 men showed that while they had slightly lower active grief levels, they had higher difficulty coping, and their despair and total grief scores were higher than women also surveyed six to eight weeks after loss.[118]

In *Coming to Term*, a father named Frank explained how the news of his partner's miscarriage 'sent me off the deep end, literally'. 'The hardest thing was that I really did see that as my daughter.' Frank started to cry. 'I was so in love with her. It was amazing for me how

strong I felt about something that didn't even exist. I felt this unbe-
lievable love bond of affection for this embryo. When it died, I really
felt a part of me died.' Frank ended up seeking counselling to help
him process his grief.[119]

The perception that men must support their partner through the
loss at the expense of their own self-care could be a major contributor
to the stress on their mental health. This combined with taboo around
men expressing vulnerability, and the fact that they're less likely to
seek medical or psychological support,[120] can result in a different set
of challenges for them after miscarriage.[121]

Paradoxically, studies have shown that this muted reaction can
mistakenly lead a birth parent to believe their partner is not grieving
and therefore affect their ability to talk to their partner and seek
support.[122] This is a game with no winners. 'Many (heterosexual, in
these specific instances) men feel they're being noble by stuffing away
their feelings and looking after their partners, but those partners are
wondering why the heck they're not feeling anything,' writes blogger
Aaron Gouveia in *Men and Miscarriage*[123], which he wrote with his
wife MJ. From her own perspective she writes, 'He could see I was
struggling with everything we went through, but I couldn't see that
he was trying to spare me, I just saw cool disinterest.'[124]

Miscarriage can also put huge stress on a relationship. A 2003
study of women who experienced miscarriage found that one year
post-loss, only 23 per cent claimed to be closer interpersonally with
their partner and six per cent sexually. But 32 per cent and 39 per
cent respectively said they were more distant.[125] 'Those who claimed
their sexual relationship or interpersonal relationship or both were
more distant at a year post-loss were more depressed, anxious, angry,
and confused.' The study authors note that this combined with prior
research showing 'men tend to keep to themselves after miscarriage,
deny their own loss, engage in avoidance, distract themselves through
work and if highly self-critical experience greater despair and difficulty, suggest that couples may need coaching in how to best care for
each other after miscarriage.'[126]

But it's not just straight couples for whom early pregnancy can cause relationship fractures. 'I told Mojo she didn't understand, she didn't have to feel it in her body,' writes Frankie Van Kan – a Melbourne-based queer writer, sex worker and performance artist – in *Archer*. 'I didn't stop to think about what it would have been like to watch someone you love go through it. To know you couldn't take away someone's pain while simultaneously trying to deal with your own. Our communication slowly broke down as we struggled to deal with the fallout in different ways. The grief peeled away in layers. Our relationship became entangled in one of those layers and eventually peeled away as well.'[127]

Many couples benefit from counselling, either to give them tools to cope or a neutral space in which they can share their feelings without the fear of judgement.

Aaron and MJ Gouveia experienced several losses and are very open in their book about the toll it took on them individually, as well as their marriage. The subject of toxic masculinity appears in almost every section of the book and reaches its flashpoint when Aaron finds out that the fertility issues the couple were experiencing are a result of his sperm quality. 'That toxicity is so powerful that as soon as I found out I had an issue, I automatically labelled myself as defective and pathetic and crawled into my shell of self-loathing at the exact time that my wife needed me so we could form a plan of attack and get to where we needed to be.'[128]

The late, great bell hooks wrote, 'The first act of violence that patriarchy demands of males is not violence towards women. Instead patriarchy demands of all males that they engage in acts of psychic self-mutilation, that they kill off the emotional parts of themselves. If an individual is not successful in emotionally crippling himself, he can count on patriarchal men to enact rituals of power that will assault his self-esteem.'[129]

After the births of their two older children, Tom's wife experienced a hydatidiform mole, also known as a molar pregnancy. This kind of miscarriage is complicated by monitoring required after surgical removal as the placenta can become a rare form of cancer called choriocarcinoma. Tom's wife had to wait for eighteen months for the confirmation that she was not at risk of cancer and didn't need chemotherapy (she later went on to have a third living child). Given the nature of her third pregnancy being totally unviable and its evolution into a long-term battle for his wife's health, Tom didn't see the loss as a miscarriage, he described it as a 'total misfire'. But this was at odds with his wife's perspective, which he didn't realise until he spoke to her before our interview, ten years after her diagnosis.

'I realised, chatting to Rachel before I came to talk to you, she's not over that,' Tom said as he choked back tears. 'I took a very clinical approach with "Well, we don't have a child and now we have a problem". But she still thinks about that fourth kid. And I just have never been able to think about it in those terms.

'In my mind, it's an incomplete egg and it doesn't form properly and never forms into a baby but it multiplies. So this isn't even near a baby, we've got a problem. That's how I thought. But for her, she had pregnancy symptoms. It was a pregnancy. She was experiencing everything to do with pregnancy, while also knowing there is no baby at the end of it.'

Wearing all the shoes

Jane has a unique perspective on pregnancy loss, having been both the person having a miscarriage and the person supporting a partner experiencing miscarriage. She has been with her wife for six years. When they talk about each other, it's with a powerful sense of love and respect. The kind that runs so deep, every other couple around them feels just a little bit jealous.

While many roads to having a baby are difficult, the road for female couples is laid with speed bumps. IUI or IVF is needed and there are legal hurdles around sperm or egg donors. When you add pregnancy loss to what is already a difficult road, it feels particularly unfair. But Jane's struggles to have children started long before she met her wife.

When I talk to Jane, she's forty-three, but when she was in her late twenties, she was in a relationship with a cis man. While the relationship wasn't by any stretch perfect, they had decided it was time to start a family. Jane got pregnant relatively quickly, but at her nine-week scan she was told things weren't progressing as they should. The baby's heart rate was slow and the growth wasn't where it should be. At ten weeks and two days, Jane miscarried at home, sitting on the toilet. 'It was a lot of bleeding and cramping and I just remember sitting there for ages,' she says quietly.

Later, Jane and her partner decided to try again, and again got pregnant reasonably quickly. This time they made it to twenty weeks, but when they attended their scheduled scan they were devastated to be told the baby had died at seventeen weeks and two days. 'At the time, sitting in the waiting room, I was on my own and I remember because, at that stage, I could feel that I was pregnant,' she explains. 'And I remember sitting there holding my stomach. And then I remember being in the chair, and I don't think I felt super positive, but I don't think I thought there was something wrong with the baby, I think it was just that life wasn't great at that point.

'I remember just the radiologist saying, "I'm sorry, there's no heartbeat." That's where my memory stops, my detailed memory. I remember feeling like my jaw go numb, the way it does when you're nauseous. And I went into shock.'

Jane has epilepsy and she believes the loss was caused by a seizure she suffered during the pregnancy.

After the scan, she remembers lots of paperwork, talking to a doctor, talking to a second doctor for a follow-up opinion and then having to work out when she was going to come back to give birth. That happened two days later. 'I have a recollection of being at home and wanting the fetus out of me,' she says. 'It was a very quick turnaround between wanting to be pregnant and wanting it out of me. It was like whiplash and at the time was incredibly hard.' Jane was also frustrated that she had to give birth, without the option of a general anaesthetic. 'I couldn't reconcile that,' she explains. 'I remember being really confounded that I still had to go through birth.'

But the aspect that weighed on her mind the most was how to convince her partner to let her do it alone. 'I had to carry him a great deal and I couldn't conceive of how I would manage his grief as well.' Jane gave birth alone, in line with her wishes. She held her baby but describes feeling 'uncomfortable'. She was in shock and struggling to connect. Later, passing comments compounded that grief.

'I was having an argument with my sister, because I talked about a stillbirth at seventeen weeks, but she said, "That's a miscarriage," and I said, "I gave birth, it's still a baby".' Now Jane finds herself in a very different position, as the wife of the woman who is carrying her child.

Jane and her wife's first three pregnancies all ended in miscarriage. Jane says that when she experienced her own losses, she was horrified at her former partner's ability to pivot out of loss and function. Something she just wasn't able to do. And she learned from that. 'We can look to our partners for solace and we can look to our partners for comfort and we can look to our partners for shared experience. But I was acutely aware that I couldn't stop her pain or her grief, and I couldn't make it better,' she explains. 'I also had the ability to understand that the time would come and if I could just sit with her, sit with her grief, and not try and fix it, and not try and rush it and just sit with it . . . I knew that that is what was needed.'

She didn't expect her mind to turn to her ex as she navigated recurrent miscarriages with her wife. 'I was surprised to feel empathy for my ex. I was surprised. But it is very hard.' Looking back, she believes her partner was relieved to be asked not to attend when she gave birth. 'Weirdly enough, being the non-jurisdictional partner on the other side of a pregnancy, where it's not happening to my body, I have some empathy for how that's possible,' she explains. 'I didn't realise at the time . . . it is very hard to wrap your head around.'

Jane has a very clear sense of her role when her wife – who at the time we spoke was thirty weeks pregnant – experienced loss. 'I see my role as to do all the things that she doesn't want on a day-to-day basis,' says Jane. 'Regardless of whose task it normally is, it's mine. I am trying to stay a couple of weeks ahead of her pregnancy experience in terms of what I'm reading and what I'm thinking about, so that when she arrives at a particular place that I'm in, a place where I can just sit quietly and listen. And then have either preparedness, solutions or alternatives. She's not reading a lot. Because of previous losses, she wants to stay in her body and I think that's fine.'

In terms of Jane's experience with pregnancy, both as a partner and as a birthing parent, it has changed some of her perspective of the world. 'I'm white, I'm fairly middle class and it was an absolute tragedy, but it wasn't enacted upon me,' she explains. 'It was just something that happened. It was like a growing up moment, realising that we'll lose our parents, you lose your siblings, you lose your children. For some people they're part of an ongoing inequity. It didn't make me feel better. But it made me feel more like I was sloughing into society, in the spectrum of society, these things happen.'

Most LGBTIQ+ couples have navigated discrimination of themselves and their relationships. If they haven't experienced it on a personal level, they certainly experienced it at a national discourse level during Australia's disgraceful 2017 marriage equality plebeshite. This is just one of the disenfranchisements that can become apparent and contribute to grief when there is a miscarriage. As with all LGBTIQ+ relationships, we are moving to a place of acceptance, but we are far from being universally accepting. One of the earliest challenges in family planning within same-sex or gender-diverse relationships comes from societal pressure to justify a desire to become parents, amid belittling of their relationships. Another challenge can come from deciding which partner will carry the baby or whether a surrogate will be used. These can be long and complicated journeys.

In a book chapter entitled 'Silent Miscarriage and Deafening Heteronormativity: A British Experiential and Critical Feminist Account',[130] the authors contend that many medical providers need to 'demonstrate awareness and sensitivity to women's relational contexts and ensure, in the case of lesbian couples, that parents are acknowledged and actively included in consultations.'

Ashley Scott is Executive Director of Rainbow Families. The organisation, which works to reduce discrimination and disadvantage faced by LGBTIQ+ parents and their children, introduced their own antenatal classes, because allowances were not made in mainstream classes for the experiences of LGBTIQ+ people. 'A friend and her partner tried to fall pregnant and her partner had a number of miscarriages. And then they swapped and decided that my friend would be the carrier for the next pregnancy and the next pregnancy was successful,' he explains. 'At the antenatal class they went to, the group was divided into mums over in one corner and dads in the other corner and they said, "And now what we're going to do is stick balloons up our shirts and pretend we know what it feels like for your wife to be carrying this baby." Can you imagine the trauma and emotions that were brought up for that woman who had experienced miscarriages?'

The grief can also be compounded when it comes at the end of an IVF journey. Months, possibly years of fertility treatments, only for the pregnancy to end and be faced with the proposition of getting back on the roller-coaster, let alone the burden of the costs involved.

For couples who are using a surrogate, the experience is different once more. Social worker Jill Johnson-Young explained to the *Washington Post* how miscarriage differs for her clients who are pursuing parenthood via surrogacy.

'They just get a phone call [if the surrogate suffers a miscarriage] and they don't have a baby anymore. Their world is turned upside down. They have each other and their role is to help each other with this loss that few people see as a real loss.'[131]

Ashley Scott, who had children with his husband via surrogacy, knows several dads whose international surrogates have experienced miscarriage. 'It's a really, really horrible time, because you feel extremely isolated. You're not part of the community yet. The Rainbow Families community sort of happens once you have that baby. And though a lot more queer people are having children, we were the first of our friends to do it. There isn't a community of support around for queer people experiencing pregnancy loss.' Often in the case of surrogacy, a pregnancy loss can also represent the end of a journey to become parents. 'International surrogacy is super, super expensive. So for a lot of people that can be the end of their parenting journey, because they can't actually afford to go through the process again. So that's really sad for those families.'

The oldies

Grandparents are an interesting proposition when it comes to pregnancy loss. Among the people I speak with, there seem to be two primary reactions. The first are the grandparents who are shattered, either because it is painful to watch their child grieve or because they've had their grandchildren or the dream of grandchildren snatched away (at least for the time being). The second are the grandparents who don't view it as loss and are therefore dismissive, or those who, due to generational differences, don't feel comfortable discussing it in polite conversation. Read: don't talk about it at all, just move on and get pregnant again.

An Australian study published in 2020[132] examined the themes that arose for mothers whose children experienced pregnancy loss and made several recommendations. The first was that grandparents need early access to guidance and information, as well as peer support. Interestingly, many of the grandmothers interviewed said they wanted to also have or make memories of their lost grandbabies. So another recommendation was that the 'involvement in memory-making activities could reduce ambiguity and disenfranchisement'.

When it came time to look at the feelings or needs of grandparents, I thought, who better to talk to than my mum? The first thing I noticed was that my mum (who by the way is one of the smartest, most generous people I know) was very much able to compartmentalise my pre-twelve week losses. She had not bonded with them at all.

'It wasn't about me. I wanted my child to be happy and fulfilled and have what they want.' And she experienced a lot of trauma, in watching me suffer. 'It was horrendous,' she says. 'My great fear was that the loss and pain was going to go on and on. And who knew if there was going to be a happy ending? It was very frustrating. When your kids are going through stress or challenges or ill health, you want to find a way to help and support.'

Recently another family member that my mum is close to experienced a miscarriage, after a round of IVF, and my mother supported her through at least some of the grief. When I asked Mum what she'd said in the circumstance, I was so proud of the words she chose and way she framed her support. She had come a long way from the way she talked to me about loss. I asked her if she had learned anything from the process.

'I tend to focus on glass half full rather than glass half empty and that's a personality thing,' she explains. 'I thought the way to encourage and support was to look at the positives. But I think you have to allow the person the space to grieve in their own way and if they are feeling negative at that phase you have to allow for it.'

Little people

Some years ago I was lucky enough to interview Yuin author and educator Bruce Pascoe. The interview was about his just-released book, *Found*. The story somewhat unintentionally had parallels with the experience of Stolen Generations. Given members of my husband's family had been stolen, I asked him for some advice as to when parents should begin truth-telling with their children. His response was unequivocal. 'Six months of age. Lay it all out there,' he replied. 'I never talk down to kids, they're rugged little individuals and they do get upset by the inequities and misfortune in the world, but I think it's possible to talk to them about it. And I don't think you destroy their hopes, or their happiness, by talking about the realities of the world. It's the way you talk about it. That is important.'

It is a cataclysmic challenge when younger siblings know about a pregnancy in its early stages and are then unprepared when the pregnancy ends prematurely, without a living sibling. Equally, it is important for children to understand from an appropriate age that not all pregnancies end with babies. The key is preparation. When you tell a kid they are going to be a sibling, perhaps have a plan in place as a backup if things don't work out the way you intend.

There are a raft of books about grief and loss available for kids, some of which use metaphors and some of which are more literal and direct. It is for each parent to decide what approach they want to take.

Louise had a threatened miscarriage (with a vanishing twin) and later a termination for medical reasons (TFMR), in addition to her living children. The first person to notice she was pregnant was always her daughter. During her threatened miscarriage, she had prepared her seven-year-old daughter for the possibility of a loss. It was important emotional groundwork, because Louise's subsequent pregnancy ended in a TFMR when her daughter was ten. 'We had talked about this a lot, about how sometimes babies don't grow right or they can't keep growing and that is sad, but it does happen quite a lot,' she explains. 'So she was already emotionally aware of that as a possibility and, because we'd been through all the testing, she was super aware that the baby that was born in the end, it might not keep growing. In the other pregnancy I explained about how the baby can't keep growing and the best thing was to take it out. She was upset at the idea that it was still alive at that point, but she understood the rationale. She's a particularly emotionally mature child.'

The other perspective comes from Liz, whose parents had several losses due to chromosomal issues in her family, one of which was a later miscarriage when Liz was around six years old. 'I remember being really confused, because I remember seeing Mum visibly pregnant,' she recalls. 'I don't remember being sat down and told: "This is the thing and it happens." But I do recall her being upset and just quieter than normal, and Mum is quite a bubbly, happy person. I remember later when she didn't look pregnant anymore, there wasn't a baby.

I remember being really confused, because I'd experienced the birth of my brother and him coming home and him being there. But this baby was not there. And that's not how it's meant to happen.'

Liz still thinks about the baby that didn't come home. 'I'm sad for my parents. Particularly Dad, that he didn't get the third child that he really wanted.'

With a little help from my friends

When my best friend got pregnant at forty, I was a mess. I was so incredibly happy for her – borderline ecstatic – but I was paralysed with fear. Pregnancy over forty comes with much more risk. Not just miscarriage risk, lots of them. A whole bunch. For the most part, she managed any anxiety she had well, though she's pretty unflappable at the best of times.

Around her eleven-week mark, she was waiting on the results of her NIPT and we were chatting. She asked me about some of my less than ideal results from an NIPT test during one of my later pregnancies. I stopped, paused, thought it through and then told her in no uncertain terms that we wouldn't be discussing that until we had reason to and we had to focus on staying positive.

Later, talking to my psychologist, I broke down. Not just a little. A lot. I was howling, tears rolling down my cheeks, my whole body shaking. I don't think I spoke more than a few words the whole session. I was absolutely overwhelmed with feelings of guilt. My friend is the kind of person I call when I'm in trouble. She drops everything to be by my side and I do the same for her. But doing that for me through eight pregnancies, cost her something. It cost her the ability to go into her own pregnancy naive and happy, not considering for a moment that something might go wrong.

I realise there are, of course, benefits to knowing something can go wrong and being prepared, but ultimately there is a cost involved with supporting someone through the darkest days pregnancy has to offer, in some cases the darkest days they'll ever see or know.

Equally, it costs some friends dearly that when they are pregnant, they have to keep their happiness muted for the sanity of others around them who may be struggling. In some cases, these tensions are just too much. Danna Lorch writes in *The Atlantic* about how 'the intense pain of losing a pregnancy can overshadow any ability to express genuine happiness for a friend's childbirth, even if that happiness exists deep beneath the surface'.[133]

'For some people, realising that they can't become biological parents easily or at all reorients their entire life – including their relationships,' she explains.

Throughout the period when I was losing pregnancies, I was genuinely happy for those around me who started or added to their families. But going to baby showers or namings was sometimes challenging. It wasn't because I didn't feel their joy, it was because I couldn't face the reality of what I'd lost. The persistent whisper of 'Why isn't this me?' running through my brain. One friend was kind enough to reach out to me and suggest that if it was too much to come to her baby shower, she would understand. It meant the world to me that I didn't have to make an excuse, that she understood and offered me a gracious way to stay away.

It's important for your friends and family to understand that, but too often they don't. 'Why can't you just be happy for us?' is a refrain we hear far too often. In most cases we are happy for them, but it's muffled by an overwhelming grief that allows no other feelings the air to breathe.

Another important factor to remember is that not everyone wants to talk about loss. I remember being perplexed when talking to someone who hadn't told anyone about their miscarriage when it had happened and I asked them why not. Her response was that 'every time I opened my mouth to tell someone, no words came out'.

9 to 5

Returning to work after a miscarriage can be incredibly challenging or a welcome relief. Personally, I took off very little time after my first miscarriages and later worked through almost all of them, other than the time it took to attend scans and check-ups. This really comes down to whether you are physically well enough to return to work and whether you need to sit with your grief or be distracted. For me, I needed to chip away at my grief in small increments, and being at work, focused on something else, enabled me to do that in a controlled way. For others, sitting in grief and addressing it head-on is the way they choose to process. There is no right or wrong answer.

In an Australian study, the vast majority of respondents reported taking a median leave period after miscarriage of seven days.[134] Among those people who told their boss or colleagues about their loss, reasons included needing support and understanding and avoiding triggers in the workplace such as discussion of pregnancy or babies. Among those who didn't disclose, it was because they felt it was too personal and too painful and people 'don't know what to say and inadvertently say things that are hurtful'.[135]

Ultimately, workplaces are a microcosm of broader society and you can expect a range of different reactions upon disclosure. Some will offer you sympathy. Some will offer you nothing. Being prepared for this in advance is advisable.

Not all workplaces are safe spaces for personal disclosures of this kind. Pregnancy can be seen as weakness and result in fewer opportunities, with the perception that the employee is going into a 'family phase' and will therefore be a less reliable or focused worker. Hello patriarchy!

Six Feet Under

I rushed into the tiny toilet at work. I knew before I got there but it still felt like a slap when I saw the bright red specks on the pad. I could almost feel the sting of a handprint on my cheek. And then the process started. Again.

A call was made to the specialist. An urgent ultrasound referral sent by email. A rush down to the clinic on level two. Miscarriage confirmed. Text boss. Get in the car. Drive home.

I walked into the bedroom. My husband was lying on the bed.

'What are you doing home?'

'Another miscarriage.'

'What?'

All the symptoms had been there. They were the strongest they had been. I couldn't keep food down. My breasts felt bruised. All my joints were aching. I was bloated. It was never going to be enough.

As I started to change out of my work clothes and into my griefwear (my most worn trakky daks, an oversized t-shirt and one of husband's hoodies), I felt a new reaction to this loss. One I hadn't felt before. Incandescent, uncontrollable rage.

Now, anyone who knows me will tell you that I have quite the impressive temper. My mum bought husbo a t-shirt that says 'My wife is fragile, not fragile like a flower, fragile like a bomb.' But this was different to anything I'd ever felt before or since.

This was red hot lava of emotion spewing out of me. I was shouting, screaming, throwing things. 'It's not fucking fair, it's just absolutely not fucking fair!' And just like that, I was broken. My legs gave way and I sank to the ground in front of the open wardrobe, the carpet burning my knees as I hit the floor and slid onto all fours.

Husbo jumped off the bed and wrapped his huge arms around me, as I sobbed, 'I thought this was it, I thought this was the one.' And the pain of hearing his whispered reply, 'I thought it was too,' tore my heart clean in two.

IIIIIII

I stood in the shower, the water as hot as I could physically bear it. It flowed down my entire body.

'Why did you do this? Why didn't you just grow?' I shouted downwards, berating the dead baby inside me. The baby, simultaneously there but gone.

And then I stopped, racked with guilt. And I whispered, 'I'm sorry. I'm sorry.'

And I cried.

IIIIIII

It wasn't long after that, husbo asked if we could stop trying. The answer, for me, was simple.

'No. I will not stop trying. My family, our family, is not complete. There's a black hole. I know there's another child waiting to meet us and be ours. I can feel them out there, somewhere. If you want to go, I respect that, but I will expect you to honour the agreement we made to give me sperm so that I can have a second child.'

He never explicitly said he was going to stay.

But he did.

IIIIIIIIIIIIIIIIIIIIIIIIIIIIIIIIIIIIIIIIIIIIIIIIIIIIIIIIIIIIIIIIIIIIIIIIIIIIIIIIIIIIIIIIIIIIIIIIIIIIIIIIIIIIIIIIII

8

I Wanna Be Sedated

We've long known that pregnancy loss is 'strongly associated' with anxiety, depression and suicide, so there's really no excuse for how bad we are at treating the mental health of parents.

Kelly's voice cracks as she says, 'Three days. Three days difference. That's all it was.'

When she lost her baby girl in 1996, Kelly already had two sons, the first born in 1991 and the second in 1993. She then proceeded to have five miscarriages, the first four before twelve weeks gestation. But the last one ended at nineteen and a half weeks. She had just one ultrasound, but a week later she went to the doctor because she couldn't feel the baby moving. She had surgery to end the pregnancy. Kelly happened to know one of the theatre nurses personally and asked her to divulge the baby's gender. 'She told me it was a girl. And she said the baby was perfectly fine, perfectly formed and everything, just stopped breathing.'

Kelly pushed for them to find a reason for the loss but was dismissed. She went back to her GP and asked for a referral to a counsellor who had experience in dealing with miscarriages. 'He said, "Oh, I don't think anyone does." And then he said, "Well, you know, it's just nature's way."' When Kelly went to a psychologist, she was similarly dismissed. So she 'shut it all down, and didn't deal with it at all'.

Eventually her relationship broke down and she separated. Her husband had custody of the kids most of the time, because Kelly was working. Then she started drinking. 'I was trying to drown shit,' she explains. 'And then, at the age of thirty, I got stood down from work because they said I had turned up drunk and was rude and abusive.' They took three weeks to investigate the alleged breaches of policy and during that entire time Kelly was drunk. At the three-week mark, she attended a meeting with her union rep, drunk. She was told other staff were scared to work with her. She doesn't remember anything else, because she blacked out.

An hour and a half later she was driving home and she decided to teach them a lesson. 'On my way home, I bought three bottles. I got home, put all my paperwork out, set it on the table so that people would know where to get my insurance payout and all that sort of stuff. During that time, I drank two bottles, I took the last bottle to the car with me, I connected the hose to the car, taped it all to the windows, got in my car and [put] the ignition on and proceeded to drink the rest of it. I came to after they woke me up really groggy, police and ambulance and neighbours everywhere.'

She was put on stress leave from work and, as part of the return to work program, had meetings with psychologists. It was the first time she talked about the loss of her babies, but in particular, her little girl. 'So that's how I ended up speaking to someone who actually understood about miscarriage, because it came up when I was in hospital. They sent a report back to my employer to say that I really needed to talk to someone that can deal with this other issue that was deep-seated, that has never been dealt with.'

Ten years after the loss of her baby, a psychologist asked Kelly if she wanted to name her. Kelly named her Erica. 'All of a sudden I thought, "Wow, it's actually been validated." I felt like because I'd given her a name it was real. And I've spoken to my kids about it and told them I had given her a name and my eldest said he remembered people saying we were having another baby. But we didn't have another baby. I told him I never really realised what that meant for him.'

If Erica had been born just three days later, the loss wouldn't have been deemed a miscarriage, it would have been a stillbirth and Erica would have a birth certificate, a death certificate, and Kelly would more than likely have been offered counselling and support. 'My baby was moving. It was three days difference, you know? That's what got me.'

Kelly eventually got her little girl, in the form of a granddaughter, and when Kelly talks about her, the joy resonates in her voice. 'I've now got a two-year-old granddaughter and she's just amazing, she's gorgeous. And I think that I've managed to let go of a lot of the resentment and the anger of losing Erica, for having my granddaughter around.'

Finding the way back

When someone announces they are pregnant, it is assumed, counted upon really, that they are taking on a new role of parent. They are expected to care for the baby from conception (No sushi for you!) and start planning the baby's future (What they will be called? Where will they go to kinder? Or school? Or university? Doctor? Lawyer?). There is ritual to mark this transition or repeat-transition into new parenthood, from announcements on social media, gifts for Mum and baby, and baby showers or even gender reveals.

But what happens when the story deviates from the expectation? How is that person reintegrated into society? Do they shift back to their previous role? Is their loss acknowledged? Ultimately there is no pathway, as pointed out by Linda Layne, who notes that while there are Hallmark cards for when your dog dies, there are none for miscarriage.[136] Though since she wrote that, things may have shifted, because when I checked, out of the 6260 greeting cards on sale on the Hallmark US website, there is now one for pregnancy loss. One is an improvement on none, right? Even if it is just 0.016 per cent.

In *Archer*, Frankie van Kan describes her heartbreak after having a miscarriage. 'I went back to our shared apartment in Marchmont and cried that afternoon,' she writes. 'Not because of the loss this time, but because I was overcome by sadness that we never had a burial.'[137]

Of course, as we know, not everyone feels sad after a miscarriage, but for those who do there are common themes found across clinical research and in the hundreds of interviews I've undertaken. Emptiness, sadness, loss, anxiety, anger, frustration, disappointment . . . all the hallmarks of death and grieving. Pregnancy loss is 'strongly associated' with anxiety, depression and suicide. And these feelings can persist for extended periods of time. One multi-centre, prospective cohort study of 537 women found that nine months after miscarriage 18 per cent had PTSD, 17 per cent had moderate or severe anxiety, and 6 per cent had moderate or severe depression.[138] And the depth of the grief or magnitude of depression is not contingent on the gestation of the pregnancy.[139]

A small study of transmasculine and non-binary parents found that emotional responses to pregnancy losses 'extended beyond the fact of the pregnancy loss' and into more generalised fears around being a pregnant man, transmasculine, or non-binary person. A 'do I really want to do this?' moment of cold feet. 'Specific to this diverse population, fears related to the possibility that pregnancy might not be a possibility, and also to the potential for the recording of information about a pregnancy loss to force disclosure to other people that a participant was transgender.'[140]

One of the most beautiful things I have ever read on pregnancy loss was a poem and explanatory chapter by the Canadian educator, activist, and writer j wallace skelton entitled 'failing'.[141] The opening section of the chapter consists of one line, 'As a trans person, I am used to my body failing me', repeated eight times. In each line, certain words are struck through to create very different meanings, for instance, 'As a trans person, I am used to my body failing me'. While certainly many people experience a feeling of failure around pregnancy loss, skelton's work gave depth to the multi-dimensional theme of failure, which

I found profoundly moving. Trans people deal with a unique set of circumstances around pregnancy loss. For example, for many trans birth parents, there can be severe body dysmorphia during pregnancy, akin to what they may have experienced before transition. If the pregnancy then fails, was it all for nothing?

All questions and no answers

No matter your gender, after a miscarriage, patients are left with a raft of questions, and often very few answers. 'When did the pregnancy end? Was it moments after conception? Was it when my doctor couldn't find a heartbeat? Was it after the shot of methotrexate when my hormone level finally stopped rising? Or at eleven weeks and four days when the doctor opened me on the table? For more than a month, I was pregnant but not carrying a child,' writes Robin Silbergleid in the chapter 'Missed Miscarriage', in the book *Interrogating Pregnancy Loss: Feminist Writings on Abortion, Miscarriage, and Stillbirth*.[142]

The Australian Psychological Society has a helpful 'find a psychologist' search tool on its website. When you navigate to the homepage (assuming you have identified that you need support and can afford to seek it out), the first step in using the tool is to choose a speciality area of practice. There are lots of lists and categories, including hoarding, psychosis, abortion, family violence, infertility, pregnancy support (interestingly filed under 'personal', rather than 'health'), trichotillomania . . . The list is seemingly endless. But it doesn't include pregnancy loss.

In 2017, 2122 people – comprising patients who have experienced miscarriage, partners, family, friends, colleagues and healthcare workers – did a survey[143] to prioritise miscarriage research areas. In the list of top ten research areas nominated by the respondents in order, number two was about the emotional and mental health impact of miscarriage on both the birth parent and partner, and number five was around what emotional support is most effective.

In Australia there are several organisations that offer counselling and support services to those who have experienced a bereavement, but they are woefully under-funded and therefore under-resourced and under-promoted to the people who need them. And some of them have a long way to go before offering a service I would even begin to describe as 'adequate'.

Anne, who is German, met her Australian husband when they were both travelling in Argentina. They had their dream wedding in Thailand before moving to Australia to start their family. But after getting pregnant, they experienced a traumatic, badly managed miscarriage. Being so far away from home, Anne realised she needed some help coping. She attended a support group through Sands (now part of Red Nose), but it didn't cater specifically to women who'd experienced early pregnancy loss. 'I found that really confronting because a lot of the people that I met there had lost babies much later in pregnancy. They were talking through that experience, and in a lot of detail, which gave me a lot of anxiety. I never went back.'

Attendees of merged support groups can include patients who've experienced a miscarriage, stillbirth, termination for medical reasons or molar pregnancy. Red Nose CEO Keren Ludski – who herself experienced both miscarriage and stillbirth – said Red Nose is moving to change that. 'The way we are moving now is to having pretty much predominantly loss-specific groups,' she explains. 'You do have to understand the complexities of it.'

Despite most people associating Red Nose with Sudden Infant Death Syndrome (SIDS), it was already working in this space before its merger with Sands and is now positioning itself as being able to offer support for losses from conception all the way through to early childhood. In 2020, a huge 34 per cent of its referrals were for losses under twenty weeks. What's interesting is that a large proportion of those, 30 per cent, were 'self-referred', meaning the patient had sought out support themselves and not been referred by, for instance, a GP. In fact, just 20 per cent were referred by health practitioners, but this figure is expected to increase as awareness grows of Red Nose's role and services in this space.

Equally, the support groups don't always hit the mark, with really serious consequences. Cara, in her thirties, and having already had two miscarriages, called one large, well-known group after undergoing a termination for medical reasons. She was told they didn't know what to say to her about her termination (which took place due to chromosomal abnormalities), despite the organisation promoting itself as offering support in that circumstance. The peer support worker said someone would call her back, but they didn't. It led to Cara, who had a history of drug dependency, falling off the wagon. It simply shouldn't be like this.

For those with existing mental health conditions, a pregnancy loss can be another stressor that means they are in acute need of psychosocial care. When Natasha and her husband decided to get pregnant, she had to go off the medication she was taking for depression and ADHD. She also had a diagnoses of bipolar and a borderline personality disorder. When she had her first miscarriage, Natasha was offered a referral for counselling by a sympathetic obstetrician at the hospital who had taken the time to get to know her more than some of the other healthcare professionals she had seen and was aware of her history of suicidal ideation. Her second miscarriage was much more stressful, due to mismanagement by the hospital for her appointments and a number of administrative stuff-ups, and yet she was not offered any counselling. 'Perhaps I should have taken up a miscarriage counsellor. I don't know how much help it would have been. I don't think that they routinely get the psychologists or counsellors on board, which they probably should, because I am psychiatrically disabled, but I reckon it should be for everybody.'

Online support groups for miscarriage have blossomed on social media to fill a vacuum in the real world, both in care and information provision. Thousands of people make use of these forums every day, predominantly on Facebook, desperate to connect with peers who have had or are having similar experiences. Patients share their feelings about their lost babies, their partners, their lives. It's a veritable smorgasbord of peer support, sympathy and empathy, as well as suggestions for coping strategies. It can also be a treasure trove of information about fertility, testing regimes, medical system navigation, 'cures' and next steps.

I have been an active participant and observer for a number of years in several Australian, American and UK groups, and while some of these groups are incredibly helpful, I do have some concerns. In an area of medicine that is misunderstood, under-researched and so rarely talked about openly, there is much conjecture. What works? What doesn't work? Everyone is looking for a miracle cure or prevention. Grief can lead to desperation and superstition. Sometimes the peer-provided information is based on old wives' tales, outdated or just plain wrong. Many of these groups have grown organically and are moderated on a volunteer basis, which makes the task of management onerous, leading to risky propagation of 'fake news' that ultimately goes unchecked. Similarly, some online support groups run by non-profits simply don't have the resources to monitor every post, when there are hundreds of posts and thousands of comments being published each day. As well as information not getting sense-checked, posters who are really struggling are not offered referrals to professional counselling that may be very much needed. For me this constitutes a dereliction in the duty of care.

An example of this is the use of fetal dopplers at home. A doppler is a small electronic device that sells for as little as $100 and enables you to hear a baby's heartbeat. Its usage is aimed at soothing an anxious parent's mind, especially if they've previously experienced loss. Doctors, midwives and specialists almost universally condemn using these devices at home, because (especially in the early stages) the heartbeat can be difficult to find. But dopplers are discussed and encouraged in many of the online support groups. Ironically, in a situation where parents are looking for solace, they run the risk of extreme panic when they can't find the baby's heartbeat. Parents may also accidentally think they've found the fetal heartbeat, when in fact they're monitoring the birth parent's heartbeat, meaning that if there is an issue with the baby, they don't realise. Perhaps if patients were given support or referrals for assistance in coping with anxiety in pregnancy subsequent to loss, or if the system allowed for regular ultrasounds, 'workarounds' like this could be avoided.

Another example promoted in support groups is a strategy whereby you do a cheap pregnancy test every day to ensure that the positive line is darkening – an incredibly imprecise, unscientific method for determining if your hCG is rising. You guessed it: another attempt to alleviate anxiety. As mentioned on page 116, this is something I did for almost all my losses. It gave me comfort, even when it showed that things weren't going to work out. The sooner you know, the sooner you can begin the process of grieving and try again, right? Ultimately, some form of comfort is what so many of us are seeking. Even if this particular tactic is not recommended by doctors.

Superstition can be strong in the groups, but that is not necessarily a bad thing. People wish 'baby dust' upon each other and share photos of rainbows they see when out and about (rainbows representing live children born after loss) and wishes that the sightings represent good omens. Live children born after rainbow babies are called pots of gold. The ones who leave too soon are called angel babies. All of these words invoke magic or spirit, which in itself is comforting, but more importantly they bind together the community with its own language, expression and most importantly: compassion and understanding.

Memory

In Japan, parents who experience loss commemorate the souls of their babies with Jizo statues, which are small stone statues made in the image of Jizo Bosatsu, the Buddhist god of children and travellers. They wear small red caps and capes. Jizo statues have caught on in certain Western circles now too, for parents looking outside their own (sometimes non-existent) customs for methods of commemoration. In Jewish law, *aveilut*, formal mourning, is not undertaken after miscarriage (or for that matter even stillbirth). But immersion at the ritual baths (*Mikvah*) is obligatory by Jewish law. The reason given is that it is 'an opportunity for spiritual and physical transition'.[144]

One of the key symptoms of PTSD is memory loss. As noted by Bessel Van Der Kolk in his seminal text *The Body Keeps the Score: Brain, Mind, and Body in the Healing of Trauma*,[145] 'memory loss has been reported in people who have experienced natural disasters, accidents, war trauma, kidnapping, torture, concentration camps, and physical and sexual abuse'.[146] Van Der Kolk explains in his book that due to certain areas of the brain shutting down during traumatic events (and during recollection), 'the imprints of traumatic experiences are organised not as coherent logical narratives but in fragmented sensory and emotional traces: images, sounds and physical sensations'.[147] I didn't realise until I came to write this book how many of my memories had failed to take root in my brain, were muddled or incomplete. It gave me comfort to speak with so many other people who've had similar experiences. Having keepsakes to trigger memories that you want to retain can be an important part of processing.

Many parents and families I speak with keep their ultrasound photos, if they've been able to have any before their loss. In some situations, patients might not want copies of an ultrasound photo, for instance if they've decided to undertake a termination for medical reasons. In my view, where they exist the images should be kept on the patient's file, should they change their mind down the track.

It is also becoming more common to hold and be photographed with your lost baby or after your loss, sometimes with a partner, in the hospital. When American celebrity Chrissy Teigen miscarried her son in 2020 (though two years later she redefined it as an abortion) she announced it by posting photos to her social media channels of her and her husband John Legend, pre- and post-delivery in the hospital. She was roundly attacked for both taking the photos and posting them. In a response on *Medium*, she was able to explain very clearly why she ensured photos were taken at every step of the journey.

'I had asked my mom and John to take pictures, no matter how uncomfortable it was. I explained to a very hesitant John that I needed them, and that I did NOT want to have to ever ask. That he just had to do it. He hated it. I could tell. It didn't make sense to him at the time. But I knew I needed to know of this moment forever, the same way I needed to remember us kissing at the end of the aisle, the same way I needed to remember our tears of joy after Luna and Miles. And I absolutely knew I needed to share this story.'[148]

The second purpose served by memorialisation is marking a baby's presence on Earth. Helping the grieving parents to prove, both to themselves and others, that their babies existed. While this has been the case for decades within support groups, it has now transformed into an industry of sorts, albeit one geared more towards later losses. There are tattoo designs, jewellery makers who incorporate hair/breastmilk, art, memory boards, memory boxes and the list goes on. All Australian states now have miscarriage memorial or commemorative certificates available through offices of births, deaths and marriages; they don't act as a legal document but do offer a form of recognition. Some hospitals offer group memorial services to families, though these often have Christian religious elements that at best don't appeal to everyone or at worst can be exclusionary.

In her thesis *Women's experiences of pregnancy loss: An interpretative phenomenological analysis*, Esther Lea Kint points out that there are 'various behaviours representative of "unresolved" grief'. Examples of these behaviours include buying mementos on special occasions or anniversaries to acknowledge an absence or refusing to part with the possessions of someone lost.[149] That might include baby goods that were already in the home before the loss happened. I've heard terrible stories of people who have experienced loss coming home to find nurseries packed up and put away by well-meaning family or friends and this compounding trauma, because they were not items with which the parents were ready to part as they made them feel close to their lost babies. In an alternative perspective, I'm still finding maternity wear hidden all over my house, because after each loss I couldn't even bear to look at it. Another reminder that every loss and every reaction to it is different.

The final purpose in memorialisation and commemoration is book-ending a chapter and moving forward. Rabbi Deborah Brin writes, 'Rituals are creative uses of the medium of time. Think of the ritual as an elongated moment, a moment squeezed for all it is worth to make a memorable distinction between what came before and what comes after.'[150] As noted earlier in this chapter, when a person is pregnant, society already sees them as a parent, responsible for caring for that baby. But when they lose that pregnancy, there must be the option of a pathway to reintegrate back into society. To mark the loss and to move forward in whatever way is appropriate for them.

All that is left

You might remember Elsa from chapter four. She miscarried her fifteen-week-old daughter Lucy in the shower at home after leaving her local hospital's emergency room, after hours of waiting with no information. In a panic, she put Lucy in a container and put her in the freezer.

This was not Elsa's first loss. She gave birth to her daughter Emma at fourteen weeks, when doctors found Emma had a genetic condition not compatible with life. Elsa was offered genetic counselling, support from a social worker and Emma was cremated. Thinking that Lucy should also be cremated, Elsa and her partner turned up at a funeral home and explained the situation. They were turned away at the door and told they needed a certificate from the GP because the funeral home 'couldn't confirm they hadn't committed a crime'.

Australia needs to have a serious conversation about disposal of remains, something that can and should be done better. In 'Respectful Disposition In Early Pregnancy Loss',[151] the paper's authors argue that when discussing the disposition of remains, nurses must understand the concepts of personhood, place and protection. We have already addressed personhood. Place is about the fundamental human need to have a place in the world. Place is also about the parent(s) having a place (whether that is within a home or elsewhere) to go to mourn. Protection can relate to several factors in the wake of loss, including the perception that the body is supposed to protect the baby and how safe and respectful handling in death can extend this protection in the mind of the parent, where they may feel their body has failed them.

'Nurses stand in the unique position of both caring for women experiencing an early pregnancy loss and advocating to create processes that ensure respectful disposition of fetal tissue and remains. Through assessing current disposition practice, reviewing local disposition ordinances and state legislation, and collaborating among all involved clinicians, nurses can subsequently implement change that honours the meaning of the pregnancy loss for the woman and her family.'[152]

Another reason we need to address what happens to remains is within the context of genetic testing, meaning testing the pregnancy tissue to establish if there was a chromosomal abnormality that caused the loss. From a psychological perspective, there is huge benefit in getting the testing done, because confirmation of genetic abnormalities can be instrumental in a patient being able to move forward and let go of any self-blame they might be harbouring. From a medical point of view there are also benefits, with the early capture of abnormalities that would be considered more likely to repeat, or in the case of fetuses that are chromosomally healthy, to start investigation as to why the miscarriage has occurred.

In the public system, it is standard practice to have testing done when you've had three miscarriages in a row and are therefore considered to be a recurrent miscarriage patient. Even in the private system, where patients are able to foot the bill, many doctors rarely offer the option or explain how to capture and store tissue if you're seeking answers as to why a miscarriage has taken place. There can be logistical and storage issues when collecting the tissue yourself, though if a D&C is taking place, tissue retrieval and analysis is more straightforward.

'This is one of the reasons that I try and persuade my patients to undergo a [D&C] as soon as they are confident in their own minds that the pregnancy has died,' writes Professor Lesley Regan, one of the world's leading miscarriage clinicians and researchers. 'Although this is unlikely to be at the top of your priority list when you have just received the sad news, I promise you that when the initial shock wears off, you will want as much information as possible about your pregnancy and why it miscarried.'[153]

In earlier chapters we touched on the physical issues that may arise if there's a delay in being able to get a D&C, but the psychological implications can be even more acute. Many of the people I interviewed talked about their urgent need to have the pregnancy be over, once the miscarriage was confirmed. It's a feeling often described as being a 'walking coffin'. For this reason, if a D&C is delayed, it can create significant mental anguish. This is far too often misunderstood by some medical professionals, who see procedures solely through a physical lens.

It's a similar situation with ultrasounds, where patients request ultrasounds in the case of threatened miscarriage. Medical providers say that this is not useful because if there is a problem during the first twenty weeks, it's rarely able to be remedied. They don't understand that alleviating the patient's anxiety with an ultrasound could have hugely beneficial effects on their psychological well-being, which can in turn benefit the patient's physiology.

Get to work

In 2021 there was a strong push from within certain sections of the miscarriage support community to introduce bereavement leave for people who experience early pregnancy loss. It was given a boost by our friends across the ditch, with New Zealand introducing three days of bereavement leave for birth parents and their partners who experience miscarriage. India and China both have miscarriage bereavement leave after introducing it in the 1960s. But despite it being in place for a number of decades, take-up is almost non-existent. In Australia, two days of paid miscarriage bereavement leave were eventually added to the *Fair Work Act* in 2021.

Sophia is a high-profile Australian television personality. She was forty when she decided to have a second baby and got pregnant. But at the eight-week mark, things started to go wrong. She didn't feel any pregnancy symptoms, which she thought was odd, and then she started to bleed. She was at work and due on air. 'All of my immediate bosses, all the way up the line, were middle-aged men. So basically, I was at work, knowing that I was miscarrying and we're getting closer and closer to going on air. My boss is a nice man but I thought he'd freak out. I didn't want them to call an ambulance or something. So I just went ahead and went on air. After that, I went and miscarried in the ladies' toilets,' she says. 'I've gone into that toilet cubicle probably two or three times a week in the two decades I've worked here since. And every single time I think of it.'

After a miscarriage, it's not as easy as simply walking up to your boss and saying, 'I need miscarriage bereavement leave.' Not everyone is comfortable sharing such an intensely personal event and not everyone's organisation has an HR department where confidentiality is assured. Data also shows that fear of discrimination is not unfounded. In 2014 Australia's Human Rights Commission (HRC) released its report 'Supporting Working Parents: Pregnancy and Return to Work National Review'.[154] HRC did a first-of-its-kind survey that showed half (HALF!) of mothers reported experiencing discrimination in the workplace at some point during pregnancy, parental leave or on return to work. There were terrible examples of blatant disrespect shown to women returning to the workplace after early pregnancy loss and clear professional ramifications.

'Since returning to work I have had no support from either my boss or from management. In fact I believe I have been almost forgotten about,' said one.[155] Many employees feel that by being open about their loss, they may be divulging an intention to get pregnant and will then be passed over for promotion, shifts, work, or will be treated like they don't have their 'heads in the game'.

When Enid had a surgical procedure at the hospital to complete her miscarriage, she was given some time to recover in a curtained-off area before being moved to the general area where all day procedure patients went before discharge. 'As I walked with a nurse into the seated area I saw a junior colleague from work was also sat there. I hissed at the nurse something pretty unintelligible that I knew that man and didn't want to sit next to him and she managed to quickly understand what I was saying and sat me at the other end and pulled the curtain around me,' Enid explains. 'No one at work knew we were trying to have a baby and I was up for promotion at work and didn't want anyone in my team to know.'[156]

Cheryl has three invisible disabilities, and another two chronic illnesses, and therefore needs workplace adjustments to be able to work. Twenty years ago she had several miscarriages, before losing her daughter Emily during childbirth. She suffered a severe depressive episode and tried to take her own life. 'When I returned to work a month after that, I was advised that because I was "unreliable", my responsibilities had been transferred to someone else, my hours reduced, and that, basically, I had been demoted,' she explained. 'It didn't matter that I had worked there for five years without incident, that I had been promoted twice and they had been happy with my work before I needed a month off work. All that mattered was that I was now seen as "unreliable" and "mentally unstable".'[157]

When looking for something to which we can compare bereavement leave, a good example might be family and domestic violence leave, which was introduced in Australia in 2018. While there are clearly differences, they share some themes of sensitivity, trauma and (misplaced) self-blame or shame. At the time of writing, workers in Australia are entitled to five days of unpaid domestic violence leave as part of Australian National Employment Standards. There are moves under way to make this ten days of leave, which are likely to be in place by the time you read these words.

When I started asking contacts within the domestic abuse space, it became very clear very quickly that these entitlements are not often taken up. One union official I spoke to told me the pattern was predicted, with uptake rates expected to be low because 'the proportion of workers in any given workplace who are both experiencing family and domestic violence and have the confidence to seek assistance in the form of paid leave will be quite small'. I was also told that 'uptake rates vary from workplace to workplace depending on various factors, but are generally quite low across the board'. Campaigners in the space have said repeatedly in interviews that it's as much about 'sending a message' as practical support.

While I applaud the concept and idea of miscarriage bereavement leave, practicalities around take-up are yet to be addressed. One of the first corporate organisations to come forward and offer miscarriage bereavement leave was a large Australian bank. I contacted the organisation to ask if they had a plan to overcome some of the barriers to this leave actually being taken up and the simple answer was no. They said HR could handle sensitive leave requests. But the person I was speaking to also acknowledged that the reason for leave would, in some form, be conveyed to managers.

Interestingly, in a small-scale study released in October 2021, and led by the exceptional Dr Melanie Keep of the University of Sydney, the argument is made that flexible working arrangements should be addressed by workplaces in the context of returning to work after loss. This has not been raised at all during the move to introduce bereavement leave,[158] but it could nevertheless make life much easier for grief-stricken parents.

Wrong time, wrong place

As you sit and wait for an ultrasound to confirm whether or not you're having or have had a miscarriage, or even to see a doctor because you're bleeding and you're scared, it's a time of immense anxiety and pain. Desperate for good news, but preparing for the worst. If a miscarriage has already been confirmed, you might be in shock, or grief may have already set in. As you look across the crowded waiting room and see heavily pregnant patients – they might be discussing baby names, laughing with a partner or friend, or doing inane, everyday things like taking work calls – you wonder: Do they realise how lucky they are? Are they laughing at me? Do they know? Do they pity me? And the worst question of all . . . why them and not me? Being put in this position can be utterly devastating and cleave your heart into pieces. It's not 'rational'. Grief, loss and pregnancy hormones are the arch nemeses of rational thinking. But when you're losing a baby you so desperately want, what does rational mean anyway?

The complaint from people experiencing miscarriage around being seated in public waiting areas with pregnant people must surely be among the most common complaints within the support groups I frequent and one we touched on briefly in chapter four. This is despite it potentially being so easily remedied with a small separate, cordoned-off waiting area that could be offered, even by a screen or divider. When I ask the people I interview to tell me about their recollections and memories of miscarriage, the pain they experience when put in this position features heavily and frequently.

In a very similar way, when a later miscarriage means you're going to have to birth the baby, it's incredibly traumatic to have to do it in a labour ward. At fifteen weeks, Marie was told her daughter had died in utero. Her voice shakes as she describes arriving at the hospital to give birth. She was walked through the entire maternity ward before being put in the ward's tearoom while awaiting access to the birthing suite.

'I was by myself, in pain, surrounded by posters about breastfeeding, pre- and postnatal support, an entire wall of pictures of babies and thank you cards, while mums are walking up and down the hallway with their new babies, their partners are getting them cups of tea . . . It wasn't the place I needed to be at that point, when I'm about to lose my kid.'

Another parent I spoke to, Sally, described to me how it felt to regain consciousness after her D&C in the labour ward to the sound of babies crying. She put her hands over her ears, rolled up in a ball under a blanket, inconsolable and crying as she tried to block out the sound of babies that weren't hers.

In August 2021 the Scottish health service agreed to institute an area separate to maternity wards where patients could give birth in cases of stillbirth or miscarriage. The move was a result of two years of campaigning by Louise Caldwell, who lost her baby at thirteen weeks in 2019. She told the BBC, 'Like many, many women, I will be haunted by the labour ward for the rest of my life. I have spoken to women who fifty, twenty-five years later are still haunted by the labour ward.'[159]

Equally, words matter. When June experienced an ectopic pregnancy, she was rushed to emergency and told it would be removed with a laparoscopy, where the abdomen is inflated and then a surgical procedure takes place. 'It's where we blow you up with gas as though you're at forty weeks,' June recalls the attending male registrar explaining, in between cracking jokes with the attending nurse. 'It just seemed tone deaf at the very least,' June says, 'if not actively cruel.'

While there are many terms that doctors tell me are for clinical use only and not used in front of patients – for example 'spontaneous abortion' and 'products of conception' – I have heard these and many others used in clinical contexts, research papers and within education forums for clinicians, both experienced and in training. I remain deeply concerned at some in the medical profession who don't seem to understand the power of language and the negative effect this can have on the well-being of their patients. I think this disconnect stems from both a lack of education, a slowness to adopt cultural change and an inability to take a patient-centric approach to well-being.

Because miscarriages are often confirmed by ultrasound, often it comes down to ultrasonologists (sometimes obstetricians) or radiologists to deliver bad news. Monica Dux wrote of her ultrasound experience, 'She turned the screen towards me so I could see for myself and said bluntly, "There's the sac. No heartbeat, no nothing. It's dead." And so ended my second pregnancy.'[160]

Adverse findings in ultrasound are far too frequently delivered in a clumsy or even outright disrespectful manner. Or not delivered at all if the clinician has been instructed that news can only be delivered by the referring medical practitioner, creating a sense that the practitioner is not being honest with the patient. Or at least that they're obfuscating the truth. In their defence, very little training in how to deliver bad news in obstetric contexts is offered as part of ultrasound qualifications.

This is something Dr Samantha Thomas of the University of Sydney is trying to change. A sonographer whose PhD was on the topic of communicating adverse findings to pregnant patients, she was inspired to approach the Australasian Society for Ultrasound in Medicine (ASUM) to initiate the guidelines' development. Together they convened a multi-disciplinary team comprising medical professionals, sonographers, patient advocates and academics to complete the project.

'Many sonographers were stressed because they did not have any training or consistent departmental protocols which encourage a collaborative approach and gave them the support needed when faced with unexpected or adverse obstetric findings,' she told me for an article published in *Guardian Australia*.[161] They were trialled in a pilot rollout in Perth and Sydney, with ASUM reporting a 'high rate of parent and clinician satisfaction'.

'Sonographers are on the frontline conducting these scans and parents are telling us delayed communication from the day of the scan until the next time they see a doctor concerns them,' says ASUM's Chief Executive Lyndal Macpherson. 'This is not only about communicating findings with parents but also equipping sonographers to share their communication with the reporting doctor so there is a clear understanding of the information being shared across all professionals in the care team.'

It was an important and much-needed development when the guidelines were launched in 2022. Let's hope they continue to find their way into the reality of practice.

We Are Family

I typed the name into the search bar. Bolgraaf. It's Dutch. There are no other families in Australia that share my paternal nana's maiden name that we know of, at least with that spelling. So I was surprised when the cemetery's website pulled up three extra gravesites I didn't know were there.

Taking care of myself while writing this book has been a challenge. Revisiting my story, sharing in so many others . . . I could put a deposit on a beachside holiday house with the money I've spent on therapy bills.

I welcomed the distraction when I fell down an ancestry.com rabbit hole. The catalyst was a seemingly innocuous question I asked my dad about how my nana and pop (his parents) had met, when Nana was in Sydney and Poppy in Melbourne.

'Nana came to Melbourne for the Jewish sports carnival,' Dad explained. 'She was a gymnast. Poppy was at the party for the athletes.' I started to wonder whether there was any press. A quick search found an article in *The Age* on 3 January 1938, on page four no less! The headline read, 'Happy garden party for Judean visitors'. And just like that I was off and running.

Being an obsessive researcher at heart, it wasn't long before I was rifling through war records, birth and death records, putting in applications for death certificates and piecing together the hugely colourful history of my dad's family. There were twists and turns and sadness and hope and all the makings of a damn good novel. Fact is stranger than fiction, right?

I was beyond frustrated when I hit a dead end with the leads that ancestry.com served up through its intricate, winding algorithm. I was going to have to do some work to find another trapdoor down the rabbit hole.

I was hurtling from genealogy site to genealogy site, throwing in search terms relating to my dad's family, thinking as laterally as I could to rustle up that one little thread I needed to set me back on my path of discovery.

Rookwood? It rang a bell. I clicked on the link. Oh yes, Sydney's Jewish cemetery. I had been to this site before and seen the gravesites of several of my nana's siblings buried there. It was doubtful I'd find anything I hadn't already seen, but my need for a lead overtook my doubts and I moved my cursor up to the search bar. B–O–L–G–R–A–A–F, tapped my fingers, outpacing my brain.

Up popped all the names I knew both from my research and from the stories my family had told me over four decades. So many names. Among them my great-uncle Maurice and my great-uncle Charles. My great-grandmother Leah and my great-grandfather John Nathan.

And then, at the very bottom of the list, I saw it. 'Unnamed Bolgraaf'. Unnamed Bolgraaf? Was there something wrong with the records? Confused, I clicked on the entry.

I could see from the attached photograph it was a very old part of the cemetery. The writing on the graves to the left-hand side were almost unintelligible due to decades and decades of wear. There was a big tree in the background and the sun was shining down on the gravesite. Well, I assumed it was the gravesite. There was no gravestone, so it was difficult to tell.

I went back to the master list and scoured the entry for clues. Who did this grave site belong to? But there was nothing. Then I scrolled down a little further and saw it. A second entry. Also labelled 'Unnamed Bolgraaf'. I scrolled down. A third!

The 'plot', as they say, thickened.

||||||

Every Jewish community has a Chevra Kadisha – Jewish burial society – or at least some iteration of one. They perform the rituals associated with death and keep fastidious family history records. Sydney's Chevra Kadisha had to be my first stop. I picked up the phone and dialled the number.

I explained my confusion to the kind woman at the other end of the line. She listened carefully. I gave her the spelling of the name and the plot and row numbers of the three stoneless gravesites. And then I hesitated, nervous to articulate my suspicions out loud.

'I strongly suspect they could be babies.'

||||||

Leah Gruzman was born in 1889 in Russia. She was travelling on a boat to Australia with her sister Fanny, when they met two Dutch brothers, John Nathan and Solomon Izak Bolgraaf. They arrived in Australia around 1914 and Leah married John and Fanny married Solomon. By 1918, John Nathan had signed up for military service, perhaps not realising World War I was drawing to a close. Or perhaps he did.

Leah, his wife, started having children in 1917, kicking off proceedings with my great-uncle Maurice. He was followed by my nana Sophia in 1919, then by Eva (1921), Rachel (1923) and Charles (1924).

John Nathan ended up working in the pub trade and by 1930 had finally managed to purchase a pub license for the Royal Mail Hotel in Woolloomooloo. He was a gambler and an alcoholic and my nana used to recount the stories of the regular beatings doled out to her mother. Leah died at just forty-five years – according to her death certificate her death was a result of arteriosclerosis (hardening of the arteries that carry blood to the heart) and a cerebral haemorrhage. John Nathan died one year after her at just fifty-two years.

Meanwhile, Fanny and Solomon also had Simon and Sophie (1919), plus Michael, or Mick The Barber as he was known (1928). Sometime between 1919 and 1928, she had two other children, Maurice and Rachel.

The Unnamed Bolgraaf graves were created in 1915, 1923 and 1928, so they could have been born to either couple.

Were they my great-cousins or my great-aunts and uncles? Were they twins or singletons? Did the two sisters comfort each other as they experienced their losses? Or was it just one sister who carried the burden of grief?

||||||

Unfortunately, despite scouring the records at the burial society, the lady at the Chevra Kadisha couldn't find me the answers I so badly needed. The never-ending questions continued to swirl around in my mind, plaguing my quiet moments and playing cat and mouse with my imagination.

'I'm struggling to get information for you because the passings away were a long time ago,' read the email. Time, it seemed, had stolen all my answers. My suspicions were confirmed, at least in theory, by the researcher, who agreed that, with no name and no tombstones, the most likely answer is that the gravesites contained babies.

While Jewish observances vary by community, my family of that generation were Orthodox Jews. It is likely that they abided by the tradition that you don't mourn a baby's death until it is thirty days old, even though a Jewish naming ceremony traditionally takes place eight days after birth. It's highly unusual not to put a gravestone on a gravesite; indeed it is considered very important to erect one.

The discovery of these babies weighed on me. I had a fistful of questions to which I knew I would never find answers. But whether I knew the details or not, I knew in my heart these gravesites represented some form of loss. And all losses have commonality. I felt a strange link form, far beyond bloodlines, tying me to these powerful ancestors I had never met.

|||||||||||||||||||||||||||||||||||||||||||||||||||||||||||||||||||||||||||||||||||||||||||||||||||||||||||

9

More Than Words

What loved ones say or do in the wake of a loss can provide the greatest of comfort or deepen torment and grief. Here are some dos and don'ts.

I've truly lost count of the number of times I've been contacted by friends, family or acquaintances to ask some variation on the following question: 'My friend/sibling/partner/colleague had a miscarriage. What do I do, what do I say?' Equally, some of the most common complaints in support groups are around dismissive, hurtful or downright shitty things people say to someone when they've had a miscarriage. I ran a meme series on my Instagram account called 'Fuck This Shit', about the stupid things that people say to people in the wake of loss. And when I asked for submissions, I got the same submissions over and over. For months.

With the confusion around whether or not loss before twenty weeks is in fact a loss, often people seem unsure what to say. This combined with the discomfort society has for sitting with or addressing grief means many are totally unable to find the words. Or, at least, the right words. The first thing I always recommend is to call it by its name. You would be surprised how moving it can be just to have someone offer acknowledgement with the simple words, 'I'm sorry for your loss.' I personally usually follow up with, 'Life can be such a shit sandwich.'

If you are speaking directly to the person who has experienced the loss, their partner or their family, ask them how they are. Ask them if there is anything they need. Ask them how they are feeling. Here's the important bit though: listen when they respond. Give them whatever time they need. And pay close attention to how they refer to their loss. If they call it a loss, you call it a loss. If they call it a baby, you call it a baby. You get where I'm going with this, right? If you are not talking to them directly, drop off some flowers. Or a homemade casserole. Or some meal delivery vouchers. Do whatever you would do with someone who is grieving; their grief is no different to anyone else's.

It's also very important to take cues or ask permission before grand gestures. You can never ever assume that you know how someone is going to react to grief and loss or what they will want or how they will behave. Ask if there is anything they want you to do.

Also, if that person has lots of support, perhaps wait a week or two or even a month and then check in. There can be a level of shock in bereavement. Sometimes when the dust has settled and everyone else has moved on, it can be the hardest and loneliest time and you need a friend.

If someone close to you decides to try again and becomes pregnant, make sure you check in on them from time to time. Pregnancy after loss can be an overwhelming, anxiety-laden or harrowing time for some parents.

Now for the don'ts. If someone told you their parent had passed away, would you say, 'Oh that's sad, at least you've got another one!'? No. I didn't think so. Sometimes life is shit and there isn't a 'silver lining'. For someone who has just lost their baby, pointing out a silver lining is, to put it mildly, not helpful. I really do try not to judge people, but 'Oh well, at least you can drink now' is a totally inappropriate response to someone's miscarriage. Don't point out their age ('You still have heaps of time!'). Don't point out their luck in already having kids ('Oh well, focus on little Rufus, at least you've got him, be grateful!'). Don't point out all the good things in their life ('You've got a great job, a lovely house, a great partner, it'll happen when it's time!'). Just say you're sorry and listen. And for chrissake, don't ask them if they're going to try again. They may not know. They may not want you to know. Ultimately, it's really none of your business.

If you are pregnant, be prepared to give the person some space, and don't under any circumstances be offended if they don't want to see you, rub your belly, come to your baby shower or go over your baby names list. It's not about you. Or their happiness for you. They may need time to process. Do you want them turning up to your baby shower and sobbing in a corner? Surely it's in no one's best interests to let that particular scenario play out.

All the grief, anxiety and fear of early pregnancy loss can be amplified when it comes to recurrent miscarriage. In *Coming to Term*, Jon Cohen writes, 'Anderson felt alone, isolated. "The first loss, I got flowers," she said. "The second, third and fourth, I got nothing." Her supportive husband could not turn her depression around. "Men want to fix things," she said. "And they can't." Her friendships felt the strain too. "No one – and I have lots of friends – gave me what I needed," she said. "To just say, 'Oh my God, that's terrible.' That's all I wanted someone to say."'[162]

Linda Layne also writes about the difficulties of recurrent miscarriage. 'Perry-Lynn Moffitt (1994) reports that after her first miscarriage "people responded by sending flowers and notes of condolence. Others stopped by for brief, but supportive visits," but when her next pregnancy also ended in miscarriage, "most [of our friends] didn't want to talk about it. There were no notes or flowers this time".'[163]

Certainly this is something I experienced when my miscarriages started to rack up. I craved support and love, but I also didn't want to be a burden to my friends. Who wants to be the 'sad one' who brings down the mood because you're on miscarriage number whatever. There was an elephant perched in the corner of the room whenever I saw anyone, except it wasn't an elephant, it was an ever-growing pile of dead babies I never got to meet.

The Way We Were

'Isabelle is medically well and there are no concerns regarding her plans to conceive.'

'Isabelle is yet to experience any significant pain or bleeding.'

'I am still very optimistic for Isabelle's chances of having a healthy pregnancy given that she and her partner have one live-born child.'

'Just a quick note to update you that Isy's NIPT returned a high-risk result for T21.'

'It's certainly pleasing to see her again so soon after her previous miscarriage.'

'She had an ultrasound that demonstrated the miscarriage was complete.'

'Suction curettage for missed abortion.'

'I'll see mum and baby at the six-week postnatal check.'

'Isy opted for a STOP which was performed . . .'

I'm angry at my memory. Did it lie? Did the doctors not tell me the truth? Did it create what it thought were pillowy buffers to soften the blows that came time after time, week after week, month after month, year after year?

Sometimes the scrawled handwriting or notes swiftly typed between consultations help me place the flashbacks for which I have no door. Other times they prove to me just how scrambled they are, my recollections. My thoughts. My memories.

They're mine. So why are they not in my head, but in these notes?

And then I'm back to being angry. Angry at my mind, my memory, my body, my trauma.

Few people are given the opportunity to read these pages. But I'm not few people. I'm me. They are my notes. I need them. They tether me to my truth. Even if it's a truth I don't yet comprehend. Will I ever really understand? At night, alone, I trawl them, mine them looking for answers.

When you drop a Jewish prayer book, a Siddur, you pick it up and you kiss it. Maybe it's an apology. Or maybe reverence. Because within it is the name of g-d. When my rabbi taught me this tradition, I don't think I ever asked why. We were all too busy to ask questions. We were giggling, kissing the Siddurim, over and over, even though we had never let them fall.

I thought of this memory as I stood in the queue to get my 172 pages of notes bound in clear plastic, with a black, spiral, plastic spine. I wanted something colourful, but they didn't have anything except white, black or grey. So now it looks like something funereal. It irks me every time I pick them up. They're not about death, but hope. Hope for what?

Sometimes when the trauma overtakes my mind and my brain feels like it's floating inside my head, I need my spiral-bound, funereal notes. Notes to prove to me that it happened. That it's not an invention. That it's over. That I have lost them and I have the right to grieve, feel lost, feel sad, miss them, for a little while.

As I was getting ready to walk away from the printing desk, I panicked. I had two more sets of the notes printed. Three sets in total. Five hundred pages of someone else's recollections of my memories. Three carbon copies so I can always find them when I need them. So I always have the answers.

Well, not all of them.

||||||||||||||||||||||||||||||||||||||||||||||||||||||||||||||||||||||||||||||||||||||||||||||||||||||||||||||||||||||||||||||

10

Papa Don't Preach

There is a perceived tension between being pro-choice and mourning a pregnancy loss. This has led to a shameful lack of advocacy and support from within the feminist movement.

Back in January 2021, the ABC ran a story about a woman who miscarried on the side of the road in New South Wales while trying to make it over the border to her home in Adelaide[164] amid Covid-19 restrictions on travel. She was four weeks pregnant. I wrote a Twitter thread about the subsequent outcry, addressing a perception that the story was blaming the miscarriage on bumpy, rural roads. To me the story suggested border closures were having a terrible impact on those who needed medical care or to be with family. Either way, in the middle of the thread, someone tweeted back at me, 'Miscarriage? At 4 weeks? AKA a period. Fuck off and stop taking the piss.' Assuming the poster to be a troll looking to cause distress, I responded, 'Stop looking for reax and publicity you absolute stain.'

Several months later, I saw a friendly Tweet interaction between that user and an acquaintance. Surprised, I approached the acquaintance privately and asked how well she knew the user, who we'll call Justine. The response really surprised me. 'I think you'd like Justine because she writes a lot about feminism.' I was flabbergasted. How could someone who strongly identifies as a feminist send me that tweet?

More on that later.

The fight within

When the overwhelming grief and shock of my first miscarriage started to subside and my brain emerged from the fog of pain to resume some semblance of analytic function, I found myself battling two opposing positions in my own head. On one hand, the pain I felt was real. I had no doubt it was a baby I had lost. How could I feel this way when I was and am so militantly pro-choice? How could I feel this all-encompassing sense of loss over something I know is the size of a sesame seed? Or a blueberry? Something I would never biologically or medically classify as a baby? While I'd never had to seek an abortion myself, I would never have hesitated to, whether it was a question of need or just want. Through my twenties I had encouraged, accompanied and supported several friends through terminations. I had marched past the protesters, screaming back at them that they could shove their 'Jesus loves me' bullshit. They had no idea how to react when I declared I was Jewish and not the least bit interested in Jesus or any of his opinions.

But with the pain of my loss, there came a tension I didn't understand and didn't want to discuss with anyone. I felt like a hypocrite and a fraud. It was a painful situation and I gladly walked away from it as quickly as I could in order to focus on getting pregnant again.

When my pregnancy journey was complete, I was catching up with a friend. We sat in the garden of a cafe, eating breakfast, sipping lattes and catching up on everything we'd missed since we last spoke. In the course of the conversation, she got a little teary and said, 'There's something else.' She confided in me that she'd had an abortion, back when I was navigating my run of miscarriages. I felt a sudden surge of (unfair) rage, which I managed to (mostly) swallow. I told her as gently as I was able that her reproductive decisions had absolutely nothing to do with my reproductive challenges and that I would never ever judge her for taking control of her reproductive future or fertility. Privately, I was bitterly disappointed and heartbroken that she, or maybe my lost babies, had denied me the opportunity to support her through the decision or the procedure, given the way she had supported me unwaveringly through my challenges, with so much care and love.

As the weeks crawled by following that conversation, I was comforted by the knowledge that my beliefs in choice and abortion access hadn't changed. That conversation had reinforced in my own mind that I was still militantly pro-choice. I was still the same person, with the same fundamental belief system. And yet, I didn't know how to reconcile these two seemingly contradictory positions. Someone who mourned a pregnancy that ends at six weeks, but also would support anyone's right to have an abortion for whatever reason and at whatever gestation they want to have it. It felt like an internal battle that I needed help to resolve.

Mercifully, I found the answers I needed in the first book I purchased when I started my research to write my own book about miscarriage and failures of care. (Yes. This one.) In *Motherhood Lost: A Feminist Account of Pregnancy Loss In America*, which I have referenced in previous chapters, Linda Layne explains at length the concept and perception of fetal personhood. We addressed this in chapter six, when we were looking at why some people mourn miscarriages while some are unaffected or less affected. I came to understand that my losses were not babies in the medical sense, but more the promise of babies. A memory of things yet to come. It's a small distinction, but incredibly important in this context. Layne declares that 'in retaining a studied silence on pregnancy loss, feminists have not only abandoned their sisters in hours of need, they have contributed to the shame and isolation that attends these events, and have, de facto, surrendered the discourse of pregnancy loss to anti-choice activists'.[165]

The cultural and historical reasons that abortion and miscarriage are intertwined have resulted in real-life, contemporary consequences for patients. Examples include restrictions around what are known as the 'abortion drugs' (misoprostol and mifepristone). One or both are used in medical abortions, terminations for medical reasons and in some cases of missed miscarriage. In Australia, misoprostol is routinely prescribed in the case of missed miscarriage to prompt the bleeding to begin. However, according to medical research published in *The Lancet* in 2020, in losses pre-fourteen weeks, the combination of misoprostol and mifepristone – much more commonly used in abortion – results in better outcomes. 'Women with missed miscarriage should be offered mifepristone pre-treatment before misoprostol to increase the chance of successful miscarriage management, while reducing the need for miscarriage surgery.'[166] So why aren't both being prescribed and why aren't they available more widely? In terms of why both are not being used, I think the answer lies in delays to implementation of newly recognised best practice. But in terms of broad availability, there are other issues.

According to Marie Stopes, which runs the accreditation for GPs to prescribe the combination, as of July 2022, only 3441 GPs had the qualifications to be able to prescribe the drugs nationwide, out of an estimated 35,000 practising GPs. According to the Royal Australian College of GPs, 'it remains unclear how many are actively providing this service.'[167] And there appear to be several disincentives for GPs to provide the service of prescribing the combination, either for abortion or miscarriage.

The first is the perception that there are barriers to getting accredited. Some doctors told me it was very difficult. It's not. It's an online training module that takes between two and three hours and it's free. Though I acknowledge that given the workload GPs are working under, this might seem like just another thing that needs doing. Obstetricians and gynaecologists don't need any additional accreditation.

The second reason is that the course of treatment is time intensive with little remuneration. One GP I spoke to told me, 'Well, I do it because, yes, I want to help people', but the time required means she has to charge an $80 gap (compared to $433 or higher with Marie Stopes).

'It takes heaps of time, typically several appointments' worth, and often phone calls,' she explains. 'I know that there's a hotline, but patients tend to want to speak to me, if they run into problems. Then there's also follow-up, which I bulk bill.'

And then there's the third reason – and it's a key reason many doctors simply don't want to take it on. 'I've had hate mail to work, and threats to my kids at work,' the GP told me.

Roe vs Wade

Around the world, reverberations of fear and disgust have been felt as the US winds back abortion rights in the wake of Trump's America and the legitimisation of extremism. Perhaps if American feminists had watched the creeping attacks on patients who experience miscarriage they would have seen the rolling back of these rights coming. It was formalised in 2022 when, to the shock of the entire world, the Supreme Court repealed Roe vs Wade, the 1973 legal decision that found the US constitution conferred on all Americans the right to have an abortion.

In the past several years leading up to that crucial blow, America had seen a spate of manslaughter prosecutions of women in America – almost always women of colour – after miscarriages.[168] A bill was introduced in Ohio that would have required doctors to implant surgically removed ectopic pregnancies back in the uterus or face abortion murder charges.[169] Just to be clear: it's a medical procedure that doesn't exist in science.

In the same way that the backbone of the first wave of feminism was suffrage, the second wave of feminism was centred on abortion rights and access to contraception, because, as we know, people with uteruses can never be equal or free without reproductive control. But in the quest for abortion rights, second wave feminism has shown an inability or unwillingness to advocate within the space of pregnancy's most common complication, or indeed other aspects of reproductive freedom, such as the freedom to conceive or parent. American academic Loretta Ross writes, that '"choice" as conceived by white feminists, focused almost entirely on a woman's ability to prevent conception and motherhood'.[170]

I have personally found it incredibly frustrating that since the overturning of Roe vs Wade in America there has been such a strong media focus on the importance of D&Cs or the use of misoprostol and mifepristone in miscarriage management, given the prior absolute lack of interest or engagement on the topic.

Amanda Allen is a senior counsel at and the director of the Lawyering Project in the US, which uses the law to improve abortion access. Cari Sietstra is a co-founder and principal at Cambridge Reproductive Health Consultants, an American non-profit dedicated to improving reproductive health worldwide. They write, 'Anti-abortion policies frequently ensnare miscarriages and funnel women who lose wanted pregnancies into sub-standard treatments that can lengthen their pain and suffering.'[171]

In relation specifically to early pregnancy loss, the feminist focus on such a narrow view of reproductive freedom has left a vacuum that is, indeed, filled with the language and imagery of the pro-choice movement. Take for example Professor Leslie Reagan (no relation to Dame Regan, by the way). When she experienced a miscarriage at eleven weeks, she received a card from the hospital midwives with their sympathy and some additional medical advice. 'The stationery featured baby footprints on each page,' she writes. 'Those footprints for an eleven-week pregnancy still make my stomach turn. This material was not just helpful medical material, it was sympathy with a vested political interest. Baby footprints are one of the symbols – along with roses and foetuses in jars – of the anti-abortion movement.'[172] The loss of a baby before it's recognised medically as a baby is the domain of pro-lifers only and it's where we subliminally reach for imagery and comfort, even if it's not remotely where we sit politically, morally or ethically.

Kate Parsons writes beautifully of the tension between the feminist movement's rejection of personhood, which forms the basis of the pro-choice movement, and her own work to situate the grief of her miscarriages within her feminist and pro-choice beliefs, in a process startlingly similar to my own. Parsons argues it is not important to determine whether a fetus is a person, but why the person experiencing the loss may feel they need to categorise it as such. 'In doing so, we can interpret the pleas of the women who insisted that they had lost a baby/child not simply as a metaphysical insistence about the beings they may have lost, but perhaps, alternatively, as an insistence that their pain be recognised, socially, as a loss that is significant and worthy of grief.'[173]

She agrees with Layne that if feminists don't address this tension, we are surrendering the discourse of miscarriage to the pro-life movement. She points to a study showing that one third of pro-life activists have experienced some form of parental loss. But Parsons also issues a 'crucial cautionary note'. 'As feminists work to negotiate the following interlocking projects: on the one hand, we must be able to recognise pregnancy losses as potentially morally significant, and offer greater support to those women who are deeply affected by their miscarriages; on the other hand, we must frame our political positions so that we recognise each individual woman's right to embrace or to reject development of a fetus in her own body.'

I contacted one high-profile commentator, considered one of Australia's foremost feminist thinkers, asking to interview them for this book and outlining some of the issues Layne had raised with the feminist project and its silence around miscarriage, for fear of upsetting the abortion applecart. A reply popped into my email inbox within a few hours, but it was to decline the opportunity, saying they were far too busy. What followed was a bizarre, protracted rundown of all the reasons everything I'd inquired about should be summarily dismissed without discussion. 'I really hope that you do not take too much notice of Linda Layne. I am afraid that Americans' view of abortion – even feminist Americans, often especially feminist American women – that it is just not worth taking them seriously.' Nowhere in this one-page provocation was there even a mention of miscarriage, the actual topic of my book. Instead I found myself working through a diatribe against the rolling back of Roe vs Wade in America, a take-down of American feminism and a misreading of some questions I had posed about fertility windows. 'Sorry for the rant,' they wrote. Point, as they say, made.

The kids are all right

I don't think it would have been possible to have a better feminist role model than my mum. She is, in every sense, my hero. Born in 1950, she is a true second wave feminist. She marched in the street for abortion rights and the pill. She marched against the Vietnam war. She was one of the first women in Victoria to do a double university degree with honours. She supported my barrister dad financially by doing French tutoring when he went to the bar. She kept her maiden name when they got married, much to the consternation of, well, everyone. She marched to demand an end to the criminalisation of homosexuality. She waited until her career was established before having her first child, me, at the 'elderly primigravida' age of twenty-eight.

But when, as a teenager, I confided in her that I was having sex, her response absolutely floored me. 'You need to go on the pill,' she said. 'Okay, no problem,' I replied, 'but that won't stop me getting AIDS, a condom will.' It was the first time I saw a clear delineation between her feminism and mine, a generation gap emerging in real-time, influenced by the specificities of the period in which we came of age.

I was surprised when my mum later admonished me for telling people I was pregnant before I hit twelve weeks. She never asked me why I was telling people before twelve weeks, to which I would have responded that I felt each pregnancy should be celebrated and that if I was going to have a miscarriage there was no shame in it and I would need support. She just saw it as 'oversharing', never stopping to consider why it made her uncomfortable. Perhaps because in her day, these were things we didn't talk about. Just like periods. Or STDs. Anyone with knowledge of systems like patriarchy or racism know that they're insidious and very difficult to shake off, even when you want to.

But as I extend further into my forties, it's a grim reality that each of us will eventually become the generation at which 'OK, boomer' epithets are launched, sucking our teeth at the music young people are listening to, wondering about all the new-fangled rubbish and lamenting how things 'used to be'.

'There's a real age line around feminism,' explains Claire Pullen, who was the chair of the (successful) NSW community campaign to decriminalise abortion. She goes on to give an example. 'Leaving aside the race, class and disability pieces, which come up a lot, if there's a group of feminists my age and younger – I'm forty – a discussion around whether a trans woman is a woman just doesn't come up. But for older women who identify as feminists, that's a huge fracture.

'I do want to be appropriately respectful of how driving a problem it was, having children you didn't want to have, for that generation of feminists,' she explains. 'But you're absolutely right in identifying that there's a complete lack of nuance or sophistication about how some feminists engage around the politics of pregnancy.'

Pullen notes there is a unity to be found in these issues and we have to differentiate between people who do feminism imperfectly and the feminist project. 'There's a commonality of interest there, but the problem is that you've got people whose feminism has not developed over time, and those people have the biggest soapboxes and the biggest platforms and their understanding is essentially being preserved.'

Nowhere can the generational fractures within feminism be seen more than in the #metoo movement, during which high-profile second wave feminists, including Margaret Atwood and Germaine Greer, accused their younger counterparts of 'victimising men' and 'making it impossible to flirt'. It fuelled a new round of debate around the generational divide and gatekeeping in the movement that continues today. There also seems to be a pervasive view on some topics from older feminists of, 'Well, we dealt with it and it didn't kill us, so . . .' Or maybe, 'Your boss only pinched you on the bum, it's not a big deal, just tell him to fuck off.' In 2018, Laura Hudson, then a journalist for *Verge*, tweeted, 'I have great respect for the contributions that many older women made to the feminist movement, at times when it was harder than I have ever experienced. It is also time for them to listen, to learn, to step aside.' It created a furious backlash online and the tweet has since been deleted.

Author, academic and advocate Jackie Huggins, in her book *Sister Girl: Reflections on Tiddaism, Identity and Reconciliation*, famously called feminism in Australia the 'white women's movement'.[174] Her 1987 paper *Black Women and Women's Liberation* extrapolates on this description. 'Unfortunately, despite all the rhetoric about sisterhood and bonding, white women are not sincerely committed to bonding with Black women to fight sexism,' she writes. 'They are primarily interested in drawing attention to the oppression they consider they experience as white upper or middle class women.'[175] Not much has changed. There is, however, a growing, mainstream chorus of voices criticising a failure to include a range of experiences – people of colour, trans and non-binary people, those from lower socio-economic backgrounds, people for whom English is a second language or those with a disability, just to name a few – in the feminist project.

We know for an indisputable fact that people from all of these groups experience higher rates of miscarriage and adverse pregnancy outcomes (which I'll be addressing further in the next chapter), and also more barriers to quality healthcare more broadly. Yet even within campaigns around abortion, Australian second wave feminism rarely addresses the issues around equitable access to services for those marginalised demographics, including geography, cost or referral pathways.

The illusion of control

For me, gender equality is about choice and control, within a frame-work of equality. Choice, for instance, around whether you want to have a family or a career or both. Control, for instance, over when you have that family or that career or both. And equality between all genders within that context, so there is equal opportunity for those things to be achieved.

As the fight was waged for reproductive rights, not just abortion but also access to the pill, we have seen the emergence of what some might call a misunderstanding, if we're being generous. In truth, it's a fallacy. And that is the misnomer that we have total control over our reproduction. In the quest to control our ability not to have children, people have come to believe that you can choose when to have children. The truth is that you can decide you would like to start a family, but that doesn't mean you will be able to or that it will be a straightforward or easy path.

As women have been encouraged to seek fulfilment beyond or instead of child-rearing and housekeeping, parenting has been pushed out into later life. According to the AIHW, the average maternal age in Australia rose from twenty-seven years old in 1979 to almost thirty-one in 2019. Since 1999, the rate of women giving birth aged forty to forty-four has almost doubled, while women in the forty-five to forty-nine age group has almost quadrupled.[176]

In speaking to obstetric experts the world over, the one thing I can tell you they agree on with absolute and total consensus is that the risk of miscarriage and other adverse pregnancy outcomes rises as parents age. Especially once they go over the current threshold for what is now considered a mother of advanced age: thirty-five. But rarely do you hear discussion of the fertility window in feminist circles. In fact, it seems to be somewhat taboo, interpreted as the suggestion that we should return to the dark ages when women were expected (and in some cases forced) to take off their shoes, get back in the kitchen and get on with the baby-making. There is consistent messaging, sometimes direct and sometimes subliminal, that you can choose to have a baby whenever you want and age is just a number. Celebrities give countless interviews on the front pages of magazines and newspapers about giving birth in their forties.[177] Others claim that if you just eat right and exercise, you too can naturally conceive and have your first child at forty-five,[178] which is just statistically extraordinarily unlikely. If you can, you're the exception and far from the rule. Actor and TV presenter Sonia Kruger was justifiably applauded far and wide when she acknowledged openly that she had used a donor egg to conceive a baby at almost fifty.[179]

There's also the option of egg freezing or IVF, consistently presented as get-out-of-jail-free cards. Have your cake (career) and eat it too (babies)! In America, Apple and Facebook are footing bills of up to US$20,000 for female employees to freeze their eggs, as they devote their prime childbearing years to building their careers. The idea may now be taking off in Australia. In 2021, *Guardian Australia* ran a story headlined, '"Very pragmatic": 42 per cent of Australian women are open to egg freezing as a work perk'.[180] It's what I would describe as a 'long read' at thirty-seven paragraphs. But it's not until the third-last paragraph that we get a dose of reality, where the journalist finally points out that UK statistics show a 'birth success rate of around 18 per cent for women using their own eggs'. Additionally noting, 'According to IVF Australia, egg freezing is "unlikely to lead to a pregnancy" in women older than thirty-eight. "Because you have frozen eggs does not mean that they will lead to pregnancy or the number of children that you desire."'[181]

When I speak to younger friends about their intentions (or not) to have children – a common topic they raise with me when they are around my own children – often a response I hear is, 'Oh I'm not even thinking about it, but if I have any issues, I'll just have IVF.' Success rates in IVF are improving, but are still extremely confronting. Best case IVF success rates in patients under thirty-four years old are around 30 per cent. Nowhere near a done deal. Rates of success decline each year after that, before hitting five per cent when the patient is forty-three or older. IVF is also not a guarantee against miscarriage.

No one is saying people who don't feel ready to have children (whether for lifestyle, financial or other reasons) should rush into baby-making; I certainly don't want to see women back in the kitchen, barefoot and pregnant at seventeen, unless of course that's what they choose. But presenting egg freezing or IVF as fail-safe insurance policies is misleading.

During my own journey to parenthood, uncovering these facts, I have more than once felt betrayed by the feminist movement. I did everything I was supposed to do: forged a career, cracked the glass ceiling, created my own financial independence, feathered my superannuation nest egg, travelled the world. None of that helped me when I was on miscarriage number seven at the age of thirty-nine, running out of time, looking at statistics, wondering whether to spend $15,000 on IVF with a slim likelihood of success, staring down a future with a family that isn't complete for me and wondering why in the fuck no one told me how sharply my risk profile rose with each passing birthday dinner. A 2022 study showed female surgeons have a 'significantly greater' incidence of miscarriage, infertility and pregnancy compilations. This is in part due to the stress of their jobs, but also because many delay having children. Quite astoundingly, of the 4533 female physicians who completed the survey, only 8 per cent were aware of the risks of delaying pregnancy. The study concluded that 'the culture of medicine and surgery must continue to evolve to better support women with family planning during their training and careers'.[182]

Parents are also having children later because the costs of raising a child have ballooned. Everyday bills like rent and food are sky high and have totally outpaced wage growth, let alone social security payments for those unable to work. At the time of writing, Australia's unemployment benefits are some of the lowest rates in the OECD.[183]

Perhaps if we focused on equality in the home, both in terms of labour and income, wage parity, driving down the cost of childcare or indeed making it free, better social security payments that reflect a living wage and other supportive measures, parents and families wouldn't have to wait quite so long to start their families, miscarriage rates would go down and fewer families would need help from unreliable and incredibly costly artificial reproductive technologies. Just a thought.

That which shall not be named

If there is silence around miscarriage, termination for medical reasons (TFMR) exists in an underground, lead-lined room with sound-absorbing foam. Such is the taboo around TFMR that it is usually carved out into separate support groups, because some of the participants in miscarriage support groups find it too traumatic a topic.

TFMR is when a parent chooses to have a termination, rather than progress with a pregnancy, because it is likely the baby will die before or soon after birth or be born with significant disability, affecting their quality of life. These issues can be identified by ultrasound, NIPT, amniocentesis (testing amniotic fluid) or chorionic villus sampling or CVS (testing placental cells).

There's something otherworldly and profoundly antithetical about voluntarily ending a pregnancy when it's a baby you want. We're consistently taught that abortion is empowering and gives us choice. So it's a strange juxtaposition to be faced with a decision that feels less like empowered choice and more like the best of a raft of truly shitty options.

'There is a deafening silence,' agrees Red Nose CEO Keren Ludski. 'Families coming to see us because of TFMR make up a significant percentage of the families seeking support.' She says the reason for this is because there's so much guilt and shame. 'People feel the need to justify their decision-making and I don't think it's about justifying it to others, I think it's justifying it to self.'

In my experience, TFMR was my option when there were no other reasonable options. I didn't want to bring a baby into the world if there was a risk that baby would have a significantly reduced quality of life.

In the UK a survey of 1300 people who opted for TFMR found that almost three quarters didn't feel they would get the same compassion as stillbirth or miscarriage. After their terminations, 87 per cent felt guilty and 80 per cent felt isolated.[184]

There are so many questions. Have I made the right decision? Have I made the wrong decision? What if the tests are wrong? What if the scans are wrong? Does this mean I don't love my baby? Does this make me a terrible parent?

Some parents choose not to screen for genetic abnormality. Some parents do the screening and decide to proceed with the pregnancy anyway. Some parents choose to end pregnancies in which there are chromosomal abnormalities. All of these decisions are intensely personal and all are correct; there is no wrong answer. But there's no question that these are decisions that exist in a strange twilight zone of choice, duty, obligation, blame and personal ethical frameworks. Some feel it is a moral obligation to bring that child into the world. Others feel it is a moral obligation not to.

It is incredibly frustrating that thousands of patients across Australia are offered NIPT testing (something the government should be funding for all patients), but when those results are not what we hope, we are not supported to discuss it. We are judged for the decisions we make. I resent that feminist pro-choice movements rarely represent TFMR in their advocacy. It adds to the grief, isolation and shame for dealing with a situation in which, truly, no one is a winner. People increasingly feel comfortable acknowledging abortion, whether with close friends or family or more broadly. Activists in the space loudly proclaim it a lifesaver. But you don't hear many activists giving interviews about how a TFMR saved their baby from stillbirth or a lifetime of pain. Or marching with a placard in the street, for that matter. Ultimately, parents deserve choice, and that choice is theirs alone to make. If you are pro-choice it applies in all circumstances. Not just the ones in which you are comfortable.

I have cared for the most beautiful babies and children born with chromosomal issues. I know many families who cherish those children. While I am grateful in some respects that the decision to proceed with a TMFR was made for me by virtue of the fact that my baby was not compatible with life, these are not situations that are cut and dry, black or white. Risk has to be quantified and evaluated. And that in itself is an incredibly painful process for any parent. Whatever decision they make is the right decision.

Better together

The more I explored the topics of feminism and miscarriage, the more my mind wandered back to my interaction with the 'internet troll' Justine, who I talked about at the start of this chapter.

After many weeks of rolling the exchange around in my mind, I decided I had to approach Justine and I sent her a message that went exactly like this:

> *Hi Justine, I am writing a book about miscarriage and I've thought a lot about this tweet that you sent me back earlier last year. One of the chapters I'm writing about is feminism and miscarriage. I note that you write about feminism and you identify as a feminist and for this reason, I'm really interested as to why you would have written this tweet to a woman who has experienced seven miscarriages. I'm not looking to cancel you, or have a fight with you, I'm hoping to have a genuine discussion about where this came from. There are some academics who argue that there is a perceived tension with being pro-choice and mourning early pregnancy losses. I'm wondering if this might be a factor? We have a lot of mutual followers, and, I suspect, friends. I hope you can spare some time to speak with me. Isy*

Justine agreed to speak with me and, over Zoom, we had a long and wide-ranging discussion. It turned out that Justine is ten years older than me and at fifty-one she has two children, the first she had at twenty-seven and the second she had at thirty-seven. She sees herself as nestled between the second and third waves of feminism.

'I don't actually understand how you can know you're pregnant until you've had a period after four weeks,' Justine said. I explained that a blastocyst can implant up to a week before your period is due and once it implants, high sensitivity pregnancy tests or a blood test can pick up early levels of hCG. This happens regularly if someone is actively trying to get pregnant, has experienced previous losses or is doing IVF and is testing very early and very regularly. Ultimately it is absolutely possible to know you're pregnant at four weeks.

'I was wrong. And I didn't even know that before you hit twenty-eight days and had a missed period it was possible to even tell you had a pregnancy. So that was an uninformed comment by me,' Justine apologised. 'I've noticed this a few times where I have been picked up or called out about things and I realise how limited I am, and possibly all of us are, by our own experience and by the absence of certain experiences. So yeah, I made an uninformed and ignorant comment, essentially.'

She also acknowledged without hesitation that she had read the tweet through a pro-choice lens and, while reading back she could see it wasn't an abortion issue, she doesn't doubt that her reading affected her reaction. 'There is a systemic and structural fear that if we give an inch, then that's grounds for us to be wound back a mile.'

Despite owing me nothing, she was quick to apologise to me and we will definitely stay in touch. 'I've got a 24-year-old daughter and part of handing on the baton is being humbled by ideas that are different to yours. I'm so glad we've talked.' I was glad too.

I am grateful for the work and the labour that my mother and previous generations of feminists expended and the gains they reaped that benefited all of us. But there is more work to do to extend these gains, especially among people of colour, people in lower socio-economic groups and those who are gender diverse. The baton must be passed, not just ceremonially or in spirit, but in practical, visible, tangible ways. And conversations must take place beyond the sphere of toxic social media, where there is no nuance, and tone and intention get lost along the way.

Seven Wonders

'Hey Isy, it's Dr Lovely.'
    'Oh hiya! How are you?'
    'Hey, where are you?'
    'I'm just at my desk at work.'
    'Can you go somewhere private?'
    'Why? What is it?'
    'Please can you go somewhere private?'
    'Just tell me. It's okay. I can take it.'
    'Can you at least sit down? Are you sitting down?'
    'Fucking hell, you're scaring me. Tell me what's going on.'

||||||

I was serving brunch. I can't for the life of me remember what we ate. I remember Sam brought pastries. Delicious pastries. But I don't remember if they were sweet or savoury or what else we had on the table. Her husband Connor was pacing the pavement outside, on an urgent work call. We were all still getting to know each other, but we had lots in common. Each couple had one child, both sons, and they were more or less similar ages; we were all interested in writing and current affairs. Sam and I had bonded over motherhood, the joys of being on the peripheries of the Jewish community rather than knee-deep in the borscht belt and how many wines it took to decompress after long days of parenting.

Over brunch we were telling our birthing stories. We compared notes on our obstetricians. I sang the praises of Dr Lovely. And Sam revealed she had given birth with the Cervical Celebrity. Husbo asked who the Cervical Celebrity was. I explained that he was one of the most sought after obstetricians in Melbourne. 'Why didn't we see him then?' queried husbo.

    'He's super expensive!' I laughed.

Later, after they'd gone and I was loading the dishwasher, I couldn't get that conversation out of my mind. I started to wonder. How much was this baby worth to me? Why hadn't I gone to see the Cervical Celebrity if he was so amazing? I didn't want to break up with Dr Lovely, I absolutely adored her. But I needed to make a decision about whether we were going to keep trying to conceive or move to IVF, and I wondered if a fresh set of eyes would be just what the doctor ordered. So I got a referral and off I went across town to see the Cervical Celebrity. I was still bleeding from the most recent loss when I walked into his office. And we all know how that appointment went.

While empathy clearly wasn't his strong point, he was an excellent, experienced medical physician, and he did something I'll be grateful for, for the rest of my days. He refused, point blank, to refer me for IVF.

He told me IVF was for people who can't conceive and conception definitely wasn't part of my problem. He told me that the outcome with IVF was not guaranteed to be any different, apart from the high cost and trauma of the procedures. So I made a decision. We would keep trying naturally until I turned forty and then we would move to IVF.

In August 2018, at the ripe old age of thirty-eight, I found out I was pregnant for the seventh time. I had notched up six miscarriages and one living child. I knew I was pregnant as soon as the blastocyst attached itself to the wall of my uterus. I had been under the care of the Cervical Celebrity after seeking his second opinion, so I called his office. The receptionist organised a referral for a blood test, even though they said based on my ovulation dates I couldn't possibly know I was pregnant. The good doctor called me himself to tell me, seemingly awed. 'Your hCG is only thirteen. How did you know?'

'I always know.'

Once the pregnancy was confirmed, I transferred back to my Dr Lovely. The pregnancy was as gruelling as the others, but each time the anxiety rose a notch. Wake up. Check for blood. Go to the toilet. Check the toilet paper for blood. Go to work. Go to the toilet every hour, on the hour, to check for blood. Each night before I went to sleep, I whispered a prayer to my body: please, please don't bleed. And for the first time in my septet of pregnancies, it didn't. Maybe this was it. The little girl I so desperately wanted. My daughter.

'Hey y'all! Just a question for all the pezzas who've experienced multiple miscarriage, when do you tell people you're pregnant? Twelve weeks? Twenty weeks?' My post went up in my favourite Facebook support group.

'None of us know if or when each pregnancy is going to end,' came a reply. 'Enjoy each one for as long as you can. Tell people when you want to. There are no rules.' So that's what I did. I told everyone I was pregnant. The guy at the market who sold me an egg and bacon roll. The woman who checked out my shopping at the supermarket. Everyone at work. All my besties. And each day I pleaded with my body, 'Please don't let me down, please don't bleed.'

To celebrate my pregnancy getting to twelve weeks without bleeding, Mum and I booked a weekend away. Daylesford! We would shop for Art Deco things we didn't need, eat dinner and just have some time for the two of us. Mum and daughter time. Something all mums of daughters need, right?

||||||

'It's the NIPT test. It's come back as high risk of T21,' said Dr Lovely.

'That's Down syndrome.'

'Yes.'

'How often are the tests wrong?'

'I've never had one that's wrong. They're 99 per cent accurate.'

'How quickly can you fix it?'

||||||

I walked back into my office. My two closest friends at work had seen me run out into the foyer on the phone. They knew it wasn't good. I walked into our meeting room and closed the door after they walked in.

'Downs,' I whispered.

'Oh no, Isy,' said Bron and her eyes filled with tears. Peter visibly paled, not sure what to say.

And then, just for a split second, I stopped thinking about how to manage the situation. My brain flicked the auto-pilot switch off for just long enough to think beyond the pregnancy I was in.

'Oh fuck. I'm going to have to start again,' I spat out. 'Oh fuck. Oh fuck. Oh fuck. Oh fuck.' I couldn't stop saying fuck. It was like whatever needle was playing my internal monologue got stuck and there I was. Repeating it. Over and over.

The beginning. Ovulation. Conception. Making it through to twelve weeks. The whole gruelling slog. But this chapter wasn't over yet. Not even close.

Then I had another thought. I was supposed to be going away with Mum to Daylesford. To celebrate this baby. We were due to leave that day after work.

||||||

I dialled the number. She didn't pick up. I dialled again. She didn't pick up. I dialled again. Finally my friend Kristen answered.

'Hey, I'm at work. Three calls, are you okay?'

'No, I'm not okay, I need to talk to you right now.'

'Okay, hang on, I'm walking outside.'

I told her everything. The likely diagnosis. The likely outcome. Expected next steps. Kristen was mostly silent. And then came the reason I called her.

'So, I have something to ask you.'

'Yes, anything.'

'Do I go to Daylesford this afternoon? Is that weird? To go away for the weekend right now? What is the right thing to do? Can you just please tell me what to do?'

||||||

I thought I was an expert on pregnancy. I used to joke that I knew more about pregnancy than any obstetrician I'd ever met and my obstetrician would laugh and agree with me. But just when you think you know it all, the universe sends you an Earth-shattering lesson to teach you that you know absolutely nothing about, well, anything.

Despite an NIPT having an accuracy of over 99 per cent, it's still not what you'd call 'diagnostic'. Which means you have to have more tests to confirm a T21 diagnosis. The most common of these is a CVS, which is very large needle inserted into your belly to extract some placental cells. But it was too early to do the test. So . . . eleven days. Eleven days I would have to wait.

In the meantime, husbo and I talked. We talked about Down syndrome. We talked about what we wanted. I'd cared for children with Down syndrome. I knew it was a spectrum in the sense that there are people with T21 who can live independently and hold down jobs. There are also some who are so severely disabled that they need constant support and care. I knew they were often born with heart issues. I knew 60 per cent of Downs pregnancies end in miscarriage. I read every word I could get my hands on. And I waited.

||||||

I remember every meal we had in Daylesford, and how there wasn't a single one where I didn't cry. I sobbed during breakfast, lunch and dinner. I cried myself to sleep at night. I had to nap each afternoon because I was so utterly drained. Mum rubbed my back as I sobbed. Wait staff avoided our table. Could I drink wine? I was still pregnant after all. We shopped for distraction. We bought presents for everyone back in Melbourne. I convinced Mum to buy a huge Art Deco liquor cabinet. I bought husbo some cute socks. I bought some vintage tin toys for the Didgerijew.

It was a blessing to be away from my son and be able to mourn wholly and fully. And even though I didn't think it was possible, it brought my mum and I closer together.

||||||

'I don't think you need to have a CVS,' the obstetrician/ultrasonologist said gently as he did the scan.

'What? Why?'

Eleven days were up.

'See that fluid around the baby's body? That's called hydrops. It's a build-up of fluid. It means the organs aren't working properly. Your baby's nuchal fold is 9 millimetres. That's one of the biggest I've seen. This pregnancy is not going to result in a live birth. The CVS would really only be for your peace of mind.'

The scan over, I pulled down my top and he gestured to his desk in the corner.

'Would you like your ultrasound pictures?'

'Yes, please. Thank you.'

He passed them across. It was obvious he wanted to ask me a question, but he was hesitating. After a pregnant pause, the words finally left his mouth.

'Would you like to know the gender? You don't have to.'

Unlike him, I didn't hesitate. Maybe I should have. Either way the journalist in me won that battle and I blurted, 'Yes.'

'It's a girl.'

||||||

'Hey I need to have an abortion. Can you please come with me?'

'Of course I will. You don't want Jack to go with you?'

'He can't. He has something on and I don't want him to miss it. Roy will go and stay with my mum and dad for a few hours.'

'What time do I need to be at your place?'

||||||

A private Facebook message dropped in with a ping. It was the admin from my favourite support group.

'Sorry, you're going to have to delete that post.'

'What, why? How come?'

'We don't allow any discussion of termination for medical reasons in the miscarriage support group. There are groups specifically for TFMR support, if you do a Facebook search.'

'Oh, okay, why is that?'

'Because in the miscarriage support groups, there are women who are hurt that you would choose to abort your baby when they can't have one.'

Choose. What an interesting word to use.

||||||

'I can't do it here. This is a Catholic hospital. I'll do it tomorrow at the other hospital. If I can find an anaesthetist. Hang on.'

I was sitting in Dr Lovely's office on a Friday afternoon. She had rushed in to meet me in her gym gear. And now she was calling every anaesthetist she knew, asking them to help her terminate my pregnancy tomorrow. A Saturday.

She gave me the name and details of the hospital where the procedure would take place. She also gave me some tablets to take on the morning of the procedure. She explained it all very clearly but I didn't take in a word she said. It was like she was talking to me from under water. She wrote down the time I needed to take the pills on a piece of paper, so I wouldn't forget.

'Can I ask you a question?' I asked her once everything was set.

'Of course, anything.'

'Are you rushing to do this termination because this pregnancy is risky?'

Dr Lovely had two young children. Saturday was her day off. It was bad enough working in obstetrics and not knowing what time of the day or night you'd be summoned for a delivery or a complication.

'No. There's no medical reason. I just want this to be over for you as soon as it can be.'

||||||

I sat in the waiting room. The pain was coming in waves now.

'It almost feels like contractions,' I whispered to the nurse.

'The pills you took,' she said quietly, her voice full of sympathy. 'They soften your cervix for the procedure. You are having contractions. Wait a second and I'll get you a heat pack.'

||||||

The surgical nurse wasn't in any way rude, but she was harried, stressed and to the point.

Name?

DOB?

Reason you're here today?

'Well, I'm having an abortion because my baby has severe Down syndrome and isn't compatible with life.'

She jerked as though a small surge of electricity had shot through her body and looked up from her clipboard.

'I . . . I am so, so sorry.' As she said it she placed her hand on my foot, which was under a white waffle hospital blanket, and she squeezed it gently.

'That's okay. I don't blame you.' And I tried to smile.

But instead I started to cry. I looked up at my friend who had accompanied me and tears were coursing rapidly down her own cheeks. It was bad enough I had asked her to give up her Saturday to come with me. She didn't need this.

So I balled my hands into fists, took a deep breath and I just . . . stopped.

||||||

I am wheeled into theatre. Dr Lovely is there. The anaesthetist is too. I grab his wrist and I look him in the eye and thank him for coming in on a Saturday at late notice. He smiles kindly. I look past him at Dr Lovely.

'Why are you wearing that stupid hat?'

'Excuse me, this is my favourite scrub hat.' Dr Lovely, wearing a ridiculously stupid rainbow unicorn scrub hat, laughs.

'I don't like it. I'm going to get you a new one.'

Everything goes black.

What feels like seconds later, I wake up.

My friend is standing next to me with her hand on my shoulder.

Dr Lovely is at the foot of the bed.

'It's over?'

'It's over.'

||||||||||||||||||||||||||||||||||||||||||||||||||||||||||||||||||||||||||||||||||||||||||||||||||||||||||||

11

Who Are You?

Identity – and its varying facets – can and does dictate the way you are treated by the medical system and the care you receive.

In the summer of 1994, a group of Americans calling themselves Women of African Descent for Reproductive Justice ran a full-page ad in the *Washington Post*. It had over 800 signatures from Black activists, scholars and thinkers. It launched a movement and concept called Reproductive Justice, a combination of the terms 'reproductive rights' and 'social justice'. The ad was created to respond to the Clinton administration's proposed Universal Health Care Plan. It stated in no uncertain terms that the group would not approve a plan that didn't enable free and equal access to abortion services. However, it went further. It also said universal healthcare coverage must cover all people, irrespective of income, health or employment status, age, location and affordability, without deductibles and co-payments. 'All people must be covered equally,' it read. And then it went further.

The package should cover when people didn't want to have babies (abortions and contraception), but it should also allow everyone equal access to medical technologies to have a child. And be able to safely provide for and parent that child.

In other words, true control over fertility for all patients, whether they wanted or didn't want children. This included all relevant healthcare services, including diagnostics, treatments, preventative options, long-term care, mental health services, prescription drugs and pre-existing conditions. 'All reproductive healthcare services must be covered and treated the same as other healthcare services,' the ad read. 'This includes pap tests, mammograms, contraceptive methods, prenatal care, delivery, abortion, sterilisation, infertility services, STDs and HIV/AIDS screening and treatment.' And then, you guessed it, it went further. They also called for discrimination protection for all women of colour, the elderly, the poor, people of any sexual orientation and those with disabilities.

Three years later, sixteen organisations came together in America to form the SisterSong Women of Color Reproductive Justice Collective. SisterSong sought Reproductive Justice, centring people of colour, including Black, Indigenous, Pacific Islander, Asian, Arab, Middle Eastern and Latinx women, queer women and trans people. Within those groups, the organisation further centred those with low incomes, young mothers, those who have been criminalised, sex workers, people with disabilities and those living with HIV/AIDS, recognising the inherent role of intersectional layers of disadvantage in caregiving.

This movement pushed far beyond white-driven, second wave feminism's wholesale focus on abortion. It included abortion, as of course it should, but progressed into a new space, with a vision of everyone having total control over their fertility; the right not to have a child, the right to have a child and the right to parent children in a safe and healthy environment.[185]

I'm going to pause for moment and ask the question: why would you centre marginalised groups in a movement like this? Why would you not make it universal? Good question.

Layers of injustice

Leading American critical race theory scholar and civil rights activist Professor Kimberlé Crenshaw defined the concept of intersectionality through a framework that reveals the compounding disadvantage experienced by Black American women. In her seminal essay 'Demarginalizing the Intersection of Race and Sex: A Black Feminist Critique of Antidiscrimination Doctrine, Feminist Theory and Antiracist Politics',[186] Crenshaw described how 'dominant conceptions of discrimination condition us to think about subordination as disadvantage occurring along a single categorical axis'. She explained that 'this focus on the most privileged group members marginalizes those who are multiply-burdened and obscures claims that cannot be understood as resulting from discrete sources of discrimination.' This results, she notes, in the marginalisation of Black women in feminist theory and anti-racial politics, and this can be said for many other groups of marginalised people.

Professor Bronwyn Fredericks, Professor Odette Best and Dr Mick Adams also describe this gap in their book *Yatdjuligin: Aboriginal and Torres Strait Islander Nursing and Midwifery Care*, 'In the same way, when the women's health movement speaks in broad terms about women's health, it tends to minimise the urgency of addressing the health status of Australia's Indigenous women. A focus on the health discrepancies between Aboriginal and Torres Strait Islander women and other Australian women could lead to concrete change.'

They point out no one should be coerced into trying to unravel intersecting facets of their identity. 'Aboriginal and Torres Strait Islander men and women should not feel as though they have to make a choice between gender issues and Indigeneity when they are trying to gain access to services. They should not be asked to separate their gender from their culture. At the same time, they should never feel that they cannot have culture without gender (whether they opt for manhood, womanhood or some other kind of personhood).'[187]

Let's consider for a minute the metaphor of triage. When we walk into an emergency room, it's not about who walks in the door first, it's about who has the greatest need. In terms of medical care, medical attention and patient-centred approaches, white, middle to upper class, cis women do not have the greatest need. So it makes absolute sense that while we're all in the queue, the people most in need have to be placed at the front. Then change will trickle upwards, because we sure as hell know it ain't trickling downwards to the people consistently at the bottom of the list.

The Inverse Care Law was coined by Julian Tudor Hart in *The Lancet* in 1971 to describe how 'the availability of good medical care tends to vary inversely with the need of the population serviced'.[188] Simply put, the people who need medical care the most (those on low incomes, those doing high-risk, physical work, non-English speakers unable to navigate complex medical systems and so on) are the least likely to get it. A *Lancet* editorial in 2021 celebrating the fiftieth anniversary of the law's publishing depressingly noted that it is as relevant today as it was when it was written.[189]

Choice is great in theory, but just because services exist doesn't mean access is equal. And if access isn't equal, the idea of choice is a fallacy. In Australia, we can see this demonstrated by the number of people who can't access IVF, or multiple rounds of it, because it's far too costly. And we can also see it in the geographic and cost barriers to abortion.

One of the founders of the Reproductive Justice movement, Loretta Ross writes, 'Clearly many women lack the cash to pay for these choices, including motherhood, and thus face what might be called choiceless choices.'[190]

These conversations have been going on in Australia among Indigenous academics and activists for decades. In her groundbreaking text *Talkin' Up to the White Woman: Indigenous Women and Feminism*, Distinguished Professor Aileen Moreton-Robinson writes, 'For Indigenous women all white feminists benefit from colonisation; they are overwhelmingly represented and disproportionately predominant, have the key roles, and constitute the norm, the ordinary and the standard of womanhood in Australia.' She adds, 'White women are not represented to themselves as being white; instead they position themselves as variously classed, sexualised, aged and abled.'

I'm an educated white cis woman, with private health insurance. No number of traumatic miscarriages or pregnancy losses change that, or the fact that I view healthcare and my treatment through a privileged lens. But there are experts in this field writing with staggering insight, knowledge and understanding about inequities of healthcare access. Scholars and academics doing integral work, none more so than those doctors who are themselves part of marginalised demographics. So where am I going with this? It's a book about miscarriage, right? Not equity of healthcare access. But any book on the topic of medical care needs to address inequality, because the two are inextricably linked.

It is incontrovertible that worldwide, people of colour, those with lower levels of education and those from lower incomes are more likely to experience adverse pregnancy outcomes, including miscarriage. One American study showed Black women are twice as likely as white women to miscarry after ten weeks of pregnancy,[191] while a Danish study showed patients who had lower levels of education, were from lower socio-economic groups or were on disability pensions experienced elevated levels of miscarriage.[192]

Queer writer and activist Miriam Zoila Pérez quotes queer immigrant writer and activist Verónica Bayetti Flores explaining how a Reproductive Justice framework must take into account, 'whether a gender non-conforming person can feel safe from the threat of discrimination or violence while accessing such gendered care; whether a person has a clinic nearby or whether they have to travel a significant distance; whether there's an immigration checkpoint along the way; what access to transportation looks like; the economic impact for a person who does not have paid sick leave of taking several days off due to long-distance travel and waiting periods; whether the clinic is wheelchair accessible, and on and on.'[193]

A study in preconception behaviour among low-income, minority women in America found that just 12 per cent of the women planning to get pregnant were taking a multivitamin or folic acid.[194] How can you afford it when you earn less than $20,000 a year? They were also practising 'negative but modifiable behaviours' like drinking and smoking. The study's authors called for better education for those in low-income groups who are of childbearing age or planning to get pregnant.

One study that investigated how patients experiencing miscarriage are treated in American emergency rooms found that Asian, Native American, Native Hawaiian, Native Alaskan and mixed race, uninsured and Medicaid-insured patients were more likely to be admitted than white and privately insured patients. This might sound good, but again, this is about paternalism and control. We can see that by the second suite of data: this same cohort is more likely to have surgery instead of non-surgical treatment for ectopic pregnancy. Surgical sterilisation is used in 20 per cent of sexually active Black and Latinx patients who want contraception, compared to 16 per cent in white patients. All groups of non-white, Medicaid-insured or uninsured patients are far less likely to receive pain medication compared to white and privately insured patients.[195]

Research in Australia has also found that there is a geographic inequity of healthcare service provision for miscarriage patients.[196] And while we will be examining the Aboriginal experience of miscarriage in finer detail in the next chapter, it is worth noting here that in Australia, Aboriginal and Torres Strait Islander peoples face the worst health outcomes of any marginalised group. They are more likely to experience chronic disease and die young. In 2018 the overall death rate for Aboriginal people was almost twice the rate for non-Aboriginal Australians. They are also the most incarcerated people in the world and they are 16.5 times more likely than white Australians to die in custody.[197]

'The routine reporting of persisting racialised health inequalities doesn't appear to have inspired a race-critical research agenda; instead, the statistical story of Indigenous health inequality has become a routine of health discourse in Australia,' write Professor Chelsea Watego, Dr David Singh and Dr Alissa Macoun.[198]

In 2015, of those under sixty-five living with a disability in Australia, 38 per cent had difficulty accessing medical facilities,

13 per cent who needed help with healthcare activities had no source of assistance, 19 per cent didn't see a GP because of the cost, 27 per cent didn't see a specialist because of the cost and 30 per cent waited longer than they thought reasonable to see a medical specialist.[199]

Those within the gender-diverse community are more likely to have psychological co-morbidities like depression, anxiety, PTSD, personality disorder and psychosis. They are also more likely to be on the autism spectrum and experience eating disorders.[200] Despite the risk of pregnancy reigniting feelings of body dysmorphia, more trans and non-binary people are (wonderfully) choosing to have babies. 'For those who do not identify as the gender they were assigned at birth, who do not ascribe to the gender binary or who have body dysmorphia as it relates to their identity and/or sexuality, this feeling of bodily betrayal is often compounded,' writes American psychologist Jessica Zucker. 'From being misgendered by medical professionals to the physical signs and symptoms of pregnancy warring with their gender identity, the body becomes something of a minefield.'[201]

'Some trans men, trans women and people who self-define as trans-non-binary encounter Reproductive Justice issues that the larger society generally does not acknowledge, does not understand or rejects,' writes Ross.[202] Unsurprisingly, Australian research shows that trans parents are having extremely similar emotional reactions and devastation when faced with early pregnancy loss, but they're not being offered tailored support services, which recognise their need for safe spaces, both for the patient and their partner (where there is one).[203]

Speaking the same language

In 2021 American Professor Jill Wieber Lens – a leading expert on legal recognition and treatment of stillbirth and miscarriage – wrote a paper for the *Washington Law Review*, addressing how Reproductive Justice could apply to pregnancy loss specifically and how it could improve care within that context. The paper is wide-ranging and fascinating, unpacking several aspects of the movement, for instance the rejection of the individualistic notion of choice, based on the intersecting and complex nature of experience. But she notes that the movement has the potential to highlight the related rights around loss.

'Those rights include a woman's right to prenatal care that will help prevent the undesired end to her pregnancy,' she writes. 'She has birth justice rights to give birth to her stillborn child as she desires and to be fully informed of her treatment options in case of miscarriage. She also has a right to culturally appropriate mental and emotional health treatment after miscarriage or stillbirth.'

She concludes, 'Expressly adding these rights to the Reproductive Justice framework properly recognises miscarriage and stillbirth as meaningful reproductive experiences that marginalised women are especially likely to experience.'[204]

While it couldn't be argued that the movement has taken meaningful root in practice in America, which continues to experience high levels of structural racism and discrimination in its medical systems, the fact that we're not even beginning to have these broader discussions (beyond abortion) in Australia should be of deep concern.

In addition to nosebleeds and masks, the Covid-19 pandemic also gave us something else: a stark case study into inequality in healthcare. Australian Bureau of Statistics (ABS) data as at the first half of 2022 showed that where data on country of birth could be obtained, 907 people who died from or with Covid-19 were born in Australia, compared to 1640 born overseas.[205] People were also more likely to die if they were from disadvantaged socio-economic groups; the figure was over three times higher in those from the most disadvantaged socio-economic groups.[206]

My friend Dr Mariam Tokhi is a GP in Melbourne at Utopia Refugee and Asylum Seeker Health. She has seen and helped her patients navigate barriers to healthcare for years. She explained the layers of difficulty faced by people who are newly arrived in Australia and for those who don't speak English or have lower levels of proficiency.

'Often people who don't speak English, or new immigrants, face a completely new healthcare system that often works quite differently to wherever they're from, and that's very varied,' she explains. 'And then the question is, what sort of reception do they get when they turn up?

'The fact of the matter is that Australian general practice is currently predominantly set up to cater to a wealthy, middle class population who can advocate for their needs and communicate those needs quickly. Because the current Medicare Benefits Schedule model incentivises and remunerates practitioners to work fast; you earn the most if you see a patient in under six minutes.'

Treatment for pregnancy loss can be complicated, delicate and requires discussion of both physical and psychological care. That can be incredibly challenging when the practitioner and the patient can't speak the same language.

'For someone who doesn't speak English, they're going to need longer consultations and, ideally, we should be seeing patients with interpreters. From my own experience working in mainstream general practice, it's really hard to find someone to come into your clinic.'

There are other barriers that make providing culturally safe care difficult. 'There was some research that was done in the northern suburbs where I worked with the Assyrian community that I got to review and it addressed the language barrier. But also patients were asking, "Why doesn't the doctor look at me?", because the doctor was looking at the computer screen the entire time. We're trying to multitask all the time and, honestly, I think we now know that multitasking isn't effective in any sphere of life.'

Dr Tokhi also points out that without the time to listen to patients – really listen – it's difficult to have empathy or understanding of their personal circumstance. 'Yesterday I saw a patient and it took me an hour. It was someone in early pregnancy who was having a lot of issues around hyperemesis (severe morning sickness). There was a medical component to it, but she happened, very luckily, to be accompanied by a friend who pulled me aside and said they didn't think she was telling me the whole story and filled me in on her history of intimate partner violence and family violence in the background that was exacerbating all of the stuff around the nausea and vomiting.'

She summarises, 'If we don't understand the context in which a patient is living and what their life history is, we don't know, and we can't treat and engage with our patients effectively, and the fact is that medical doctors still tend to come from a reasonably privileged part of society.'

Background and context are hugely relevant factors in determining the care a patient receives. There are many demographics for whom taking the first step to seek care can be a huge challenge. One example is the disability community, which has historically faced appalling eugenics-driven population control measures in this country. But did you know it's still happening? As recently as 2012, Australia's Human Rights Commission said action was needed to stop coerced or forced sterilisation of people with a disability.[207] Often, this is enacted after miscarriage (or pregnancy), when it is apparent that the individual is sexually active.

Reproductive Justice addresses the rights of all to have and parent a child, or not. For the disability community and other marginalised groups, this includes the right to have all available investigations should miscarriage occur, or access all relevant fertility treatments should they be required. In a 2016 position paper on sexual and reproductive rights, Women With Disabilities Australia (WWDA) called on the federal government 'in consultation with people with disability and their representative organisations, to develop a national strategy to improve access to, and implementation of comprehensive, equitable, accessible, and disability-inclusive sexual and reproductive health education and information, with a particular focus on improving the access to such information for women and girls with disability, regardless of the setting in which they work, live or study.'

While much of this chapter has explained the origins of the Reproductive Justice movement as it was developed in America, Aboriginal and Torres Strait Islander academics and activists, especially women, have been fighting for the same rights since colonisation.

In the colony known as Australia, this battle is especially relevant in the context of self-determination, which has been shown repeatedly since the development of Aboriginal-controlled health services in the 1970s to be incredibly effective in achieving better outcomes for Indigenous peoples.

'It is the right of Aboriginal and Torres Strait Islander women to determine for themselves what their health system will look like,' reads the National Aboriginal and Torres Strait Islander Women's Health Strategy published back in 2010. 'Aboriginal and Torres Strait Islander women and their organisations must have a pivotal role in consulting, designing, developing, implementing and evaluating health services for Aboriginal and Torres Strait Islander women.'[208]

If this is supported by state and federal governments, as encouraged in successive *Closing the Gap* reports, it may alleviate some of the dangerous spaces that Aboriginal and Torres Strait Islander parents find themselves in, both in terms of early pregnancy loss, but also parenting more broadly. 'Indigenous females, especially those who live in rural and remote areas, often do not have access to culturally safe comprehensive primary healthcare services – one consequence is that girls and women are not adequately screened for cancers impacting their sexual and reproductive health,' writes Professor Pat Dudgeon, a Bardi woman and psychologist. 'There is a consensus across the health literature in the field that access to culturally informed, culturally safe health services is vital to the strengthening of Indigenous women and girls' sexual and reproductive health.'[209]

Biripi academic Dr Tess Ryan says relegating health and science to a set of diagnostic criteria is reductive to the structural processes that allow inequality to affect an individual's health and well-being and 'for First Peoples we know that inequity can be deadly'.

Redemption Song

I was totally and utterly spent.

Each and every loss had left a small, baby-shaped hole I didn't know how to fill. I was resolute in my resolve to keep trying, but holy hell I was tired. And for the first time after a loss I felt the need for closure. A way to bookend that chapter and start anew. When I went to Dr Lovely for my check-up after the D&C, she asked me how I was doing and I told her as much. Dr Lovely is also Jewish and she suggested a visit to the *Mikvah*, the ritual bath, a place of renewal and purity.

My father's family was *frum* (religious) while my mother's family was completely secular after losing so many relatives during the Holocaust, before they arrived here from Europe. Within my family we practised Orthodox (traditional) Judaism, but while we were observant, we were not religious. For many women, their first visit to the *Mikvah* is when they get married. Because I had not had a traditional Jewish wedding, I had never been. But I knew enough about it to know that it was exactly what I was looking for. Something to mark the end of a chapter and the start of a new one. Dr Lovely knew the Rebbetzin (the Rabbi's wife) who ran the *Mikvah* and offered to reach out.

When I went in for my next appointment, Dr Lovely looked stricken. She had spoken to the Rebbetzin to facilitate my visit to the *Mikvah* and had been told in no uncertain terms that I was not welcome, because my baby was born out of wedlock; my husband wasn't Jewish and my marriage unrecognised. The Rebbetzin didn't reach out to me, offer me an alternative or even attempt any pastoral care. Dr Lovely handed me a prayer card that the Rebbetzin had given her to pass on, apologised profusely and said she was really shocked and disappointed.

So that's how I found out that, for some members of my own community, I was Jewish enough for my family to die in the gas chambers, but not Jewish enough for care, consideration, sympathy or empathy at my greatest hour of need.

I didn't have a true community in Melbourne; the Jewish community here is very insular. If you're not in it, it's difficult to be in it, so to speak. I made the decision that never again would I be part of an Orthodox community. But I did want to find a new spiritual home. After years educating myself about my husband's Aboriginal culture, cognisant that I live on stolen land, and ensuring that my son was connected to his Country, I realised that I had neglected my own tribe.

I sat down and wrote a long email to the then Rabbi of my progressive congregation. I knew his name and I knew the congregation well, having attended a few *simchas* (celebrations) and funerals there. The email opened with these two lines, 'I have a question I would like to ask you. I apologise for the long email, but I have a bit of explaining to do.' What followed was nine paragraphs of raw grief; for my baby, my Judaism and anger at the way I had been treated by the Rebbetzin who oversaw the *Mikvah*. I explained I was looking to join a new congregation, but wanted to know from the outset whether my family would be welcome in his fold. The email was sent on a Friday, at 4.09 pm, on the cusp of the Sabbath, to a man I had never met.

He called me twenty minutes later, as I boarded a tram on the way home from work. He told me that he could feel the pain in my words and that he didn't feel it was sufficient to email me in response. He wanted me to hear him speak the words.

He told me that I was welcome at his congregation. He told me I was loved and that my children are a blessing and that the community would greet them and me with open arms, as well as my husband, in whatever capacity he desired to be included.

Tears ran down my cheeks as he embraced me with his words and showed me a warmth that I so desperately needed at that point in time. I am so proud to be able to call this man my friend and my Rabbi. He brought me back to Judaism, helped me find my way and steered me out of grief.

||||||||||||||||||||||||||||||||||||||||||||||||||||||||||||||||||||||||||||||||||||||||||||||||||||

12

Gagil Marrung

Lead author Cherisse Buzzacott, Arrernte midwife and mother, and Isabelle Oderberg

Colonisation and Australia's history of racism have led to very specific challenges for Aboriginal and Torres Strait Islander peoples in almost every aspect of their lives, including around pregnancy and loss.

Miscarriage or pregnancy loss is challenging for anyone to navigate in terms of ongoing support, follow-up and treatment, intensified by having to side-step questions from family and friends who may or may not understand the experience. Consider then Aboriginal and Torres Strait Islander peoples who face a variety of negative encounters within a healthcare system not designed to be inclusive of their culture, language, identity, and familial needs, while overlooking the very barriers that are cemented in the foundations of that system. Racism, racial abuse, criticisms of misunderstood 'lifestyle choices', medical manipulation and coercions are just a short list of the experiences of Aboriginal women in hospitals or seeking medical care.

This chapter, Gagil Marrung – meaning 'becoming well' in the Gathang language of the Birpai nation – will explain the specific and violent challenges faced by Aboriginal families when navigating early pregnancy loss. Ultimately the system can only be made better by health professionals – midwives, obstetrician, advocates, and Aboriginal women themselves who have experienced pregnancy loss – informing a direction towards the decolonisation of healthcare settings for Aboriginal parents.

While Australia has a high success rate overall when it comes to maternal and child health compared to other countries, Aboriginal families do not experience the same positive outcomes. The experience of a healthy, complete pregnancy relies on the physical and psychosocial health of the individual and their community. As outlined previously, we don't have data on early pregnancy loss in Australia, but it is highly likely that Aboriginal patients are experiencing miscarriage at much higher rates than the rest of the population.

We can make an educated deduction that this is the case, because many of the factors that raise a patient's risk profile are disproportionately represented in Aboriginal communities. Many of these are the markers of generational trauma and include lower incomes, lower levels of education, higher rates of domestic violence and sexually transmitted diseases and more.

Worimi woman Dr Marilyn Clarke was Australia's first Aboriginal obstetrician and gynaecologist and agrees that while health services with self-determination at their core are leading to some excellent health outcomes in community, it is very likely that miscarriage rates among Aboriginal and Torres Strait Islander peoples are higher.

'For example . . . tubal scarring can be a risk factor for ectopic pregnancy and we do see more chlamydia in certain communities,' she explains. 'So if you extrapolate, there are possibly more ectopic pregnancies for example. And we know the risk factors that contribute to some of these adverse outcomes, like smoking and drinking. I think getting accurate, identified data would be helpful.'

Although shocking, when discussing these issues with Aboriginal women, it's not surprising. Most women have a family member, a friend or colleague who has experienced early pregnancy loss and the long-lasting effects it can have on well-being and planning for the future. Aboriginal families tend to be a lot larger and a core part of a bigger, broader community, consequently the effects of one miscarriage can cause widespread grief and enduring feelings of loss.

Gathering data in Aboriginal communities comes with a new raft of challenges beyond those outlined in previous chapters. 'Research is a dirty word in a lot of communities, the perception that people just take and then don't actually give anything back, or community members don't see the actual results or benefit from research,' explains Donna Weetra, a Narungga woman who works as a researcher at the Murdoch Children's Research Institute and was part of the Aboriginal Families Study. 'When non-Aboriginal people want to come and sit down with Aboriginal people, there are language differences straight away. People don't want to step outside of themselves and actually acknowledge where they are and the skills and resilience that come into many of those communities where they're sitting.'

Family ties

Back in 2021, Cherisse Buzzacott wrote in *IndigenousX* about the pressure on Aboriginal women to have babies and the importance of family in our culture. 'In my experience in the Aboriginal family context there is silent expectation to raise children. Culture relies on the expansion of our families to carry on our practices, families, obligation to care for land, or to care for our Elders, and us when we grow old. I come from a relatively small family, in comparison to most, with a larger extended family. My grandparents had tens of siblings, they each having tens of children, and so on.'[210] When we put this to Melanie Briggs, a Gumbangirr and Dharawal midwife with Waminda South Coast Women's Health & Welfare Aboriginal Corporation, she agrees.

'There is an expectation, you're right, I did feel that growing up as well,' she said. 'There is a bit of an expectation on us to continue our Songlines from our old people, and that's because they're full of pride. Where I live, they weren't allowed to practice culture, they weren't allowed to speak language. Everything was taken and their children were taken from them and that's why they push us to have children and to practice and do all these things.'

The role of a woman is key to most Aboriginal communities but can differ across diverse population and language groups. In Cherisse's experience, women hold equal power and knowledge of Country, songs, are caretakers for animals and Country, and protect all else that their people value. Their role is central to the continuation of thousands of years of livelihood and knowledge sharing. Women are caregivers, providers, they hunt as well as gather, traditionally hunting smaller animals and collecting plants and seeds to make bush medicines. They hold special positions for children, husbands, and Elders. All that is sacred with being a woman is held by women in an important part of culture known as Women's Business.

Women learn as girls the importance of Women's Business, and their roles and responsibilities are taught by their mothers, sisters, aunts, and grandmothers from a young age. Traditionally, Aboriginal girls were taught how to craft tools and learnt about their roles in hunting, harvesting and ceremony. Aboriginal women Elders hold knowledge and customs to support pregnancy and birth, and methods to support strong mothers and babies, along with responsibility as a caretaker of Country, protecting women's only sacred sites.

The ability to bear and birth children is an expectation, very often vocalised, in a society where children are the future, a major player in the ability to learn and maintain culture, knowledges and language. The value of children counts on the success of Aboriginal women to bear them.

Having a baby in an Aboriginal community, you receive an unspoken affirmation and respect. For Cherisse there was never a real pressure to have children, but it remained a silent expectation, that as she got older was echoed by senior women in her family. There were occasional, casual questions like, 'When will you make me an aunt/grandmother?' at family functions, and comments made about women's weight and whether it might indicate they were pregnant.

This is likely a worldwide phenomenon experienced by many different girls and women at a certain age, thanks to the social construct of women's roles in the home, as caretakers with a natural ability to nurture all contributing to the idea that a woman's place is as a mother. In Cherisse's experience within Aboriginal culture, women were equally a party to decision-making and stood alongside men, with authority over dispersion of food, water and tools. They also had decision-making responsibility over cultural knowledge and skills.

Miscarriage can lead to a myriad of problems for any Aboriginal woman. Cherisse has seen instances where a pregnancy resulting in miscarriage has gone undisclosed to family and friends for fear of the backlash of the result of that pregnancy, with the wider community believing the woman to be at fault. Concealing pregnancies can be medically challenging in terms of follow-up for issues like excessive bleeding to even miscarriage management. Due to fear a previous miscarriage may be talked about by health staff in the presence of family members, a patient may seek care later in her next pregnancy, missing crucial opportunities for antenatal screening and testing.

Stigma around miscarriage in Central Australian communities can be exacerbated by specific mindsets around a patient's behaviours or the behaviours that led to the miscarriage, and even if not physically responsible, questions may be asked about decisions the parent made in the lead-up. These might be comments about wrong skin pairings or marriages, referring to the Aboriginal skin name systems that have been passed on through generations, which allow Aboriginal people to form relationships. Avoidance of people and any activities outside of those skin names can result in bad feelings or outcomes. Other Aboriginal women in desert communities may be afraid to face their communities, including Elders and family, expecting to receive blame and backlash for their miscarriage.

The internal shame of having a miscarriage can deeply affect a woman's feelings towards herself and her ability to become pregnant, possibly leading to her questioning her role within her own family system. This can increase the risk of creating feelings of worthlessness, guilt and shame.

In any case, Aboriginal women who are unable to bear children will often raise other children within their own family to fill a societal role as caregiver. If someone does have issue with infertility or recurring miscarriage, it is not unusual to raise a baby that is not theirs, likely children of siblings and parents' siblings. This kinship care is accepted by family, with the child being wholly aware of their biological mother.

The difference between remote and urban communities

There is a misconception that the majority of the Aboriginal population in Australia lives in remote communities, most commonly identified as the Northern Territory, Western Australia or Far North Queensland. This is not the case. The largest collections of Aboriginal people are in and around the urban cities of Brisbane and Sydney. In fact, according to the 2016 census, 81 per cent of all Indigenous people (including Torres Strait Islander people) were living in 'non-remote areas', compared to 19 per cent of Indigenous people living in remote and very remote areas.[211] Health outcomes for those living in remote regions are noted to be comparatively much poorer, with higher rates of hospitalisations, chronic illness, mortality and morbidity.

Remote-living women have limited to no access to midwives or health professionals with qualifications and up-to-date experience in dealing with pregnancy concerns. This happens for several reasons, including low numbers of midwives broadly in Australia amid a worldwide shortage of midwives, increasing challenges for midwives in being able to maintain clinical knowledge and upskill, as well as the difficulty for health professionals living permanently in remote communities. Aboriginal midwives are in even shorter supply. According to Melanie Briggs, 'There is a 1.4 per cent Aboriginal midwifery workforce and then a percentage of that is non-clinical, so it's pretty dire the number of midwives.' At the time of writing there were three practising Aboriginal obstetrician/gynaecologists in Australia, with a fourth expected by 2023.

In urban areas, there are more maternal care services and choices available to Aboriginal women. These include midwifery-led services, continuity of care models, general practitioner and midwifery shared care services or hospital-based midwifery services. Midwifery Group Practices (MGP) are becoming more common and offer continuity of care to patients, though as noted previously, sometimes places in the MGP are limited and dominated by patients who are able to self-advocate for a place, rather than the high-needs patients who need the care more. Whether they are in urban or remote communities, all Aboriginal patients should have access to culturally safe, round-the-clock midwifery services, especially in the context of miscarriage.

Some of the barriers to care are not about the location of service or community, and are more complex, caused by the treatment received and the harm Aboriginal women experience during and following miscarriage. This stems from a distrust of mainstream health services, where patients or their loved ones have previously had harmful experiences, leading to a situation where they may actively choose not to access those services again.

Ngangk Waangening: Mothers' Stories is a beautiful book in which Noongar and Yamatji mothers tell their stories of giving birth, and several recount having miscarriages. Some of the Aunties writing in the book remember being treated on hospital verandas, because they weren't allowed inside. One author, Marie Taylor, notes 'It's imperative that Aboriginal people are employed within the hospital system.' She recounts her niece having two losses and nobody being there to comfort her. 'It's something I've spoken to them about – I said, "You're failing the Aboriginal women by not having a minister or somebody there in the hospital from the Aboriginal community who could've gone and prayed with the baby and the family and helped ease the situation."'[212]

While more Aboriginal healthcare workers and support staff are to be encouraged, there are other challenges to be addressed. One health worker told us, 'Like in this hospital, we have one ALO [Aboriginal Liaison Officer] and he's a man. So, for a lot of the female issues, they don't want to see him, that's not appropriate. Some ALOs might also know the family involved, so there are issues with confidentiality.'

The usual expectation for pregnant Aboriginal women living in a remote community is that they will attend the hospital for a period before their due date to give birth to their baby (commonly known in the NT as 'sit-down') and return to community within a few days or weeks with their newborn. This means women might be separated from their partners, their families, their Country or a community that speaks their first language. They might have no strong women around them to support and guide them through a challenging time. They might never have been in hospital or even into the bigger towns or cities in their lifetime. In the case of miscarriage for Aboriginal women in the areas where Cherisse has worked, they may only be sent to the larger towns if there is a risk of bleeding, infection, or danger to the woman. These women are usually sent to the hospital by plane in an emergency, or if it's a shorter distance, and there's an available service, they can be brought in by ambulance.

Cherisse has seen so much suffering in her experience working in a rural hospital that provides maternity care to remote-living women. These women experience separation and hurt from being removed from Country to receive the most basic of healthcare needs. Being in hospital, especially when experiencing pregnancy loss, can be a strange and worrying time, being given advice or information that is heavily medicalised. In the case of miscarriage this is all while processing feelings of guilt, shame, and loss, where health professionals are treating physical symptoms but not the psychological feelings that are lifelong and, in some cases, more harmful.

Perth-based Janinne Gliddon is a Regional Aboriginal Health Consultant and has worked across the maternity space. 'If a girl came down to Perth on their own, like they didn't have any support person with them at all, they would often be just very scared to be away from home, because they might not have ever been to Perth before. I think the major issue that a lot of them talked about over the years was the backlash that they might receive going back home or they should have been to Perth to monitor their pregnancy and they've lost the baby while they've been at hospital,' she explains.

Language barriers can be roadblocks to care and can make patients feel even more isolated. 'I tried to get them to the doctors and the nurses or midwives that explain things with more pictorial sort of stuff as well. And we don't have the luxury of having the interpreter services or availability of people in Perth that we can rely on. If someone comes from a different part of the Kimberleys or Pilbara or somewhere, we've got no one down here that we can call on to come and actually have that yarn to them in language, so they can fully understand.'

While patients are always encouraged to bring a support person, when a male partner comes along, there can be significant issues with accommodation and funds. 'They've got nowhere to stay down here, because they've got no money. Sometimes they come down here with just what they're wearing and no purse, no nothing. They've got no idea, they're just chucked on the plane and they come down. Sometimes that poor father has to either walk around in the streets if they can't get a hostel and pay for it himself, and usually they're all booked anyway. We've had some of the blokes sleeping in the park across the road, on a bench, because they can't get accommodation and they weren't approved for the Patient Assistance Travel Scheme. Sometimes the midwives are really lenient and let the men maybe sleep in the waiting room.'

Home to Country

Another challenge is empowering parents to take their baby or pregnancy tissue home to Country. This trauma can be intensified by hospital policies. There may be consent forms that are needed, information around storage of pregnancy tissue and the option that some women may choose to send their baby and placenta for an autopsy, all of which can be challenging to manage.

If there is limited English-language knowledge or the parents are still confused about the loss, they may not really grasp the concept of taking baby home. This could mean that Aboriginal women are very often returning to Country without their babies or pregnancy tissue. If they're not being supported by ALOs or language speakers, they will not understand the information available to them. Cherisse has seen situations where women and their families are not clear on whether babies can be registered for a funeral, or when there is no assistance for planning of a burial, the remains might be disposed of as waste, especially if the loss has occurred in the first or second trimester.

Janinne Gliddon recounts the story of one young girl who had two miscarriages; she lost her first at seven weeks and was never asked whether she wanted to take the pregnancy tissue home to Country. The second loss happened at eight weeks, but her mother, a health worker, attended the hospital. 'Her mother said to them, "My daughter wants her baby." But the look on the faces of the health manager and clinical nurse was like, "What?" And she said, "We want our baby so we can go and bury it." They asked her, "Do you realise it was only like eight weeks?" She's said, "I don't care. There was a heartbeat last week. There's nothing now. So it is our baby. We want to take my grandbaby home." But you could see the cogs turning in the wadjelas (white women's) heads, thinking, "Why the hell would you want it, it's just a specimen. It's too early." And I thought, wow, no girl gets asked this question, do they even actually know that they can do that?'

Janinne's mother Derryce Gliddon writes in *Ngangk Waangening*, 'At about five or six months pregnant I started to haemorrhage, so my husband Ron drove me straight to Morawa Hospital, which was about thirty minutes from Perenjori. I gave birth to a little girl and that was all I knew. Not long after she was born, they put her in a bowl and placed her on the tray in front of me, until the nurse noticed that my daughter was still there and they removed her. And that was the last time I saw my baby girl.'[213]

For those who do get through the barriers and are able to take their baby home to Country, they then have to navigate a sometimes very long journey home. If they've been sent in by their local remote health clinic, the journey home might be six to eight hours in a car or a longer bus ride. There is an added issue of transporting the baby; women don't want to be carrying their baby in a box with their memories of their pregnancy loss and a painful stay in hospital. Other family and community members will be asking them what happened in town at the hospital and might question them about their pregnancy, putting women in a difficult spot.

Yolŋu woman Leila Gurruwiwi split the ashes of her baby Elijah, born at sixteen weeks, between herself and her former partner. 'We ended up splitting the ashes in half and he took his half to the area where he grew up near Mount Hotham at a little creek that meant a lot to him. I ended up taking my half back up home on Country, and I buried Elijah with my dad who passed away when I was five years old. He committed suicide because of the pressure. So I felt like it was nice for him to be with my dad. They never met in life, but they are now together in death and in the Dreamtime.'

Dealing with death

'I think we, as Aboriginal people, we tend to deal with death a lot better than what non-Indigenous people do,' explains Gurruwiwi. 'We give ourselves time to grieve. With us, it can be for a number of days or a number of weeks, because that person has to go on that journey to the Dreamtime and back to their ancestors.'

Culture around death can be a difficult thing to manage in a colonial setting. In Cherisse's Arrernte culture, the name of the deceased is not used and the deceased person's home and the place where death has occurred needs to be cleansed, using smoke from the burning of particular leaves in what is known commonly as a 'smoking'. This is led by family members and Elders of the community and can involve the whole family. It is a difficult undertaking when the death has occurred in a hospital. Burning or fire within a hospital can be a major issue for safety and can trigger fire alarm systems, plus the movement of a large group of people through a hospital might not be appropriate due to small spaces or shared rooms. Another aspect in a remote context is that family are not always available or present, so the smoking can't take place. Being far from Country can also cause problems for family who might want to visit to support the mother. It can also be an issue for future pregnancies, where a hospital stay is expected, but there is sadness and possible shame around being close to that particular room where the miscarriage occurred or where the mother was staying at the end of the previous pregnancy.

Aboriginal people experience grief and loss very differently. Outside the Aboriginal context, grieving takes place in the period between the passing of a person, through to a funeral, with closure once that event has been held. Some Aboriginal cultures observe a period of mourning for years and even decades, much longer than after a formal funeral service has taken place. Some Aboriginal groups demonstrate this mourning by wearing black clothing, not using the name of the deceased or showing pictures of the deceased. But experiences vary across communities.

Missy, an Aboriginal woman from New South Wales, had already had two miscarriages and two living babies when she was raped by her ex-husband. Newly single with two children, she had landed a new job and was, in her words, in 'no position to have another baby', so she made an appointment to have a termination. 'I had nothing, I was starting from scratch. I was living with an esky as my fridge, the kids on mattresses on the floor. I just landed this job that I was starting up in Brisbane, with corporate,' she explained. She went ahead and ended her pregnancy. Five years later she found love with an old friend. Together they decided to have more children, to add to the family that included Missy's son and daughter from her marriage. Together, they had a son. But when they decided they were ready for another child together, they started to have losses. All up they had ten losses in two years, consisting of eight pregnancies, two of them multiples. Missy was able to get pregnant, but struggled to get past early gestation. And that's when the guilt set in. 'Part of me thought that I was being punished, spiritually punished, because I had taken the life of one of my babies before that.' Missy also found it incredibly challenging to culturally make peace with her losses, because of how they passed. During the miscarriage of her twins, the babies passed out of her in the car.

'I was having these labour-like, strong, strong labour pains, and then I felt something just pass, while sitting in the driver's seat. I went inside work straight away and went to the toilet straight away. There was this big lump. I didn't know what to do, because I'm like, "How do I keep this?", because I wanted to do some ceremony around it, to move spirit, move it where it needed to go. And I couldn't keep it. I was just like, "Oh my God, I'm just gonna have to let this go in the friggin' toilet." Because there was nothing on me that I could put it in. Culturally we want to keep things because we go and give those back to Mother Earth. That means that the spirit is always tied to Mother Earth, it's tied to me and it's tied to Mother. We get this gift of life, which is passed to us by Mother Earth, and we have these responsibilities around it. I suppose the privilege of being able to give life can also be a massive burden as well.'

Treating the whole patient

There is a shift within the midwifery space towards a holistic approach to pregnancy, childbirth, and how to improve maternal health. Women are at the centre of their pregnancies with all other paths of well-being surrounding them. The same can be said for patients experiencing miscarriage, even more so when they are Aboriginal. Within this context, health and well-being are interconnecting and interchangeable. Health looks outwards from the 'patient view', encompassing emotional, psychosocial, and financial well-being, all underpinned by cultural well-being, and all the facets held within identity.

The lens through which Aboriginal people view health and wellbeing conflicts with colonial medical systems, which compromise the way Aboriginal women are treated and experience healthcare, follow-up or lack thereof, or all the above. Birthing on Country is an innovative service model that incorporates cultural practice and upholds traditional Aboriginal knowledge and practice, to decolonise maternity care services.

'The basis of this model of care ensures that Aboriginal and Torres Strait Islander women are at the forefront in the design, delivery, development and evaluation of the services,' write Professor Ray Lovett and Makayla-May Brinckley.[214]

Lessons for miscarriage could be learned from this movement, which allows culture and family to be central to maternal health, baby's care and well-being. It is an Aboriginal-led way of providing healthcare, driven by research, and is already providing outstanding results for women and babies, giving strength and ownership to women and building towards healthy communities.

Midwife Skye Stewart, a Wergaia and Wemba Wemba woman, describes some of the differences between Aboriginal and non-Aboriginal people, with Aboriginal people able to hold space – physical or spiritual space – that allows others to engage in active listening, something communities excel in. There is no 'right way' to implement Birthing on Country, but it does need to be driven by the community and be Aboriginal-led in all areas, from the front desk through to health professionals, maintenance workers and transport officers. 'Its success thrives on our inclusion and our governance,' she says.

Erosion of trust

The current mainstream healthcare system was set up with a white view on health, based on ideas that have been developed through a strict colonised way of thinking, developing technologies through a narrow and privileged lens. Historically the study of humans was completed on Aboriginal people by those very same 'revolutionary' health experts who 'paved the way' for health, and remain current through today's naming of accolades, awards and dedicated celebrations.

Professor Pat Dudgeon describes a model for strengthening the sexual and reproductive health of Aboriginal and Torres Strait Islander women and girls, composed of seven connected domains of well-being: Country, spirituality, culture, community, family and kinship, mind and emotions, and body.[215]

This holistic approach to healthcare through an Aboriginal perspective is totally at odds with the mainstream colonial system as it stands, which is built on a history of harmful studies of Aboriginal women, men and children, with experimentation, forced trials of drugs or surgical techniques, forced sterilisation, disembodiment and distribution of body parts all over the world for study. This desire to study Aboriginal people continues today, in the most modern of research facilities, granting health experts thousands of dollars of research grants. While they may not seek to disembody Aboriginal people now, they nevertheless work under the guise of 'helping' them to build a stronger future with self-determination. All this without truly and completely allowing Aboriginal people the control and authority to do so.

'Much more is involved in health than a simple set of diagnostic tick boxes,' explains Biripi academic Dr Tess Ryan. 'It is such things as well-being, families, effective housing and your environment that interplay with health and health management. There needs to also, within this conversation, be a situation of what Aboriginal and Torres Strait Islander people call the struggle – the struggle for acknowledgement, understanding, self-determination and humanity. And how race interplays with systems, including, sadly, the health systems we all rely on to keep us alive.'

What is happening in this colony in regards to Aboriginal maternal healthcare shares some similarities with other women and gender-diverse people of colour across the world, as highlighted in stories from Black and POC (people of colour) women accessing the American medical system. Their social construct portrays the Black woman as poor, highly fertile, and depictions of pregnant Black women are accompanied by notions of drug use, welfare reliance and teen pregnancy.[216] This is not dissimilar to some of the beliefs that are deeply-seated in Australian health professionals who have limited or no exposure to Aboriginal people outside of their regular job.

Many Aboriginal women already refuse to attend mainstream clinics due to trauma from racism when previously accessing healthcare or from hearing of incidents like this in the wider community. There is a serious issue with stereotypes around 'bad' or 'neglectful' parenting. In many instances, if a baby or a child is hurt, health professionals are quick to blame the mother, often without cause. There is a consensus that the mother was solely responsible for the illness or injury suffered by the child in question when, more times than not, it is clearly an accident. When suffering from an early pregnancy loss, parents fear the same judgement and that they would yield the blame for the miscarriage occurring.

'I was lucky that I was in a space where I had lots and lots of support, lots of different people around me,' says Leila Gurruwiwi. 'But I've heard stories of people not feeling comfortable going into hospitals or any other spaces like that because they just don't know how they're going to be treated.'

Aboriginal women already feeling the hurt and angst of having to share personal experiences with people that are not the same as them (they hold different values, have hidden biases, experience family life in a different way and may be afforded a great privilege based on the colour of their skin) can be further distressed by this experience. This is aggravated by circumstances where there are many diverse language speakers or different nationalities. In addition, their lack of under-standing of how the mainstream hospital service functions can impact their ability to make decisions about their own healthcare. Cherisse often sees remote Aboriginal women agree to a proposed pathway of care purely because they do not understand, and do not want to go against the care that is being offered by a person in power, historically a white doctor or health professional.

The failure of healthcare systems to provide follow-up care for Aboriginal patients after miscarriage is exacerbated by the same systems that prevent adequate provision of pre-pregnancy care or preconception care, both of which are crucial to identify risks to maternal and fetal health. This preparation can identify issues that might affect a baby's growth in utero, to eliminate or treat illness or disorders that may impact the success of the pregnancy. This is key to worldwide health promotion standards, but is not always possible. Some women may present for care already pregnant, missing an essential chance for preconception care.

This relates to physical well-being, mental health, social supports, financial assistance, and other areas that could contribute positively to a woman's health in pregnancy.[217] Preconception care would benefit Aboriginal women as an adverse group with well-documented risk factors such as diabetes, low-birth weight babies and higher rates of smoking than the broader Australian population. It is proven that the delivery of preconception care can be affected by the woman's understanding of the need for it, frequency of healthcare checks, the availability of midwives to deliver education, appropriate resource readiness, and reviewing of primary care processes to target Aboriginal women as a priority, given their higher risks associated with pregnancy and miscarriage.[218]

Midwife Melanie Briggs is an advocate for Birthing on Country. She describes the mainstream healthcare system's inability to provide early access to support programs for early pregnancy loss as an issue, which is carried extensively by the primary healthcare services in her community. Aboriginal women's care is not seen as an emergency, especially while experiencing a miscarriage; they are sent home with little information and a painkiller tablet and told to wait it out. The challenge, she says, is that the hospital system has no continuity of care and no woman-centred focus model which can provide 24/7 care, like Waminda South Coast Women's Health & Welfare Aboriginal Corporation where she works.

'There's no support from the hospital point of view. And even where we are now there's no early access for pregnancy programs, for early pregnancy loss or nothing like that. It's just all put onto primary healthcare out in the community and they get nothing.' Briggs says the key is better communication between hospitals and Aboriginal Community Controlled Health Organisations (ACCHOs). 'There needs to be clear communication from when the woman presents to a hospital system with a miscarriage, and they need to be able to speak to the woman and ask them who's their care-provider at home. "Can we communicate your presentation to them and can they follow you up in the home?" There's a big barrier there for communication,' she explains. 'I think if that's addressed and there's a respectful mutual collaboration relationship, a professional relationship, there between the organisations and the women, the transition will be a lot smoother and a lot easier for women to be able to access emergency care straight away and then follow up when they go home.'

Mel's experience of supporting women extends to the home, as health professionals can be called to the homes of women who have active bleeding and cramping in pregnancy, often resulting in miscarriage. This support should be standard when you consider the shift of pregnancy care, early discharge in the postnatal period and even the support of homebirth, with a wide-scale systemic preference to move towards healthcare in the home. Miscarriage should have the same consideration, but if it is already failing to be identified and treated fairly in a hospital setting, what hope is there for miscarriage support and treatment to continue in a home setting?

Equally, when Aboriginal women attend a hospital or other clinical setting for early pregnancy loss, in Cherisse's experience they are encouraged to leave hospital with some form of contraception, or plan for contraception follow-up, before they are formally discharged. This is such a common practice it could be viewed as medical coercion, especially if the Aboriginal woman is younger, has had multiple pregnancies previously and has expressed no desire to curb her fertility. It is a goal of the Reproductive Justice movement to end coercive medicine.

'Whereas feminists demand legal abortions, Indigenous women want stricter controls over abortions and sterilisations because they have been practised on our bodies without our consent,' writes

Distinguished Professor Aileen Moreton-Robinson, a Goenpul woman from Quandamooka. 'In the 1970s Indigenous medical services were using Depo Provera as a form of cheap contraception: it did not work and many Indigenous women became pregnant and suffered spontaneous abortions.'[219] Forced sterilisation of Aboriginal women is far from historic, it extends right into the modern era.[220]

A lack of investigation into the causes of miscarriage in Indigenous populations could also be seen as a new method of sterilisation of a certain population demographic, reminiscent of previous population control measures enforced on Aboriginal people by the colonial government. The battle for fertility is one that is felt by many Indigenous communities across the world. 'In our communities, it is about the right to have children,' says Charon Asetoyer, executive director of the Native American Women's Health Education Resource Center.[221]

Aboriginal and Torres Strait Islander patients are less likely to be offered investigations for the cause of their miscarriage or infertility, or referrals to artificial reproductive technologies. 'I saw a woman who was already in her early forties and had never been pregnant,' explains Dr Marilyn Clarke. 'I did a laparoscopy on her and she had blocked tubes from previous pelvic inflammatory disease. She was really grieving the fact that she couldn't have children. And I said, "When did you see doctors before this?" She said she'd brought it up with her GP. I asked whether they had ever referred her for IVF or to consider IVF and she said it was never even offered to her. I offered to refer her, but she's already lost a decade of potentially going through IVF because of the assumption that she couldn't afford it or whatever assumption they made.'

Parenting in safety

Australia's modern history is one of colonisation and violence, although some would much rather it be hidden away, given it consists of two centuries of abuse, trauma, and deprecation of Aboriginal and Torres Strait Islander people in this country. The *1869 Aborigines Protection Act*

(Victoria) was just one of the many policies implemented by the then Australian Government that permitted white settlers and government facilities like schools, churches and family welfare systems to have control over the removal of children from their Aboriginal families. These children were ordered to be shipped to the other side of the country to fill residential schools and established 'missions'. Missions were founded with a role to integrate these children into Catholicism, with complete control of their well-being and no regard for the family they left behind. These children were forbidden from speaking in their learned languages and practising any aspect of traditional Aboriginal culture. The forced removal of children came from the belief that the government could assimilate them into white families, to eradicate the 'native' blood of Aboriginal people, in an attempt to destroy their future. This while forcing slave labour onto hundreds of children and their parents. 'The Stolen Generation' era extended from the 1910s right up to the 1970s and saw the forcible removal of children as a part of 'child protection'.

Although this activity was theoretically ceased, in modern times child protection agencies, also known as 'welfare', children's services and family services are responsible for a second wave of Stolen Generation. The rate at which children are now being removed from Aboriginal families is actually higher, with tens of thousands of children being taken away from kin and Country and put into foster homes, to be raised out of their cultural and familial circles.

As at 30 June 2019, 20,077 Aboriginal and Torres Strait Islander children were in out-of-home care, representing one in every 16.6 Aboriginal and Torres Strait Islander children living in Australia.[222] The rate at which Aboriginal children are being removed from their families is 9.7 times higher than non-Aboriginal children.[223]

Reports of alleged neglect, abuse and harm of Aboriginal children often stem from the healthcare system and a misunderstanding of Aboriginal parenting and kinship care. Many Aboriginal families describe the damage that has resulted from the hospitals, clinics, and other healthcare services established to care for people with injury and illness, instead instigating the removal of children from their parents.

For this reason, many Aboriginal parents may not seek healthcare during their pregnancy, which could result in not being able to identify issues for parent or baby well into gestation and may contribute to loss. Additionally, Aboriginal women may not seek support during miscarriage for fear of future impact on pregnancies, for example if someone has a previous miscarriage or even multiple miscarriages, their recreational activities or relationship status might be reported as a risk factor, again being identified within her obstetric history.

We know from the previous chapter that the Reproductive Justice movement moves far beyond the provision of birth control and abortion, to a place where all people, irrespective of demographic, are able to parent safely and are also able to parent if and when they choose. American academic Loretta Ross writes, 'Birth justice is the right to give birth with whom, where, when, and how a person chooses.'[224]

Finding cultural safety

'Cultural safety' was defined by Māori nursing academic Irihapeti Ramsden in her seminal paper 'Cultural Safety and Nursing Education in Aotearoa and Te Waipounamu', where she explained that the onus is on a healthcare professional to provide a culturally safe space for the patient. However, only the person receiving the care can define that space as culturally safe. 'Cultural Safety is therefore about the nurse rather than the patient,' she explains. 'That is, the enactment of Cultural Safety is about the nurse while, for the consumer, Cultural Safety is a mechanism which allows the recipient of care to say whether or not the service is safe for them to approach and use. Safety is a subjective word deliberately chosen to give the power to the consumer.' Unfortunately, many hospital and clinics state publicly that they provide a culturally safe space, without ever asking consumers whether they feel this is the case.

One doctor we spoke to believes that cultural competency training should be examinable, meaning it should be tested as part of qualifications. 'Trainees generally are not going to be interested in doing anything, unless it's going to be possibly in the exams and then they'll do it,' they told us. 'A lot of health workers don't see the importance of it, so they're not motivated to do it.'

Another factor is, as Professor Odette Best points out, this training rarely looks at how the practitioner's own culture affects their outlook and their patients. 'Little, if any cultural awareness training encourages nurses to think about their own cultures, such as their ethnicity, or the nursing and midwifery cultures of the professions, or sexuality culture or gendered culture,' she explains. 'Colonial nursing and midwifery practice and its impacts on nursing and midwifery care and Indigenous Australians is rarely discussed.'[225]

As part of Skye Stewart's work at a Koori maternity service early on in her midwifery career, she spent a lot of time educating around cultural safety, creating conversations around needs of the community and learning opportunities for her midwifery colleagues. Stewart says her position was much broader than just to create awareness; she needed to have a meaningful look at the way that Aboriginal people are engaged in their healthcare and educating staff on their roles. The difficulty was the revolving door of health professionals that come through the space, all lacking in key knowledge and awareness of Aboriginal people's struggles.

In her role as a midwife, Cherisse was very often being pulled in directions away from maternity care. When she was working in a hospital maternity ward she was involved in housing, transport, social services, banking and anything else that remote Aboriginal women felt comfortable to approach her about. Aboriginal women would know the experience of leaving work and taking work home with them, as they live and work in their communities and are often sought after for responses to questions on pregnancy, birth and care of a newborn baby. She is often contacted via social media by family and friends concerned about women who are bleeding in early pregnancy or to hear worries about miscarriage.

ACCHOs must be provided with better funding so they are able to provide culturally safe spaces and support. Melanie Briggs explained that outside the Aboriginal-controlled clinics, 'there are no resources, there's not enough space, there's no early pregnancy assessment clinics, there's nowhere to take these women to support them. So here we are left relying on the Aboriginal medical services.'

A landmark study conducted in Melbourne by La Trobe University, the Victorian Aboriginal Community Controlled Health Organisation (VACCHO) and three Melbourne public hospitals showed that parents having an Aboriginal child experienced much better outcomes when part of a culturally appropriate midwifery group practice. Lead researcher Professor Helen McLachlan said women with access to midwife-led continuity of care, rather than standard maternity care, are less likely to experience fetal loss before twenty-four weeks gestation, but she noted that the availability of these models for Indigenous women is limited, and little is known about the capacity of large maternity services to implement culturally specific models.

Existing (or additional) services providing this care are uniquely positioned to provide the cultural and spiritual support that women may seek, and we must empower them to do so.

Cherisse's story

My first miscarriage was just after the thirteenth week of pregnancy. We had told people the day before that I was pregnant thinking that we were in the 'safe zone', being the second trimester. I miscarried at the hospital I worked at in my hometown. Only a few visited me there, even though most people knew why I was there. They didn't come.

The likelihood of a thirteen-week pregnancy resulting in a human-looking baby was very slim. I think at the time, most people thought it was not a big deal to lose a baby at this gestation, because it was not really that formed. I didn't care. I cried a lot that weekend in the hospital. I missed the new year fireworks as I sat in my room and cried. I still walk into that hospital room every day in my role as a midwife. During my most recent pregnancy I asked to stay in that room, where I was given a cervical stitch (cerclage) for my eighteenth week of pregnancy to keep my son inside me. I felt a connection to that very first baby I had in the toilet, as my colleagues bore witness to the whole incident. It was a life cycle of events.

The second time I had a miscarriage I had no idea that I was pregnant until I started to miscarry. I was living alone in a major city, my partner at the time was living back home in Alice Springs. A friend told me to go to the hospital. The closest hospital I knew was the hospital where I worked. I passed a massive clot on the way to the hospital and handed it over to the midwife who was collecting my medical history. I was so unaffected by the blood and pregnancy tissue as I had seen plenty of this in my role as a midwife. I had seen placentas, babies, lots of bleeding and been a part of some traumatic experiences of women in birth and on the operating table. I was numb to this moment.

My third miscarriage happened while I accepted the Inaugural Sister Alison Bush Midwifery Award, presented by the Congress of Aboriginal and Torres Strait Islander Nurses and Midwives (CATSINaM), one month before the one-year anniversary of the day I lost my daughter Senna at twenty-one weeks. I smiled with pride as I walked onto the stage and gave my speech. Meanwhile, I was masking the pain I was feeling that I couldn't hold in a baby for the fourth time in my life. I got off the plane in Canberra to my new partner, and I walked into the room of our apartment telling him that I had started cramping and bleeding. He acknowledged that and walked out. We never spoke about it again.

In 2019 when I became pregnant for the fifth time, we never spoke about the pregnancy, and we didn't tell our families until I was at least twenty weeks along. We didn't want to jinx it, so I never took photos while I was pregnant. I have one full-body photograph taken by a friend at my baby shower. I am standing in the middle of her two mothers (her aunty and her mum). I will cherish this picture of my son in my belly. I hated my stomach, I covered it every time my family was around. I hated to draw attention to my growing bump, only sharing this with my partner at different times. When my baby kicked, I didn't brag or want that awareness that this baby was growing and thriving. I felt guilty about why this moment couldn't come sooner for me, or my other babies that I had lost. I also grieved throughout my pregnancy, from the twentieth week, the experience I never shared with my daughter. The mental load was heavy. I wanted to be happy for this pregnancy and for us to finally have the full experience of being pregnant and having a baby and continuing as a family. But the feelings never came as I wanted them to; it was a constant battle to feel happy about my life being pregnant. If I could go back I would do it differently, I would celebrate myself more and enjoy every moment and share that with the people closest to me who wanted to feel and experience this with me.

No amount of time can take the pain away that I feel for my babies that were lost. They're remembered through dates on the calendar, memories, places and names, like others lost, and I believe they are in a place together in whatever form, but together and happy and always watching over me.

The ability to continue a pregnancy to full-term can rely on many different factors. Aboriginal people need to walk away from a midwife, doctor or specialist knowing that, even though they are in a state of grief, they have been informed and empowered enough to make the appropriate decisions in their care, with their bodies and their babies or pregnancy tissue. This with cultural oversight and direction and the recognised follow-up that should be afforded to all people.

Fix You

A teeny, tiny, little hand on my back.

'Are you okay, Mummy?'

I'm trying so hard to bury my sobs right down, deep in the pit of my stomach. But I'm failing.

'Why are you crying?'

I look up into those wide, almond-shaped green eyes and yet another wave of guilt comes crashing down over my head.

'Mummy, would a cuddle make it better?'

I don't want you to grow up alone. I want so badly to give you a brother or sister. A best friend. And I want to cuddle another baby as perfect as you.

'Maybe you should have some ice-cream? When I feel sad ice-cream makes me feel better.'

I've done everything they said. Every single thing they instructed, while they stood there. In their white coats. Pity on their faces. While I bled. And bled. And bled.

'Here, Mum, do you want to cuddle my bear?'

I'm running on the last fumes of hope and faith. Trying to believe them when they tell me it'll happen if I just keep trying. But instead, I keep having to say goodbye, before we've even begun.

'Mummy, do you need a tissue? I can reach the tissues, look!'

What a strange thing, to miss someone you never knew. Well, it's not strange to me. I did know you, didn't I? I was your mummy, you were my baby and he was your brother. Even if it was only for what felt like a fleeting moment in time. But no one understands the loss of something you never really had.

'Why are you sad, Mummy?'

I pull you close to me. I bury my head in your thick, red hair and I whisper to you, my love.

'We all get sad sometimes, my darling. But even when I'm sad, I love you. I love you more than the whole ocean and the moon and all the stars. My perfect sweet pea. My baby boy.'

||||||||||||||||||||||||||||||||||||||||||||||||||||||||||||||||||||||||||||||||||||||||||||||||||||||||||||||||||||||||||||||||

13

The Key, The Secret

Finding a cause for miscarriage can be like hunting for a needle in a haystack, and there's so much we just don't know. Here's what we do.

When I worked at Melbourne's tabloid newspaper the *Herald Sun*, as the decline in advertising started to accelerate and we were looking for new ways to generate revenue, we launched a project to create new content that would entice people to pay for subscriptions. Everyone in the newsroom pitched ideas and they were ranked. I was part of the team who evaluated them. One idea that was green-lit almost immediately without debate was a true crime content stream. Because everyone loves true crime, right? Real-life thrillers with clues and bad guys, motives to dissect, histories to pore over, trails to follow to find the person to pin it all on. If something bad happens, it's a natural human inclination to want to understand why. The greater the horror, the stronger the need to understand. If we can unpack why, maybe we can prevent it from happening again, right? We can find the bad guy responsible and apportion blame and hit him with a big stick to hear a satisfying thwack. But in the case of miscarriage, it's not that easy to do. There is far more we don't know, than we do.

The first reason for this is that research into conditions that affect people who aren't cis white men simply doesn't receive a balanced proportion of funding against issues that do. In the UK, 16 per cent of the population (women) will experience reproductive health issues, but it receives only 2.5 per cent of the annual research budget.[226] An analysis of funding by the US National Institutes of Health also showed a disproportionate share of resources being applied to diseases that primarily affect men.[227]

Then there's the secondary bias within reproductive health, which takes the form of a natural gravitation towards the 'issue' being the fault of the bearer of the vagina. I had seven losses, but not once was my husband asked to provide a sperm sample for analysis. Research shows that where infertility issues can be identified, half the time there is a male contributing factor. For example, DNA fragmentation in sperm (a change in the sperm's DNA or physical break in its DNA strands) is a leading cause of infertility, as are low sperm counts or motility (slow swimmers). Ground-breaking research from Imperial College London actually shows that sperm quality is extremely relevant in recurrent pregnancy loss (RPL). 'Our data suggest that male partners of women with RPL have impaired reproductive endocrine function [hormones], increased levels of semen reactive oxygen species [which can affect sperm quality and result in infertility] and sperm DNA fragmentation [which can do the same]. Routine reproductive assessment of the male partners may be beneficial in RPL.'[228]

Many of the researchers I spoke to are frustrated by the lack of attention – culturally, medically and in research – paid to the male contribution to infertility and pregnancy loss. But there are beacons of hope. At Tommy's National Centre for Miscarriage Research, Professor Arri Coomarasamy's team is running a project called The pAToMiUM trial.

'We've been investigating therapeutic options in the man that would reduce the risk of miscarriage in the woman,' he explains. The small trial of thirty men will be examining the benefits of antioxidants, vitamin and mineral supplements.

There also seems to be a reluctance to develop new treatments, which, if not properly tested, can have significant and long-lasting ramifications for pregnant people. There are two key examples of why this might be the case. The first is very well known: thalidomide, a medication that was once used to treat morning sickness. Most people would know the name and the damage it caused. It was only available for a few years, but is thought to have affected around 10,000 babies worldwide, at least 40 per cent of them dying at birth, before a connection was made between the German medication and developmental issues by Australian doctor William McBride, in a letter to *The Lancet* in 1961.[229]

But not nearly so many people have heard of diethylstilbestrol (DES). The popular miscarriage treatment was developed by Olive and George Smith, a husband and wife team, working at Harvard. A hormone-based medication, it was sold from around 1940 to 1971, on the basis that it prevented miscarriage and several other pregnancy complications. There is no proof at all that it was effective in preventing miscarriage, but what it did do was cause serious illness in the patients who took it, as well as their offspring, and even their grandchildren. DES-related diseases include breast cancer and a rare vaginal cancer called clear-cell adenocarcinoma. There is a registry for patients whose parents or grandparents took DES and they are regularly given screenings for specific health conditions. Other issues include t-shaped uteri, fibroids, breast cancer, infertility, hypogonadism, intersexual gestational defects and more. Up to 10 million patients in America took DES during the first trimesters of their pregnancies. It's not known how many patients took DES in Australia, but it's thought that up to 10,000 women were exposed to it in utero.[230] Men exposed to DES in utero have an increased risk of testicular abnormalities, some of which can lead to testicular cancer.

In relation to DES, Monica Dux argues in her book *Things I Didn't Expect (When I Was Expecting)*, 'If anything, these unfortunate experiments have firmed-up the official "there's nothing you can do to prevent it" position on miscarriage.'[231] In a practical, scientific sense, we have firmed up the ethics around studies of experimental medication, but using experimental drugs on people with terminal cancer seems a more reasonable position ethically, when compared with using experimental drugs on people who are pregnant with viable (until they're not) babies. And experiments on mice can only take you so far.

Before we enter into the world of diagnoses and causes, there are two final things to note. The first is that miscarriage can be caused by more than one risk factor. Not everything is straightforward and fits into a little box with a bow on top. Sometimes there are multiple factors at play that may or may not intersect and create a heightened risk profile. And by risk profile, that means likelihood of there being a problem. For instance, smoking may increase your risk of miscarriage, but it doesn't mean you definitely will experience pregnancy loss.

And finally, I should mention that this is not an exhaustive list of every single factor that can cause miscarriage. If you're looking for an in-depth examination of this issue specifically, I would highly recommend *Miscarriage*, by Dame Professor Lesley Regan, which I refer to throughout this chapter. Professor Regan also cautions against 'throwing everything but the kitchen sink' at miscarriage. Not just because it's unwise to be using techniques that have no basis in science, but also because if you have thrown everything at a patient at the same time, how do you know what's working and what's not?

TL;DR

In 2006 (not that long ago in medical terms, believe it or not) the European Society of Human Reproduction and Embryology updated their protocol for the investigation of the Special Interest Group for Early Pregnancy. They recommended investigations should include obstetric and family history, age, body mass index and exposure to toxins (we'll examine toxins in chapter fourteen), full blood count, antiphospholipid antibodies (lupus anticoagulant and anticardiolipin antibodies), parental karyotype and scans to ensure no tube blockages or similar issues. 'All other proposed therapies, which require more investigations, are of no proven benefit or are associated with more harm than good,' the authors wrote.[232] I think this is a good basis to guide us through. But let's dig deeper, shall we?

Implantation

When I asked Dame Professor Lesley Regan what excited her most about developments in the space, one of the first things she mentioned was the shift in view of medical professionals to understanding the importance of implantation. 'The understanding now is that the quality and depth of implantation is determined in the first trimester and that really dictates the blueprint for the rest of the pregnancy; it's a major step forward in thinking, because it wasn't like that previously,' she explained.

There are several reasons that a blastocyst might not implant properly. These include: a chromosomal issue, inflammation, microbiomes or perhaps uterine shape or the presence of fibroids, which are growths (benign) that grow on the wall of the uterus.

Cracking on with chromosomes

As we've already covered, human fertility is incredibly inefficient, with only 50 per cent of fertilised eggs thought to proceed to blastocysts that implant, and then up to 43 per cent of those fail. We've also covered the all-too-common assumption by medical professionals that there was 'probably something wrong' and that's why you miscarried.

The likelihood of chromosomal abnormality depends on what gestation you're at; a pregnancy that ends at one to five weeks has a 50 per cent likelihood of abnormality, but at fifteen to twenty weeks gestation, the statistical likelihood drops to just 20 per cent.[233] Another factor is age group. For people under twenty years old, the likelihood a miscarriage was caused by a chromosomal abnormality sits at around 37 per cent, at twenty to twenty-nine it's 36 per cent, at thirty to thirty-nine it's up to 47 per cent and for people forty and above it's 59 per cent.[234] If you're having babies when you're over forty, you're more likely than not to conceive a pregnancy with a chromosomal abnormality.

So why do chromosomal errors happen and why does it get worse with age? The answer probably lies in large part with meiosis, a word that comes from the Greek word *meioun*, meaning lessening or make smaller. Meiosis is the process (which Jon Cohen calls a 'biological cleaver'[235]) whereby an egg halves its chromosomes so that it has the right number of chromosomes when it is fertilised by the sperm, which also has twenty-three chromosomes. This means the blastocyst ends up with a final total of forty-six chromosomes, which is the right number for a healthy human. If the process goes wrong, the egg will have the wrong number of chromosomes from the outset. This process becomes less and less reliable as the eggs (and patient) age. Research shows that from the age of thirty-five, seven out of a woman's every ten eggs has 'odd features'.[236]

But as I mentioned, we know and have actually known for some time that DNA damage in sperm has a direct correlation to miscarriage, especially recurrent miscarriage. In a review of research for the highly respected medical journal *Human Reproduction*, the authors of one paper on the topic recommended that for assisted reproduction, sperm without DNA damage should be selected, while tests to identify DNA damage in sperm should be considered for all recurrent miscarriage patients.[237]

Dorothy Warburton was a Canadian scientist and a pioneer in the area of genetics and cytogenetics, with a special interest in fetal abnormalities and causes of miscarriage. She contended that when a patient who has had multiple miscarriages has testing done, it's not unusual for each pregnancy to have different chromosomal abnormalities, for instance trisomy (an extra chromosome), monosomy (a missing chromosome) or polyploidy (one or more additional sets of chromosomes). Since they develop in different ways, Warburton argues they're unlikely to be related and it's therefore 'bad luck'.

Just to note, there is one exception to this and that is structural issues within chromosomes, which are inherited from a parent with a genetic defect. This can cause repeated miscarriage. IVF can separate out those affected embryos or use donor eggs or sperm. This can also assist in cases of genetic diseases such as cystic fibrosis or chromosomal translocations, which can cause, for instance, certain types of cancer. I will address IVF and miscarriage in more detail in chapter fifteen.

Warburton goes on to say that evidence from several sources indicates that 'women with the highest risk for another abortion [miscarriage] are those with chromosomally normal spontaneous abortions [urgh] occurring in the second trimester'. She goes on, 'Such women are also at increased risk for premature births, suggesting a process interfering with the normal physiology of gestation.'[238]

Inflammation

Research has shown that dental inflammation, or periodontal disease, is one marker for miscarriage, often between twelve and twenty-four weeks gestation.[239] The primary reason for this is believed to be because the biological messengers (called inflammatory cytokines) that act on the body's instructions to create inflammation actually travel to the feto-placental unit (the whole kit and caboodle of fetus and placenta, responsible for synthesising hormones) and create an inflammatory response there too. I was recently on the website of a high-profile IVF specialist who was encouraging patients to have a dental check before they attend for appointments. But that's just one example of something that can cause an inflammatory response.

Probably the most important miscarriage treatment development in the past ten years was made by Professor Regan and her team when they discovered the connection between antiphospholipid anti-bodies or syndrome and recurrent miscarriage. The reason for this is that antiphospholipid antibodies can cause blood clots and have been associated with the development of tiny blood clots in the placenta, causing it to malfunction. 'Recent research suggests that these anti-bodies can also attack the cells of the placenta directly. By causing inflammation and turbulence of the blood flow, they disturb the normal pattern of invasion of the placenta into the maternal tissues, which is essential for successful "implantation" and a continuing pregnancy,' Professor Regan writes.[240] She notes that there are usually other factors that act as a red flag for her to investigate antiphospholipid syndrome and these include thrombosis, arthritis, skin rashes, migraine headaches and occasionally epilepsy, as well as possibly a history of thrombosis, heart attack or stroke before the age of fifty in a close relative.[241]

There are other auto-immune inflammatory diseases that are thought to be markers for increased miscarriage rates, including lupus and rheumatoid arthritis.

Another factor repeatedly raised as a risk in terms of miscarriage is weight and obesity. Unfortunately, while we live in a world that is progressively understanding that all bodies are beautiful and it takes all shapes and sizes to make the world go around, obesity has been shown repeatedly in rigorous studies to be a risk factor.[242] But why?

'Fat is not padding,' explains Professor Regan. 'It is actually an organ and it is producing all these inflammatory cytokines, and what happens is that it really affects the way the ovary ovulates and it adversely affects the way embryos implant.'

Unfortunately, the way this is raised with patients, with little to no sensitivity or support, leads to hurt, confusion, body hatred and a host of other terrible but understandable reactions, which feed into stress and anxiety, neither of which are good for the patient's mental health, future conceptions or pregnancies.

Let's get physical

It is thought that issues with formation of the cervix or uterus can cause miscarriage. These issues can be acquired (like scar tissue after surgery or benign growths like fibroids) or congenital, meaning you're born with them (for instance, a bicornuate – heart-shaped – uterus). There's also a septate uterus, where a wall of tissue creates two cavities, which can in some cases be surgically treated.

Cervical incompetence, or as some prefer to call it, cervical insufficiency, is another issue where the cervix is weak and allows the miscarriage of an otherwise healthy pregnancy. While Professor Regan does support cerclage (putting a stitch in the cervix), she will only do so if there's clear evidence of insufficiency, which she says occurs in a very small number of cases.

Infections

So what about infections? In her book, Professor Regan says that the most likely outcome of an infection during pregnancy is an entirely normal pregnancy. She also says, 'I think it's true to say that almost every viral, bacterial and parasitic infection ever described in medical textbooks has also been claimed as the cause of sporadic miscarriage.'

During a healthy pregnancy, your body relaxes your usual immunity so that it doesn't attack the baby as a foreign body (sometimes this doesn't happen and we'll address this in a tick). What that means is that you are more susceptible to certain illnesses than other folk, which is why pregnant patients are at greater risk, for instance, from Covid-19. Before you get pregnant, and while you are pregnant, I encourage you to talk to your treating doctor about vaccinations. It's the best way to protect yourself and your pregnancy. Some vaccines, like whooping cough, can be given while you're pregnant, and the unborn baby gets some benefit too, meaning they're better protected after birth.

While most infections can be treated if you tell your doctor, there are some that are associated with possible miscarriage. In the viral world, examples include chickenpox, rubella and genital herpes. In bacterial land, there is salmonella (cook the chicken through!), listeria (don't eat the sushi!) and chlamydia. Parasites might be toxoplasma or malaria.

But in a twist, Professor Regan believes that it's not a focus on infections but microbiota that might be the future of miscarriage treatment. Microbiota (*microbiome* means small life in Greek) are 'communities' of micro-organisms that live in our bodies.

'For many, many years we looked for infections and for bugs and – surprise, surprise – we never found these things, or very, very rarely,' she explains. 'We now know that the different microbiota in the vagina, in the uterus, in different parts of the pelvis and in the gut and bladder all have very specific characteristics. And we can now classify women with miscarriages in having a deficiency of the good housekeeping bugs, and then there are the nasty ones. There is emerging data to show that the placenta has its own microbiome too.'

It's not just PMT

There are several hormone issues that can cause problems during pregnancy, but the most commonly talked about is progesterone. Known as the 'pregnancy hormone', progesterone is believed to have several important functions during pregnancy, including reducing irritability in the uterus, suppressing immune responses that might encourage the body to reject the fetus, and helping thicken the uterine lining to prepare for an implantation. If implantation doesn't happen, progesterone recedes and menstruation takes place. In IVF the use of progesterone in pregnancy is standard. Elsewhere, debate has raged.

In January 2020, Tommy's National Centre for Miscarriage Research released two studies showing that taking progesterone in cases of early bleeding or previous miscarriage could lead to 8450 more babies being born each year in the UK.[243] They then called for NHS guidelines to be updated to offer progesterone to all patients with early pregnancy bleeding and a history of miscarriage. One drawback is concern that in cases where miscarriage cannot be avoided, for instance in a fetus that is not compatible with life due to severe chromosomal abnormalities, progesterone usage may artificially prolong the pregnancy by weeks, while not changing the final outcome.

In her book *Miscarriage*, Professor Regan did not support the use of progesterone upon vaginal bleeding, saying it was like closing the gate after the horse has bolted. Despite more recent research and the shift in the UK guidelines, she has not changed her view. 'At the end of the day, if the progesterone is the result of the crosstalk between embryo or fetus and mother not being correct, it is usually explained by a chromosomal abnormality,' she says. 'It's not the cause of the miscarriage, because if it was so low that it was causing miscarriage, then it's likely she wouldn't have got pregnant in that cycle. It makes no intellectual sense.'

She adds, 'If this was an expensive treatment, or if it had potential side effects, if you couldn't self-administer, and if it wasn't easy to get hold of, it [the shift in the guidelines] wouldn't have happened. Healthcare professionals, when women come to them with problems, they want to do something to help.'

But Professor Coomarasamy of Tommy's National Centre for Miscarriage Research disagrees. 'You will not find statistical significance, but the available evidence from all of the studies shows an increase in live birth. When you pool it, you get a 5 per cent increase in live birth.' For this reason, the UK's National Institute for Health and Care Excellence updated its guidance in November 2021 to recommend progesterone to reduce the risk of miscarriage for patients bleeding in early pregnancy, or those who have experienced at least one or more previous miscarriages.

It should be noted that the guidelines recommend where progesterone supplements are used, that it should continue to sixteen weeks, though again, there is debate. Professor Colin Duncan, a principal investigator at Edinburgh University's MRC Centre for Reproductive Health, argues there is no benefit to progesterone after the twelfth week of pregnancy (or possibly even the ninth week) and this aspect of the guidelines needed to be reconsidered.[244] Progesterone use is thought to come with very low risks around fetal neurological development.

Diabetes, a disease that occurs when the body does not produce enough of the hormone insulin, is not thought to be a driver of miscarriage, as long as it is well-controlled. If it isn't: Houston, we have a problem. Thyroid function is another standard test for anyone who has had more than one miscarriage, though there is still debate around the role of thyroid antibodies and miscarriage or infertility.

Patients with polycystic ovaries or polycystic ovary syndrome experience early pregnancy loss at a rate three times higher than those who don't have the condition.[245] While there is a lot of educated conjecture around why this might be, at least one reason is elevated levels of luteinising hormone. At least one study shows this can benefit from pituitary gland suppression, but other studies show that this is not helpful.

A potential pituitary gland pitfall is high prolactin levels, otherwise known as hyperprolactinemia. Prolactin affects the way ovaries function. This situation can cause a luteal phase dysfunction, which is the phase after ovulation but before menstruation.

A disease that comes up a lot in support groups is Hashimoto's. It affects mostly middle-aged women and results in hypothyroidism, or an under-active thyroid. It is associated with higher miscarriage rates and several other adverse pregnancy outcomes.[246] The good news is that it can be treated with medication.

Other matters of note

Alcohol is complicated. Some doctors will tell you that one glass of wine won't hurt, but we actually don't know how much alcohol is okay during pregnancy. I'm not judging anyone, and we all have to make our own decisions as to what risks we are comfortable taking. Certainly, high alcohol intake has been associated with higher risk of early pregnancy loss, as has smoking. Alcohol and smoking can cause inflammation and therefore issues with implantation, as well as damage to sperm and eggs.

Conversely, research consistently shows a healthy diet, consisting of fruit and vegetables and low in processed foods and meat, can be beneficial in a multitude of ways when trying to conceive.

A lot of people ask me about alternative therapies like Chinese medicine. I like to call them complementary, rather than alternative.

They're great ways to relax and feel like you're doing something while proven, science-based medicine does its job. Acupuncture was a big part of my treatment and recovery – I found that it calmed and de-stressed me and gave me something to focus on, both during gestation and in recovery. But pushing it as part of an IVF regime when it's going to foist additional costs on patients who may already be under significant financial pressure? Not cool, to say the least.

Another common claim is that miscarriage is caused by a mutation in the MTHFR gene, affectionately known by some as the motherfucker gene. Mutations in this gene affect the way the body breaks down folic acid. The spanner in the works is that around half of the population have a mutation. No doctor I spoke to believed it was a cause of early pregnancy loss. 'I used to test for "mutations" and prescribe blood thinners. Now we know that they're not mutations, they're variations that are perfectly normal. Regular old folic acid is perfectly fine. I no longer order the test,' says fertility specialist Dr Devora Lieberman.[247]

There are a number of vitamins and supplements in addition to folic acid/folate that are being routinely suggested for patients who have experienced miscarriage, fertility or conception challenges. These include CoQ10, vitamin D and a number of others. Tommy's conducted a review of existing studies to see whether there is a link between low vitamin D and miscarriage or recurrent miscarriage.[248] There does appear to be a link but Tommy's is planning further research to fully establish the hypothesis. Research by the University of South Australia examined the data of 294,970 people of white-British ancestry from the UK Biobank and found that low vitamin D could be responsible for inflammatory responses in patients.[249] And we know that inflammation is a problem.

There is also emerging research to suggest that melatonin may contribute to better egg quality, but that is far from proven science. In a field that is evolving and changing daily, it's important to speak to your doctor about any and all vitamins or supplements you're looking to take.

Patients who suffer from endometriosis – a condition in which cells similar to uterine tissue grow outside the womb – have double the risk of ectopic pregnancy. A study of 17,000 people in Scotland found endometriosis could increase miscarriage risk by up to 76 per cent.[250] There are a range of treatments available for endometriosis, depending on a number of factors. In terms of improving pregnancy rates, research shows surgical removal can be effective in some cases.

The American Longitudinal Investigation of Fertility and the Environment (LIFE) Study found an overall rate of pregnancy loss of 28 per cent, with greater risk coming from the female's age being over thirty-five, and male and female consumption of more than two daily caffeinated drinks per day. There was a positive effect from women's daily use of multivitamins.

Immunotherapy is another extremely controversial topic. These therapies commonly consist of white cell or immunoglobin transfusions, natural killer cell treatments and administration of steroids.

While many in the recurrent miscarriage community are fervent proponents of these treatments and many doctors swear to their efficacy, there is no medical or scientific evidence that they work. In fact, there are actually indicators that some can be harmful.

In rare cases where a patient has a rhesus negative blood type – signified by the + or – in their type, eg A- – and they have a rhesus positive baby, they are given an injection of anti-d to prevent problems in future pregnancies caused by anti-bodies created by the birth parent's immune system.

While there is little evidence to suggest these issues cause miscarriage in the first trimester, whether or not anti-d is needed after miscarriage to prevent problems in future pregnancies is something to speak about with your doctor.

Hi, nope

Here is a non-exhaustive list of things that don't cause miscarriage: sex, early and uncomplicated abortions, ultrasounds, microwaves, TVs, wi-fi, lifting heavy things.

No further debate will be entered into.

Fancy

I walked into the clinic. The doctor was known as one of the city's baby-makers: IVF specialists who pull out all the stops to get you viably pregnant. And no expense was spared. Well, not for the patient, anyway.

The clinic was a sight to behold. I was attending at Christmas so it was even more gaudy than usual. A set of glass doors led me into a waiting area. All the walls were pink and there were armchairs in black or pink, lush and velvet. Framed sketches of Parisian scenes adorned every wall and at the end of the row of seats there was a huge white, sparkly Christmas tree covered in pink ornaments.

The waiting area led onto a more open area directly in front of the consulting suites, where a gigantic perspex dining table was filled with specks of gold leaf. There was a bar with a hugely expensive-looking coffee machine on it. The consultation suites were decorated with motivational phrases like, 'If at first you don't succeed, fix your ponytail and try again,' and, 'Nothing is impossible, the word itself says "I'm possible".' In front of those was a pink bicycle with a basket hanging off the handlebars, filled with fake white flowers.

The consulting suites were fronted by panels of glass, with a huge, frosted strip horizontally across the middle, so all you could see were shoes at the bottom and light fittings at the top. I could see the doctor's room, as she saw a patient in her office, and waited to do my intake interview with one of her staff. The doctor's shoes were sky-high platforms in black leather with an ankle strap and a peep toe. The platform at the front of the shoe was covered in tiny gold studs.

Here is how I described it to a friend as I sat in the waiting area: 'I haven't seen the baby-maker yet. But her shoes are very high, very platform and very sparkly. And her waiting room makes me feel like I'm on MDMA and eating fairy floss at the same time. What the fuck am I doing here?' And then I forwarded a bunch of pictures with a challenge. 'Bar, restaurant, afternoon tea room or doctor's surgery. You decide.' I think the objective was to be as opposite to sterile as possible and perhaps lush enough to justify some of the extortionate fees you were about to stump up in order to try to have a baby.

First I was welcomed into the office next door to the baby-maker, where a member of staff took notes on my whole medical history on a computer. I tried not to cry as I recounted the journey that had led me here – somewhere I felt out of place and uncomfortable.

I walked back out into the waiting area and straight into my old boss, someone I consider to be a dear friend. We embraced and then I looked over at the woman sitting next to him, who was certainly not his wife. There was an awkward silence as I looked at him and raised my eyebrows. He blushed a deep shade of crimson and quickly introduced me to his business partner. He was there to do some consulting work for the baby-maker. We all laughed together. Then I told them why I was there, and everyone stopped laughing.

I walked into the baby-maker's office. She stood up and greeted me in a black cocktail dress with a skirt made of layers of beautiful chiffon forming a sort of short but demure tutu. She closed the door and sat down at the desk opposite me and said she was going to read my file. She skimmed the computer screen in front of her and then, after what felt like no more than three minutes, she turned to me and said, 'Well, I have good news, you're a great candidate for IVF!' No surprise really, given that I was sitting in an IVF clinic. In front of an IVF specialist.

'Okay, but I don't want IVF.'

She looked at me quizzically.

I told her my story. I explained the most recent loss and said I had come to see her for two reasons. The first was to establish if there was anything we could have missed: genetic mutations, diseases, hormone imbalances – anything. And the second reason was because I wanted to know if there was any research that indicated any way to improve egg quality.

The baby-maker and I might not have had the same taste in interior decor, but she was incredibly smart and one of the highest regarded

IVF doctors in Australia, for good reason. She sat down on the chair next to me and she said, 'You know, every single day I have women come in here. And they've been in these Facebook support groups and they have theories as to why they can't conceive. Or why they have miscarriages. It's because they've got Hashimoto's. Or a thyroid condition. Or the MTHFR gene mutation. Or whatever. And do you know what they all have in common? They're all over forty.' And while what she said hurt, the overwhelming feeling I had was gratitude for her honesty.

She wrote down a list of supplements and medications that were thought to have the potential to improve egg quality. They were: vitamin C with nicotinamide, vitamin D, folate, CoQ10, vitamin E, lipoic acid and melatonin.

I walked out of the baby-maker's office at approximately 4 pm on 6 December 2018. Three weeks later, I conceived my eighth pregnancy.

||||||||||||||||||||||||||||||||||||||||||||||||||||||||||||||||||||||||||||||||||||||||||||||||||||||||||

14

Toxic

There are lots of factors that can affect our fertility,
including the environment in which we live.

Look, I'm busy. Really, exceptionally busy. Part of it is being a working mum. Part of it is volunteering for causes I believe in. And part of it is never being able to say no to anything for fear that it might be the last good work offer I ever get. Imposter syndrome much? But the fact that I never have any time to myself or time to spare didn't stop me from falling well and truly down a rabbit hole investigating pollution and miscarriage risk while doing the initial research for *Hard to Bear*.

My interest in the topic of environment and miscarriage was piqued after reading a line in Linda Layne's book. 'Abnormally high rates of miscarriages are often one of the first and most visible signs of environmental crisis.'[251]

It led me to hours and hours of reading about, and trying to get my head around, concepts like DNA, epigenetics and methylation. I eventually came to the depressing realisation that there is very little doubt that the declining health of the environment in which we live is elevating all of our miscarriage risk profiles, as well as a host of other adverse pregnancy outcomes such as premature birth and low birth weights. The whole thing was really inconveniently timed, I already had a lot of work on my plate, but I couldn't stop wolfing down information on this topic. I was both terrified and fixated. I tried to move on to my next research topic, but it kept hovering there, in the back of my mind, whispering in progressively more urgent tones that it needed to be addressed and it simply couldn't wait.

Reluctantly, I called a friend who was working as a commissioning editor at *Guardian Australia* and also had an interest in women's health. I explained the whole story, complete with long-winded descriptions of concepts I was just starting to comprehend. The good news was that she agreed entirely that it was a really important story that needed to be written. Bad news was that she wouldn't let me brief one of her journalists. She wanted me to write it. So began my deep dive into 'environmental factors' and their relevance to miscarriage risk.

You're surrounded

Before we go any further, let's pause and define the phrase 'environmental factors', because, in the words of the character Inigo Montoya from *The Princess Bride*, 'I do not think it means what you think it means.'

During the 1980s and 1990s, Argentinian scientist Andrés Negro-Vilar was a leading neuroendocrinologist, based out of California. Neuroendocrinologists study the relationship between the endocrine system and the nervous system, which we'll learn more about soon. In 1983 he was appointed head of clinical programs at the Molecular Biology and Integrative Neuroscience Laboratory within the American National Institute of Environmental Health Sciences. I couldn't find any record of his death, but if he is alive at the time of writing, he is 101 years old.

In 1993 he wrote a paper about stress and how it affects fertility in both men and women, and as part of that he gave his own definition of 'environmental factors'. [252] Put simply, it is any external factor that can affect a living organism, which humans are. Negro-Vilar grouped environmental factors into five categories: chemical (man-made or natural chemicals), physical (light, temperature, altitude), biological (viruses and micro-organisms), behavioural (stress, drug addiction, domestic violence) and socio-economic (nutrition, habitat, occupation, education and hygiene).

Just like in our discussion of identity, some of these factors cannot be isolated from one another. They intersect to form multi-layered, elevated risk profiles. For instance, people in lower socio-economic groups are more likely to have experienced generational trauma that leads to drinking and smoking. They are also more likely to be in work that exposes them to pollutants and chemicals. But let's look more closely at a few of these factors.

It's all progress

When I interviewed Jon Cohen, it had been fourteen years since the publication of his brilliant book *Coming to Term* and I spent a good portion of the interview begging him to do an update. His coverage and analysis of historic incidences of environmental toxicants that are alleged to have caused adverse pregnancy outcomes and miscarriage in America is hugely important, though due to the passage of time and progress in science, some of it has been superseded.

One of the incidences Cohen discussed in the book was the infamous case of Love Canal, a planned and purpose-built community located north-east of Niagara Falls, New York. It was built on top of almost 20,000 kilograms of chemical by-products used in the manufacture of items like perfumes and solvents. In addition to a host of alleged red flags (including elevated white cell counts), it was claimed that residents also had higher rates of miscarriage. Dorothy Warburton (remember her from chapter thirteen?) was called in to investigate the results of the studies purporting to show these elevated rates of early pregnancy loss. Cohen describes her as one of the 'foremost authorities on the causes and incidence of miscarriage'. 'My reaction at the time was this was scaremongering and these were not valid scientific studies,' she told Cohen. She pointed out that the study that came to this conclusion was using 'historical controls from a different era, different racial groups, and a different location, where they defined miscarriage differently'.[253]

As much as I am a science fanatic in a constant search for evidence and proof for every claim I read in relation to medicine, there are also two caveats of which we must be mindful. The first is: just because a study is flawed, doesn't mean that something isn't happening. It just means we don't have proof that it is and the hypothesis remains just that: a hypothesis. Possibly a reasonably or educated hypothesis, but a hypothesis none the less. The second caveat is: just because we don't understand how something happens, doesn't mean it's not happening. For instance, if there are twenty workers at a chemical plant with no family history who are all are diagnosed with the same kind of rare breast cancer in the space of six months, just because we don't know how the chemical is causing the breast cancer doesn't mean that it isn't. If we knew everything, we wouldn't need science or medical research at all. Suffice to say, we certainly need both. But we are still learning and researching and we don't have all the answers.

Back at Love Canal, there were indeed serious flaws in the study, zero doubt. And there are still a lot of question marks around the health-related issues for residents. But I was as floored as Cohen when Warburton gave her response to the question of what she thought of environmental causes of miscarriage. He writes, 'Her candid response stunned me. "I spent a lot of my life, unfortunately, trying to find the relationship between environmental factors and miscarriage with completely negative results," Warburton told me. "I don't think there's any strong evidence that environmental factors cause miscarriage."'[254]

To be fair, Dorothy Warburton was born in 1934 and went into semi-retirement in 2006. She also later noted that she tries to keep an open mind, because 'we could miss things because we are so sceptical'. And there has been much progress in epigenetic research and understanding of chromosomes and reproductive science since then.

But boy oh boy, was she wrong.

Toxic(ant)

Within the environmental category of 'chemical', we have to differentiate between a toxicant, which is man-made, and a toxin, which is natural and would come from, say, plants or animals. Until I interviewed Associate Professor Mark Green from the University of Melbourne, I had no idea there was a difference. He is a leading expert in reproductive biology and Deputy Scientific Director of Monash IVF Victoria.

Green and I agree that, generally speaking, people – especially pregnant people – aren't really heading out to find cane toads to lick or brown snakes to cuddle. Admittedly, there are some other natural substances that can disrupt the way our bodies work including soy milk (because it has a high concentration of isoflavones that can bind to oestrogen receptors) but with the exception of infants drinking soy formula (which is not recommended) the high levels of intake required make soy milk a very minimal risk.

Toxicants are a completely different ballgame. A nightmare-inducing, terror-filled, danger-laden ballgame.

There are many ways in which man-made chemicals can be dangerous for human beings. For instance, carcinogens like asbestos, which can cause cancer of the lung, lung lining, ovaries or larynx. But the first issue we're going to look at is endocrine disrupting chemicals.

Endo-what?

In Coffs Harbour between 1986 and 1988, the number of children born with disabilities (including cleft palates, renal and chromosomal abnormalities) was almost 50 per cent higher than the NSW state average. In 1990, there was a very high number of SIDS cases. Miscarriage rates were also believed to be higher, though because numbers aren't tracked, this can't be confirmed. Environmentalist Dr Kate Short was quoted in the newspaper recommending people not conceive or have children in Coffs Harbour.[255]

At the time of the warnings, a number of chemicals were used in the banana plantations surrounding Coffs Harbour, including dieldrin, which is both an endocrine disruptor and a Persistent Organic Pollutant (POP). POPs are also known as 'forever chemicals' because they don't break down over time. While there were local bans put in place earlier, in 2001 Australia was one of 184 signatories of the 2001 Stockholm Convention on POPs, which effectively banned dieldrin's production and use. It is now accepted as a cause of immune, nervous system and reproductive system damage (as well as Parkinson's Disease and breast cancer). It is also an endocrine disruptor. Another pesticide called dibromochloropropane, or DBCP, used in banana plantations in Latin America is an indirect endocrine disruptor and causes male infertility and miscarriage.[256]

The endocrine system is made up of a series of glands around the body that act like a feedback loop, all communicating with each other. The central point of the system is the hypothalamus, an almond-sized part of the brain, which links the endocrine system to the nervous system, via the pituitary gland. Other major endocrine glands are the thyroid and adrenal glands, the pancreas, as well as the ovaries and testicles. The word endocrine comes from the Greek *endo*, meaning within, and *krine* meaning secrete; so basically internal secretions. Ew.

Hormones are natural human chemicals that act as messengers. They are produced in one part of the body to send messages to other parts of the body. They give instructions for what to do and feed off each other. For instance, luteinising hormone (LH) is a hormone produced by the anterior pituitary gland and regulated by the hypothalamus. A sharp rise in LH triggers egg release from the ovary (ovulation). Oestrogen, known as the 'female hormone', is produced by the ovaries and prompts the uterine or womb lining to thicken in preparation for the implantation of a fertilised egg or embryo. Such is the import-ance of hormones in the reproductive system that an obstetrician who treats infertility is called a reproductive endocrinologist. As you can imagine, any environmental factor that affects the production of these hormones – known as endocrine disruptors – can be a real problem, not just in reproduction, but in a multitude of ways.

Probably the most (in)famous example of an endocrine disrupting chemical (EDC) is BPA (Bisphenol A) which is used to make plastics. It's the reason so many of the plastic storage containers you see on supermarket shelves are proudly labelled 'BPA FREE'. Also used in plastics are phthalates (it makes plastics more flexible), which in addition to food packaging is also used in children's toys. Ironically, the plastics industry is now using chemicals that may be even more harmful than BPAs.

Researchers at the Yale School of Public Health found exposure to synthetic chemicals – perfluoroalkyl and polyfluoroalkyl substances (PFAS) – used in food packaging, many liquid and waterproof cosmetics, non-stick cookware and commonly found in drinking water supplies raised the risk of second trimester miscarriage.[257]

The list of risky exposures is long. So long in fact that if I tried to write them all down, it would chomp up my entire book's word count. But let me give you some examples. Dioxins are a by-product of the manufacturing of herbicides and paper bleaching and are often released into the environment during the burning of waste, including bushfires. Perchlorate is a by-product of pharmaceutical production and is found in drinking water. All of these have a disruptive effect on the human reproductive system. The list goes on. And on. And on. These examples are from the American National Institute of Environmental Health Sciences.[258] They are affecting the reproductive systems of all of us and they're everywhere. They're in the lining of tin cans. They're in supermarket checkout receipts. They're in plastics. They. Are. Everywhere. Meanwhile, research in 2022 showed microplastics are now in our bloodstream, potentially clogging our organs or having an inflammatory effect on crucial bodily functions.[259]

There are 50,000 agricultural, industrial and veterinary chemicals in use in Australia today[260]; 1500 are suspected to interfere with endocrine function and only a very small number of them have actually been tested.[261] In the US, more than 40,000 chemicals are used in consumer products, but less than 1 per cent have been rigorously tested for human safety.[262] 'It's a nasty chocolate box of choice to choose which of our compounds that we really want to have a look at,' Green explains. And when it comes to testing, there are several issues in research models. The first is that it's not enough to simply rigorously test one chemical. There is also the issue of how they react to other chemicals in our environment. Equally, many studies examine the endpoint effect of a toxicant (for instance resultant tumours or other cancers), but not the more subtle aspects, like changes in reproductive characteristics. Another complicating factor is that the effects from toxicants aren't just short-term. The fallout from some endocrine disrupting chemicals can take generations to show their effects, doing damage at conception or during early development of offspring.

The American Longitudinal Investigation of Fertility and the Environment (LIFE) investigated sixty-six persistent EDCs and several non-persistent EDCs. In studying 501 couples between 2005 and 2009, researchers found (among many other things) that blood lead concentration in male partners is associated with diminished fecundity or a longer time-to-pregnancy (TTP), while the persistent organic pollutants caused a 17 to 29 per cent drop in fecundity in women and men.[263]

Unfortunately, when it comes to the issue of environmental toxicants, Australia really is behind the eight ball on a number of fronts. The first is that in this country we need a total legislative overhaul around how we treat chemicals shown to have toxic effects on the health or our environment. 'Why don't we bring in some legislation at a class level rather than individual compound level to make [the government's] job easier to legislate them and to regulate them?' asks Mark Green.

Australia has lower safety benchmarks than many other countries for several classes of chemicals, including the United States. 'I looked at atrazine, which is the second most prevalent herbicide used in Australia and United States, but it's actually banned in Europe, due to the fact that it's so prevalent and they couldn't get it out of the water system,' explains Green. 'But actually Australia permits a much higher so-called "safe level" compared to even the United States, and usually the United States is the worst offender and that's quite worrying. And the Australian so-called "safe levels"? Well, most of my studies have shown they're not safe.' According to the US Environmental Protection Agency, atrazine is an endocrine disruptor and can cause restricted uterine growth during pregnancy, preterm delivery and can affect children's development during pregnancy and during sexual development.

While we don't track miscarriage rates, we do know that miscarriage rates are rising.[264] Every single doctor I asked said they believe rates are going up, including, as previously mentioned, Professor Hugh Taylor, the chair of obstetrics, gynaecology and reproductive sciences at Yale. But it just so happens that in addition to being a medical doctor and obstetrician, Taylor is also a professor of Molecular, Cellular, and Developmental Biology. 'There are so many horrible environmental toxins that I study that would lead to pregnancy loss, that it's hard to believe that it's not really increasing, but we just don't have the same level of assessment that we used to have, so we're comparing apples to oranges.'

Something fishy afoot

In 1974, Gwen Gilson and her husband bought a property in Cootharaba in Queensland. They farmed gladioli and ginger. In 1980, they decided to start farming fish. They registered the fish farming operation in 1981 and focused mainly on Australian native fish. Gilson became one of the biggest farmers of yellow belly, silver perch, saratoga and Australian bass in Queensland and was exporting all over the world, including to Germany.

Gilson claims the problems started when neighbouring farmers started spraying their crops with pesticides and fungicides. 'After the first spraying, all six ponds of breeders died,' says Gilson. 'All my land animals, which previously were so strong and healthy, started aborting their calves and my horses lost their foals.'

By 2005 she says the farmers were using larger spraying rigs and fish started dying more regularly. 'Now not only were the large breeders dying in different ponds from time to time, the fish that did spawn, the newly hatched embryos died en masse.' In 2006, all six ponds of breeders again died after spraying. Gilson got in touch with the Department of Primary Industries, but found 'no help forthcoming'. In 2007 the fish died after each spraying and by 2008 most of Gilson's horses were dead. 'Three of my mares aborted their foals, the chickens hatched with their bowels outside their bodies, the pigs went into convulsions and died, my dogs died, the ducks died and the native birds and bees started falling out of the sky after spraying,' she recalls. She also remembers one of her employees lost her first baby when he was born with similar anomalies.

Dr Matt Landos is the director of Future Fisheries Veterinary Service, associate researcher at the University of Sydney's Faculty of Veterinary Science, and also a senior lecturer at Charles Sturt University in the Faculty of Veterinary Science. He investigated the situation at Gwen Gilson's farm in 2008 and contributed to later reports. 'It was a very strange case, because the day of a spray, spontaneously all of her fish died in all of her ponds. The case history reminded me of a scene like seeing a car that's all crumpled up on a highway and one person dead. They might have jumped out in front of the car before it hit the truck, they might have had a heart attack, but probably they died in the car accident. There was a lot of compelling circumstantial evidence. However, this was far from an isolated incident at the farm. Multiple years of observations, images and case reports all pointed to the same problem of chemical spray drift impacting fish reproduction and development.'

The use of pesticides and fungicides continued. Local and inter-national media wrote extensively about the situation, but no action was taken. Dr Landos contacted the state government, deeply concerned. 'I became more involved in investigating the case, contacted the department myself and said, "Look, we do have a problem here, it does appear that it is related to chemicals, what are we going to do about it? Because continuing to do nothing appears not to be an appropriate response." They spoke to me on a couple of occasions, but then ultimately did not actually do anything.'

It was only after pressure from more media and concerned anglers noting the decline of the local wild fishery that the state government was moved to establish the Noosa Fish Health Investigation Taskforce, which included Dr Landos.

In 2007 Biosecurity Queensland sent out their Senior Fish Pathologist Dr Roger Chong, who did most of the fish pathology for seven scientific veterinary reports published as part of the Noosa Fish Health Investigation. Dr Chong worked as a vet for twelve years before moving into fish pathology and aquatic animal health diagnostic laboratory work. He worked for the Hong Kong Agriculture, Fisheries and Conservation Department for four years, then with Biosecurity Queensland for seventeen years. Through that time, he became the only qualified specialist in Aquatic Animal Health in Australia, passing fellowship examinations at the Australian and New Zealand College of Veterinary Scientists. At the time of writing, he was employed by the CSIRO in Aquaculture Research as a Veterinary Aquatic Pathologist.

His 2010 report to the Noosa Fish Health Investigation Taskforce identified six major syndromes among the fish in the Noosa River Catchment, including in the Noosa River Australian bass, Noosa River sea mullet, golden perch and silver perch at Gilson's Sunland Fish Hatchery. One of the key recommendations of the report was an investigation into the use of beta-cyfluthrin, methidathion, nonylphenol, trichlorphon, dichlorvos, methoxyfenozide and carbendazim. These are all veterinary and agricultural chemicals assessed and registered by the Australian Pesticides and Veterinary Medicines Authority (APVMA). A spokesman confirmed to me that, of the chemicals listed in the report, dichlorvos and carbendazim were subjected to reviews that were completed in 2011 and 2012 respectively. The registration of one home garden product containing dichlorvos – which the US Environmental Protection Agency classifies as a probable human carcinogen – was cancelled. Product labels were updated, but the chemical is still used.

In the case of carbendazim, which was already banned for use by home gardeners and for crops including grapes, citrus and stone fruit, it was further restricted for strawberries, pasture, clover and sugar cane. It can still be used for crops like lentils, macadamias and pyrethrum (chrysanthemum).

A review of methidathion was completed in 2019 and its registration was voluntarily cancelled in 2021. There are no products containing methidathion registered for use in Australia at the time of writing, but it is still on the AVMA's approved list as an active constituent. It is banned in the EU and USA.

No other chemicals listed were subject to review.

'Gwen developed cancer. Horses aborted. Dogs had deformed pups with no eyes. We've documented a range of things on the farm that were abnormal: frogs with abnormal-sized legs, dead honeybees, chicken with deformed feet. All these signs can align with pesticide intoxication. During the taskforce we clearly tracked the drift of the organophosphate trichlorfon into the hatchery building, and photo-graphed deformities of the larval fish hearts during development. There was a lot of evidence at that time that toxic spray drift was causing what was going on. And all that was basically swept under the carpet and downplayed by the taskforce's final report. The two dissenting views to the final report, both fish veterinarians, were those two views who had the most expertise in fish health and disease,' says Dr Landos.

'The problem hasn't gone away, in fact it's getting worse. We're seeing serious expansion in the use of agrochemicals on our landscape, ever increasing impact on the health of humans and all of the biota. Insects are disappearing and we are losing prawns from our rivers. It's unquestionably happening.'

So I asked him, why doesn't the government want to act on cases like this and so many others?

'You see there's a massive problem with government and regulators being controlled by fossil fuel interests, addicted to their profits and deeply compromised by their donations and influence. You see it with the response to Covid in the "gas-fired recovery", with the approval of more coal mines, no matter the bushfires and floods. Agrochemicals are an arm of the fossil fuel industry, the petrochemical arm. More use means more demand for fossil fuels which supports evermore extraction. As fossil fuel use in energy is priced out and replaced with renewables, there will be even more pressure to expand petrochemical use – with one of the largest users being industrial agriculture. You see it everywhere in Australia.'

Ironically, a draft Noosa River Plan was launched in 2019 to try to protect the river. It came about after a research project was launched called Bring Back the Fish, which showed there had been a 'dramatic decline' in benthic biodiversity (the small fauna that live on the bottom of the riverbed), the number falling from 9000 individuals from 150 species collected in 1998, to 1114 individuals from 50 species collected in May 2018.[265] This, along with other factors, had also driven a sharp decline in fish stocks in the river.

'The sum of effects from fossil fuel extraction is causing the planet's ecosystems to collapse. You just can't coat the Earth's surface, food and water, in biocides, that had their original conception as weapons for chemical warfare in World War II, and not cause dire health impacts,' he says. 'The war is lost. Our government sold out the future to these fossil fools. I see no sign of a government-turnaround from major party policies, and no cohesive pushback from an ill-informed society at large. It fills me with the deepest sadness to acknowledge: it is over, and a wasteland of anguish is all I can present to my son as a legacy.'

I'm a practical person and I don't like conspiracy theories. No one wants to believe that the world around them is toxic. But these are not crackpot ideas or hypotheses. We are surrounded by chemicals, dangerous chemicals; the degrading and erosion of our environment goes far, far beyond climate change. It's just that we only hear about one particular battlefront in the war.

Something in the air tonight

Just before the onset of the Covid-19 pandemic, Sydney was beset by the worst bushfire season ever recorded in New South Wales. Thick, brown air soup descended on the skyline, looking like a Bruce Willis movie involving meteors and the end of days. Friends who suffered from asthma fled the state and my family cancelled our long-awaited trip to see friends and family, fearing the effect it would have on little lungs. So, as I started to investigate the various environmental chemicals that might have an effect on fertility and fuel increased miscarriage rates, my attention turned to air pollution and bushfire smoke.

I stumbled across two large studies, one from the USA and one from China. They seemed very convincingly to make a link between air pollution or bushfire smoke and miscarriage or adverse pregnancy outcomes.

As I reported in *Guardian Australia*,[266] the study in China made a quantitative association between ambient air pollution exposure and pregnancy loss in the first trimester.[267] The second, an American study conducted in Salt Lake City in Utah, found that a 20 microgram per cubic metre ($\mu g/m^3$) increase in nitrogen dioxide (NO_2) resulted in a 16 per cent increase in risk of miscarriage.[268]

A later study from China published in 2022 also found that there was a link between particulate matter, NO_2 and sulphur dioxide and miscarriage, describing them as 'crucial associations'.[269]

By way of comparison, I approached the New South Wales Department of Planning, Industry and Environment and asked them to provide me with some data around pollution levels during the catastrophic bushfire season of 2019–20. Sydney's CBD during that period experienced a rise in NO_2 levels from $84.6\mu g/m^3$ in winter to $206.8\ \mu g/m^3$ at the bushfire peak. In Parramatta, NO_2 went from $107.16\ \mu g/m^3$ in winter to a high of $131.6\ \mu g/m^3$. These numbers are shocking. But what is even more shocking is that the NSW Department of Health issued no additional guidance for those contemplating getting pregnant or already pregnant over that period. Meanwhile, patients I interviewed who were experiencing obstetric complications were being told by their treating doctors that, anecdotally, they had seen a sharp rise in patients with adverse outcomes during the bushfire event.

It's not just bushfire-affected areas that can be risky for those who are pregnant. One of the most dangerous elements in bushfire smoke (in addition to toxic fumes) is particle matter: PM10s, which are roughly the size of a pollen grain, and PM2.5s, which are a quarter of that again. A study out of Colorado of over half a million pregnancies that were exposed to particulate matter found that exposure was positively associated with preterm birth and decreased birth weight.[270] The scary thing is, particulate matter isn't just in bushfire smoke, it's in 'regular' air pollution too. In fact, medical research has linked low birth weight, preterm birth, stillbirth, poor respiratory outcomes in newborns and children, gestational diabetes, pre-eclampsia and more to air pollution. And one Australian study showed that air pollution rates at busy intersections can be ten times worse than background levels.[271] Particulate matter is also present (along with many other toxic substances) in cigarettes, with smoking consistently being named a risk factor in reproductive issues, including early pregnancy loss.

Tasmanian obstetrician Dr Kristine Barnden assisted the Royal Australian College of Obstetricians and Gynaecologists (RANZCOG) in preparing a submission to the NSW Legislative Council's inquiry, 'Health impacts of exposure to poor levels of air quality resulting from bushfires and drought,' and says not enough information is being given to parents on the risks. She advises people to use apps for air quality and monitor them regularly.

But why is air pollution a risk? How does it affect the body? It starts with DNA methylation. This is the process whereby something alters our DNA and the way it behaves, without changing the sequencing. I interviewed Professor Jeff Craig, a lecturer in medical sciences at Deakin University for my *Guardian Australia* reporting. He studies the role of epigenetics in mediating the effects of early life environment on the risk for chronic disease. Epigenetics is the study of how environmental factors and behaviour changes the way your genes work.

'If you imagine that genes are like musical instruments, epigenetics are like the musicians who play the instruments, because they can't play themselves,' he explained. 'Together, they play the symphony of life on the genes. Epigenetics is literally on top of DNA. And epigenetics, like the musician, controls how the gene works.'[272]

Particle matter can cause changes in DNA methylation and therefore affect placental or fetal development. It also causes inflammation, a very dangerous risk factor in pregnancy.

I also interviewed Professor Sarah Robertson for the same article. She is a biomedical scientist and has worked for thirty years on understanding the immunology of pregnancy and receptivity in maternal tissues. She described pregnancy as the canary in the coal mine; a stress test of societal health. And she says we're in trouble.

'We clearly have got high and increasing rates of infertility, unexplained infertility and unexplained pregnancy loss, and increasing rates of gestational disorders like preterm birth and pre-eclampsia,' she explained, before issuing a warning. 'The future of human health and sustainability as a human race is at stake here and it's not too much to put it like that.'[273]

My feature article about risk to pregnancy from air pollution and bushfire smoke ran on 10 January 2021. On 19 July 2021, just six months later (that's basically overnight in medical terms), RANZCOG, led by Dr Kristine Barnden, issued new patient resources warning of the dangers of air pollution and bushfire smoke to pregnant people and anyone planning to conceive.[274]

Dr Barnden is a member of Doctors for the Environment Australia (DEA), a branch of the Switzerland-based International Society Doctors for the Environment, founded in 1990 with member organisations in thirty-eight countries. The aims of the groups are to publicise the relationship between the environment and human health, as well as encourage environmentally friendly behaviour.

It is now well-accepted that climate change – which would form part of the 'physical' category of environmental factors – is having real and significant impacts on human health. In September 2019, the Australian Medical Association (AMA) issued a statement calling climate change a 'health emergency'. The president at the time, Dr Tony Bartone, said, 'The AMA accepts the scientific evidence on climate change and its impact on human health and human well-being.'[275] Each year more research projects show evidence that rising temperatures can negatively affect fertility.[276] As an additional dimension to this crisis, as argued in an article in the *Medical Journal of Australia*, while the effects of climate change are worse on women, it is more amplified for 'Indigenous women, culturally and linguistically diverse women, women with disabilities, older women, and women with children, thereby also becoming a human rights and justice issue.'[277]

Infection

I won't spend a huge amount of time on infection as we've covered it in the previous chapter, but it's worth pointing out how much we still have to learn in this space.

Malaria, brucellosis, cytomegalovirus, HIV, dengue fever, the flu and bacterial vaginosis have all been associated with a higher risk of miscarriage, while Q fever, adeno-associated virus, bocavirus, hepatitis C and Mycoplasma genitalium infections are thought not to raise the risk profile. There is still more to learn about chlamydia trachomatis, toxoplasma gondii, human papillomavirus, herpes simplex virus, parvovirus B19, hepatitis B and polyomavirus BK infections, with varying study results.[278]

But even if we knew all the facts about individual illnesses, diseases can change, as seen by the evolution and variants throughout the Covid-19 pandemic and historic evolution of diseases like tuberculosis. In an article published in 2021 in *Nature* magazine, the authors suggest that micro-organisms that cause congenital disease have likely evolved to bypass the defence that allows the placenta to restrict vertical transmission during pregnancy.[279] Put in simpler terms, diseases that potentially couldn't pass from mother to child in utero now can. This is an area desperately in need of research and I suspect the reason it has been slow to be conducted is likely due to the fact that many of these diseases occur in less developed countries, which never seem to be a high priority for science.

Tricksy

When we get to behavioural and socio-economic factors and miscarriage risk, we start to get into some very tricky territory. Behavioural factors might include things like stress, drug addiction or domestic violence. Socio-economic factors might include things like nutrition, education or occupation.

In Guatemala, a large 2011 study of 1897 maternity patients presenting to a large tertiary public care hospital were surveyed to assess whether they had experienced intimate partner violence (IPV), either verbal, physical or sexual, or a combination. The findings of the research, adjusted for other factors, was that both physical and sexual IPV has a strong correlation with increased miscarriage risk.[280] But that's not where the story ends.

The study also found that patients experiencing physical violence frequently had low levels of wealth. And higher rates of violence were experienced by those with only a primary education. So here we have other potentially causal factors. If someone is on a lower income or has a lower level of education, they are likely to be at greater risk of not engaging in high quality nutrition, because that's an expensive exercise. They may not have high levels of medical or self-care literacy. They may not know it's advised to take folic acid preconception, and if they do, they may not be able to afford it. This is where multiple risk factors overlap and create a higher risk profile. And while we absolutely have to encourage more research in this area, it can be difficult to separate each input as totally independent of the next.

New Zealand – where around half of pregnancies are unplanned – announced in July 2021 that it would make the addition of folic acid to bread compulsory, in a move it hoped would prevent neural tube defects and also stop hundreds of miscarriages each year, according to the NZ College of Public Health Medicine. Australia moved to require folic acid to be added to bread in 2009, under the Australia New Zealand Food Standards Code. According to the AIHW, Australia saw neural tube defects in the general population fall 14 per cent after its introduction and a decline of 74 per cent among Indigenous women.

Meanwhile, a UK-based study found that there was a reduced risk for miscarriage among patients who ate fresh fruit and vegetables and had vitamin supplementation. Conversely, high alcohol consumption and increased stress levels (particularly highly stressful or traumatic events) elevated risk.[281]

Stress is another important risk factor in pregnancy loss. One study measured 'perceived demands' and corticotrophin-releasing hormone (known as the 'stress hormone', CRH) and found that there were elevated risks of subsequent early pregnancy loss from stress. This was even more pronounced in pregnancies of between four and seven weeks gestation.[282] But study after study has shown that people who find themselves in lower socio-economic groups (lower income or education levels) generally experience higher levels of CRH.

Epigenetic researchers have known for quite some time that stress is a factor in pregnancy loss. But research has come a long way since Negro-Vilar's paper in 1993. We also have known for some time that mental health is intrinsically linked to physical well-being. But it's not just an educated hypothesis now; we have the evidence that PTSD, trauma and significant stress can lead to changes in the way our DNA behaves. Repeated studies show DNA methylation changes in army personnel who have returned from war. They experience immune system and neurotransmission changes (the transmission of nerve impulses).[283]

Physical stress also has to be considered, not just for the carrying parent but for the person providing the sperm. An American study found a correlation between lower semen concentration or total sperm count and work-related heavy exertion, which is much more likely to be experienced in the field of manual labour, a lower-income profession.[284]

And so we find ourselves circling back to a Venn diagram of intersecting risk factors.

This isn't sci-fi

When you consider dystopian futures portrayed in novels, film or TV, infertility or reproductive challenges play a prominent role. Think of Margaret Atwood's *The Handmaid's Tale* or *The Children of Men* by P.D. James. The truth is that some of these realities are not as far away as we would like to believe.

Professor of Environmental Medicine and Public Health Shanna Swan works at the Mount Sinai School of Medicine in New York. In 2017 she co-authored a paper that showed sperm counts in the West had plummeted by 59 per cent between 1973 and 2011.[285] Her book *Count Down* was released in 2001 and predicted that by 2045 most couples would need assisted reproduction. Mark Green also points out that, in Australia, the number of rounds of IVF undertaken each year is rising by 2 to 3 per cent annually.

When Professor Swan was asked whether the patterns in her research could be attributed to social factors like patients conceiving later in life, she told the *Guardian* in 2001 it was 'not that simple'.

'When a colleague and I looked at the change in impaired fecundity [the ability to have children] we were surprised to see younger women had experienced a bigger increase than older age groups. This suggests that something besides ageing and delayed childbearing is affecting fertility. Moreover, there's compelling evidence that the risk of miscarriage has been rising among women of all ages.'[286]

There is little doubt that environmental factors are affecting fertility. So why aren't we talking about it as a matter of urgency? There are many reasons that environmental toxicity is roundly ignored by most of the general public, but I personally believe it's because it's terrifying. Sometimes it's easier to just stick your head in the sand and ignore the nightmares that haunt our sleep and keep us staring at the ceiling all night.

As Swan says, 'I am not saying other factors aren't involved. But I am saying chemicals play a major causal role. It is difficult to use that word, "cause", but it's a body of evidence. We have mechanisms, animal studies, and multiple human studies.'

This threat is real and cannot be ignored. In the words of Mohawk midwife, environmentalist, Native American rights activist, and women's health advocate Katsi Cook, 'Women are the first environment. We are privileged to be the doorway to life. At the breast of women, the generations are nourished and sustained. From the bodies of women flow the relationship of those generations both to society and to the natural world. In this way is the Earth our mother, the old people said. In this way, we as women are Earth.'[287]

Happy endings

But here's the good news. While we cannot control all the negative inputs that we're exposed to that may affect our health, there are ways to mitigate the worst of the risks. And that comes in the form of education.

Your Fertility is a coalition set up by five organisations: the Victorian Assisted Reproductive Treatment Authority (VARTA), Healthy Male, Jean Hailes for Women's Health, Global and Women's Health at Monash University and The Robinson Research Institute at the University of Adelaide. Together they launched a website that has an entire section on the effects of environmental chemicals and fertility.[288] Some of the advice includes: wash fruit and veg thoroughly to remove any traces of pesticides or fungicides; avoid using heavily perfumed products; avoid additives, preservatives and anti-bacterial agents; eat less canned and pre-packaged food; avoid plastic wrappings and cling wrap; use glass or ceramics instead of plastic (especially in the microwave) and don't use cosmetics that use parabens.

All of these things sound relatively straightforward. But they're not for people on a low income. Nor is avoiding stress, domestic abuse or some of the other behavioural environmental factors we've discussed. All we need for that is income equality, the erasure of entrenched structural racism, abolishment of disability and gender discrimination, among a few other minor things.

Trust in Me

What is trust? The dictionary says it's assured reliance on something or a thing in which we have confidence. Despite being the sort of person who always plans for the worst-case scenario in life, I was lucky enough for a long time to have a fundamental and inherent trust that things were going to work out okay. I know the exact date that trust began to erode: 7 October 2017. I was thirty-seven years, eleven months and one day old. It was the start of my third miscarriage.

But it wasn't wholesale, immediate erasure of trust in whatever it is you choose to call kismet; faith, g-d or divine intervention. Each loss represented a gradual picking away at the foundation of who I was and my experience of life. The idea that, in the end, one way or another, everything would work out fine. The notion that challenges are just speedbumps that need to be navigated. Not dead-end streets that you can't escape.

When I met my husband, we had so much in common. But we also had some intrinsic, complementary differences in perspective and outlook. I was always in a rush. He was always relaxed. And despite all the challenges he faced as a young Aboriginal man growing up in the colony, he still had faith in things working out for the best or finding a way through the dead-end streets. I leaned into that warmth and assurance. When I was anxious, he would lie next to me at night with his arms around me and tell me that everything was going to be okay. And I allowed myself to truly trust and believe it. And for a long time, it was true.

Until it wasn't.

With each loss, the trust crumbled away. At first it was just around the edges, then it went a little deeper, a little further. My nugget of trust got smaller with each passing heartbreak, each injection of grief.

It wasn't just trust in the universe. It was multi-faceted, multi-dimensional, permeating every aspect of my existence. Trust in my body. My body's ability to do its job. Trust that my babies would keep growing when I begged them to. Trust in my plans for the future. Trust in my husband's promises that everything would be okay one way or another; the promises that let me lay my head down and sleep through the night. Even trust that he would stick around to keep making those promises to me.

That core belief, in all its forms, shrank to a point where I couldn't find it anymore, even when I turned my soul inside out. The shallow waters of my anxiety started to rise. They started to flood my brain, soaking everything to the core. My mind, my body, my plans, my relationships. I expended every ounce of mental stamina to sandbag those waters and stop my thoughts from drowning me. It was a labour I didn't want, I didn't ask for, but dogged me every second of every day.

This isn't something I can fix. There is no tablet, no antibiotic, no surgery to make me into a believer again. This painful, fundamental shift in my core belief system and the way I see the world is here forever. It changed the tint of my lenses. And that is the ultimate cost of my journey.

Would I pay the price again for a second living child?

In.

A.

Heartbeat.

||||||||||||||||||||||||||||||||||||||||||||||||||||||||||||||||||||||||||||||||||||||||||||||||||||||||||||||

15

Video Killed the Radio Star

Technology. Is it friend or is it foe? Well, a little from column a, a little from column b.

Nothing epitomises the concept of a double-edged sword quite like technology. It has brought improvements to every aspect of our lives, but immense challenges too. Nowhere is this more true than in the area of fertility, reproduction and loss. Is it friend or is it foe? The answer is a little from column a and a little from column b. As Professor Lesley Regan told me, 'When you push boundaries, there's usually some payback somewhere.'

It would be impossible to look at every single technology or technological development and its pros and cons, so consider this a highlights reel.

We've already examined how the advent of better ultrasound technology and high-sensitivity, early pregnancy tests have contributed to fetal personhood and the subsequent ramifications in terms of grief and mourning. Losses that might otherwise have flown under the radar as heavy periods are now identified early and, in many cases, mourned deeply. So what are the benefits? Scans are now able to pick up a raft of both minor and serious complications at increasingly earlier stages. We're living in an era where some of these can even be remedied with surgery while the fetus is still in utero. Examples would include congenital heart defects, spina bifida, congenital diaphragmatic hernia and several conditions that affect twins. In the case of early sensitivity pregnancy tests, it allows for earlier intervention with supportive measures in high-risk pregnancy, for example administering progesterone or putting a stitch in the cervix, known as cerclage.

An extension of the at-home pregnancy test is the home ovulation kit. For those conceiving at home – whether via a turkey baster or the horizontal mambo – these are incredibly useful for knowing the optimal time for insemination (how sexy is that?). However, they mask the fact that patients with vaginas simply don't know enough about their own bodies and sexual reproduction equipment and phases (for example, ovulation). And with the technology freely available at the chemist, there's no need for us to get to know the various phases of our cycle, right? Wrong.

Power in knowledge

In 2016, ABC TV's *Four Corners* did a story entitled 'The Baby Business', examining the IVF industry. For the story, they interviewed Adelaide University's Professor Rob Norman (a leading researcher in reproductive and periconceptual medicine). He told the show that many patients undergoing IVF, well, shouldn't be. It was an astonishing statement from a man who was involved in using many of the most important developments in this area of medicine, including ICSI (Intracytoplasmic Sperm Injection, or the injection of a single sperm into an egg to overcome male infertility), pre-implantation genetic diagnosis, lifestyle programs and the development of many drugs. 'My estimate is, probably 40 to 50 per cent of people will get pregnant without IVF,' he told *Four Corners*. 'And that is by understanding their fertility window, by tracking their cycle properly, by losing weight and exercising, or having ovulation induction.'[289] Some would say this is borne out by statistics showing that one in six couples who have IVF fall pregnant spontaneously afterwards.[290]

Interestingly, when Newcastle's Hunter Medical Research Institute announced nineteen new research programs in April 2021, their new Infertility and Reproduction Research Program was on the list. It was described as 'Working to resolve the precise physical and chemical nature of what impairs human fertility and offspring health, then developing appropriate diagnostic and therapeutic measures to improve the safety and efficacy of assisted reproductive technologies (ART) and eventually do without them.'

I interviewed one of the program's researchers, Dr John Schjenken, about why they had positioned their research in this way. He emphasised that ARTs are an incredibly important part of society and give many couples the opportunity to give birth when they otherwise would not have that opportunity. 'It comes back to fundamental knowledge that we want to keep advancing and if we can develop therapeutics, interventions that will actually allow these people to conceive naturally, that would be a great step forward.'

When I tracked Professor Norman down in 2021, he also maintained that IVF is, of course, beneficial for some couples, but much can be done to encourage conception without resorting to expensive, invasive procedures. 'I'm a great believer in reproductive planning; people make all sorts of educational plans, financial plans and so on,' he explained. 'But we don't do reproductive planning.' He went on later to say, 'Most people think preconception care is going to your doctor and saying, "I'm trying to get pregnant tonight, what do I need to do to prepare for it?" Whereas, in fact, we need to think years ahead about it. A lot of that can come from education; I think we need to think how we build things. If we can do sex education in school, we need to do reproductive education.'

There have been some small shifts in this regard, with the federal government bowing to community pressure in 2022 and announcing that, from 2023, preconception genetic carrier screening would be free to access in Australia. We'll have to wait and see how that is implemented and what take-up rates eventuate.

Circling back to ovulation testing kits, the electronic version has come a long way from the old-style ten-step urine dipstick and line version. It certainly leaves less margin for error in terms of result-reading. If you can afford an electronic kit that is, because they certainly don't come cheap. And while they might seem like a good idea (and they absolutely can be a good idea in some instances), they are no replacement for understanding how your reproductive system works. For instance, they're useless if you have hormone issues like polycystic ovary syndrome (PCOS), because they can give false-positives.

So if understanding our reproductive systems is one of the ways forward that might spare us from invasive and financially crippling interventions, where to from here? Rob Norman believes more training for GPs is part of the solution. 'The vast majority of doctors are not particularly interested in reproductive issues. They may have to be prepared to do a cervical smear and give advice on contraception, but I think we probably need to get more development for GPs with a special interest in reproduction and fertility,' he explains. 'At the moment, the poor female GPs get dumped with the cervical tests and all that, because no one else wants to do it. But we really need to build that up into a discipline where you're honoured, rather than dishonoured, by having to do all that.'

Having navigated the infertility space, I feel strongly that there is a gap in the treatment chain for people who are struggling to conceive or people who are trying again after miscarriage. 'Fertility specialists' in Australia are IVF doctors and many (but not all) do have a bias to get as many patients as possible onto the IVF conveyer belt. There are very few fertility specialists who work on supporting parents to give themselves the best chance of natural conception, where appropriate.

Given we've already established that GPs carving out more time to complete additional training can be incredibly difficult, I have an alternative. A more realistic solution might be in training nurses or midwives to be fertility educators, in the same way nurses or dieticians do an additional qualification to be able to work as diabetes educators. Wouldn't that be a thing?

Telling it like it is (or not)

One of the aspects I find most troubling about IVF is the way it is promoted in peer-to-peer situations as a 'fail-safe method to get yourself a baby', either in the case of pregnancy after miscarriage or difficulty conceiving. But IVF is not an easy way out of anything. It is physically and mentally gruelling, horrifyingly expensive and, if anything, comes with a slightly elevated miscarriage risk.[291] Industry regulation of the sector is lacking and has been for years, much to the consternation of health advocates.

'It is not regulated in the way it needs to be; different countries are at different speeds on this and even within countries, different states and even within that, different doctors within the same clinic, there are different approaches,' explains Mark Green, the Deputy Scientific Director of Monash IVF Victoria.

Professor Georgina Chambers is the Director of the National Perinatal Epidemiology and Statistics Unit, a joint unit of the Centre for Big Data Research in Health and the School of Women's and Children's Health at the University of New South Wales. She is part of the team that developed a website called YourIVFSuccess.com.au, which has an IVF success rate calculator, based on information provided by a user.

I did a little experiment using the site, calculating my chances of having a baby using IVF when I was thirty-eight. My likelihood of success was just 29 per cent. When I upped my age to thirty-nine, it went down to 23 per cent. In fact, Professor Chambers told me when we met in Sydney, when the website was launched, the developers and scientists received complaints, because users found the low likelihoods of successful conception 'too confronting'.

The IVF industry has long been accused of not being transparent around success rates, which can be extremely low. 'The publicity around IVF is very misleading,' says UK-based Professor Robert Winston, probably one of the most famous doctors in the world. 'The impression is that it's a really successful treatment, but actually the European global figures, if you take the whole of Europe including Britain, you can see that after six cycles of IVF treatment, only 44 per cent of patients have had a live baby. That is not the impression that is given to the public.'[292]

In the UK, the average age of patients freezing their eggs is thirty-eight and the success rate in terms of live births is just 18 per cent.[293] The younger the egg, the better it freezes and the more likely a positive outcome. By younger, I mean under thirty.

There is also controversy over expensive IVF add-ons, such as endometrial scratching, which claims to create better receptivity to implantation (now known to be hokum) and PGT-A, which is pre-implantation genetic testing for aneuploidy, where embryos are tested before being implanted to ensure they have the right number of chromosomes. That doesn't mean the remaining embryos are sure not to miscarry, just that the ones that will supposedly miscarry are not implanted. There is also speculation that the PGT-A may inadvertently exclude or damage healthy embryos. As I type, at least one class action is being prepared in Australia, claiming that PGT-A is not effective,[294] and similar cases have been or are running overseas.[295]

The power disparity between patient and treating doctor, which I've touched on previously, means that it is incredibly important that all treatments, including add-ons, be explained in detail and that medical evidence supporting their use – or lack thereof – also be included. Presenting something as simply 'advised' is not enough to enable patients to make informed, empowered decisions. In fact, it undermines patients' autonomy and is, in some cases, actively negligent. This is even more applicable in situations where patients do not have the ability to do their own research due to language barriers, lack of access, education, time constraints or a number of other factors.

Professor Karin Hammarberg is a Senior Research Fellow at Monash University's School of Public Health and Preventive Medicine and a

Senior Research Officer with the Victorian Assisted Reproductive Treatment Authority. She conducted a study that surveyed 1590 patients about IVF add-ons: PGT-A, heparin, aspirin, Chinese medicine and acupuncture. A staggering 82 per cent had opted for one or more add-ons. 'However, IVF add-ons are not supported by high-quality evidence of safety and effectiveness, and may potentially pose risk to patients,' the study reported.[296] Another study that Professor Hammarberg worked on showed that there is 'widespread advertising of add-ons on IVF clinic websites, which report benefits for add-ons that are not supported by high-quality evidence'.[297] PGT-A costs around $800 per embryo on top of the already prohibitive costs of IVF.

IVF has long been criticised for the highly commercial nature of the business, its opacity around success rates and lapses in care and quality control in the quest for higher profit. But all it takes is for one patient using IVF with PGT-A to have success in pregnancy subsequent to miscarriage to proselytise for the treatment. Word then spreads like wildfire among their peers and any support groups in which they are active. Patients are unlikely to get any balanced view of the add-ons from the clinics themselves, or indeed on IVF, with clinicians under the pump to bring in big bucks.

I don't believe any medical treatment should be a for-profit industry. In the first instance it creates a glaring inequality between the people who can and can't afford to access the services. However I also think treatments that capitalise on the grief and desperation of patients to become parents is a dangerous status quo. These are patients who are oftentimes scared and desperate, willing to try anything if they think there's a chance it will help them become parents or avoid a (or another) loss.

But hey, don't take my word it, take it from Professor Hammarberg. 'It's a wonderful technology and it has its place, but there is the potential for exploitation, because specifically in this corporatised scenario, and we're moving more and more into that,' she explains, 'these are shareholder-owned companies, many of them, and their number one priority is to make money for their shareholders, but the patients' welfare should be number one.'

The need for speed

When someone experiences a pregnancy loss, often they want to know why. To be able to provide answers, you need to be able to get some of their fetal tissue so you can run tests. It won't necessarily have all the answers, but it's a good place to start. When a patient is given the all-too-common refrain of, 'Sorry, it was probably a chromosomal abnormality, but we don't really know, just try again,' the lack of answers can be overwhelming and cause a heavy psychological burden.

Many doctors argue that we need to be testing earlier and more frequently, both for physiological and mental health reasons.

'We don't send the miscarriage for genetic testing until after a second or third loss, which, when you think about it, is cruel to the woman going through the loss, because we know that they will probably be blaming themselves, even if we tell them that it was probably genetically abnormal,' explains Dr Zev Williams, an Associate Professor of Women's Health and the Chief of the Division of Reproductive Endocrinology and Infertility at Columbia University Irving Medical Center in New York. 'If it was genetically abnormal it gives a sense of closure to the woman and a sense of hope to the next pregnancy. If it was normal, it prompts us to do an investigation much sooner.'

Throughout her book *Miscarriage*, Professor Lesley Regan reiterates the importance of testing tissue. 'The most useful way forward is to ensure that any future pregnancy that miscarries is analysed genetically. Knowledge of the chromosomal makeup of the baby will provide you and your doctors with information that will make important contributions to your medical management. It is also likely to be a source of comfort to you and your partner.'[298]

The problems start with the collection of the tissue. If the patient has a D&C, the sample is much more easily obtained, but if they have a 'natural' or medically induced loss, more often than not the sample ends up being flushed down the toilet. Even if you are successful in collection, how should they be stored? Many patients simply aren't empowered to do it.

Not all technological developments have to be high tech. In order to overcome the issue of sample collection, Dr Zev Williams and his team altered a simple, widely available plastic toilet collection device. They put holes in the bottom to create a sort of sieve and distributed them with a storage container for the sample. A pilot study compared the tissue collected by nineteen patients at home to thirty-nine patients who had surgery and the DNA yield and integrity were similar. Participants in home collection also reported a 'high comfort level with the kit and the process of tissue collection'.[299] The kit is so low cost (which was part of the objective) that Dr Williams is able to distribute them to his patients for free.

The next problem though is that the technology used to test fetal samples is old, slow and expensive. 'Seven or eight years ago, we became familiar with nanopore-based DNA sequencing,' Dr Williams explains. 'What enticed me about it was that it was 15,000 times faster than traditional sequencing.'

The device Dr Williams has been testing is called the MinION and it is made by a company called Oxford Nanopore. It is about the size of a small stapler. The company was not marketing the product for clinical usage at the time of writing, but indicated to me that it intends to. Dr Williams says the device allows him to get karyotyping results (a full set of chromosomes) in around two hours and at a much more reduced cost of US$199.

But what if we could do the test without any fetal tissue at all?

It's in our DNA

When we have NIPT tests, the substance it screens is called cell-free DNA (cfDNA) and it's in our bloodstream. In 2020, in a study funded through Tommy's National Centre for Miscarriage Research, researchers tested cfDNA to see if a cause of miscarriage could be obtained in the absence of a sample of the pregnancy tissue. While there is more research needed, the simple answer is: yes, it can.

The study correctly identified 75 per cent of results. 'In conclusion, cfDNA can be used to detect chromosomal abnormalities in miscarriages where the "fetal fraction" [fetal DNA] is high enough; however, more studies are required to identify variables that can affect the overall results.'[300]

That same cfDNA screening technology was used in a study that showed blood from sanitary pads in the emergency room could be tested for alpha-fetoprotein (AFP are proteins produced by a fetus's liver). High levels of AFP in vaginal blood can assist in same-day detection of an active miscarriage,[301] possibly reducing the need for an ultrasound technician in the emergency department after hours.

A member of the team that conducted that study was Yale University Professor of Obstetrics, Gynaecology, and Reproductive Sciences and Professor of Molecular, Cellular, and Developmental Biology, Dr Hugh Taylor. He was awarded a grant of $8 million in 2021 to investigate whether genetic variation can result in multiple miscarriage. Or put in layman's terms, Dr Taylor and his team are going on a hunt for the miscarriage gene(s).

'For losses that are unexplainable, we're going to do whole genome sequencing,' Dr Taylor explains. 'We will screen the mother, the father and the loss and try and see if we can find something either inheritable, or that's different in that fetus that led to the loss. The idea is, once we have candidate genes . . . we'll test them in animal or cellular models to see if they really lead to developmental abnormalities in pregnancy loss.'

Taylor says developments in large-scale gene sequencing means that this is the sort of study that can now be undertaken. 'We've never really had a way to look until the last several years; we can start to look at every chain and look for sub mutations, rather than big chromosomal shifts.'

Knowledge at what cost?

Associate Professor Mark Green points out that while it can be useful to be able to offer fast-turnaround, low-cost genetic testing, this can come with ethical conundrums.

'There are lots of new technologies that are coming out making it more affordable and identifying more genes. But the problem is, what do non-experts do with that information? Because by definition, you're going to have some sort of gene abnormality – there's hundreds of thousands of genes – but how much stress does that cause? Do people know what the context is when they get that sort of information? That's what a lot of people are concerned about; just because the technology is there, is there an ability for people to understand this information in context and not panic?'

Material girl

There are many sociological, anthropological and historical studies into how pregnancy, childbearing and motherhood became so consumerised. But really, are we surprised? There's no aspect of modern life that hasn't been turned into a potential cash-generator. Advertisements for plastic toys and fast food specifically target children and pharmaceutical drugs are marketed like candy. It tells you all you need to know about the sort of world we live in. Nothing is safe.

Shopping is now a core part of the experience of impending parenthood and pregnancy. Sometimes during gestation there can be multiple events in order to allow gifting for both mother and child, a process that is repeated once the baby arrives. It's an expensive and extremely lucrative business.

Information is also in hot demand, with books, websites, forums and of course apps. There are thousands of phone apps relating to pregnancy, fertility and reproduction. They have extraordinarily high take-up in developed countries, though the information provision is totally unregulated. One study of pregnancy exercise apps found few aligned with 'current evidence-based physical activity guidelines'.[302] Another study found that users were 'not actively assessing the validity of the content of these apps or considering issues concerning the security and privacy of the personal information about themselves and their children that these apps collect'.[303]

Once you sign up to apps (or mailing lists, newsletters or online forums), they send you electronic notifications about every single aspect of your pregnancy – hourly, daily, weekly, monthly. They track your movements online and start serving you ads for pregnancy wear, baby clothes or toys. You can sync them with your calendar so that you have hundreds of alerts about when your baby is entering a leap or developing a new body part or skill. Sometimes they extend years into the future.

So what happens when the pregnancy ends in loss? How do you extricate yourself so the sucker punches stop coming when you're the in midst of your grief? Well, in most cases, you can't. Calendar events have been scheduled and you have to sort through your entire calendar two years into the future to delete them individually. Email addresses have been shared with retailers, so you start getting discount offers or special deals. When you want to log a new pregnancy, some apps simply don't understand why . . . you can't start a new pregnancy log if the old pregnancy is still going, right?

And if you have a smartphone, you'll notice changes in the algorithms that serve you content, especially advertising, on social media and other platforms. Suddenly, all the ads you're being served are for maternity wear or prams, onesies or nursery decorations, reminding you relentlessly about the baby you're not going to have.

Lara Freidenfelds also argues that constant updates about what's going on in your body, when in fact you may be on a path to loss, can be very confusing for the end user. 'The twenty-first century has seen the rise of websites, pregnancy apps and regimens of self-care and education that mandate heightened attention, early emotional investment and round-the-clock concern,' she writes. 'Although more medical attention to pregnancy has no doubt saved the lives of many women and children, and enhanced the health of many more, the current state of intensive monitoring has also encouraged women and their partners to become highly invested in early pregnancies destined to fail. Too often it has given women a false sense of control over the outcomes of pregnancies that cannot come to fruition, no matter how conscientiously a woman cares for her expected child.'[304]

While the apps and other similar services have extremely high take-up, issues have also been identified in their lack of accessibility for non-English speakers. One study found that women from culturally and linguistically diverse backgrounds, low incomes or who are unemployed have a much lower uptake of digital pregnancy resources. 'This suggests that the existing pregnancy and early childhood parenting apps available in the market may not be meeting the demands of these population groups.'[305]

So what's the fix then? I don't expect that any app developers or retailers want to willingly expend time or energy caring for the welfare of the people who sign up to these services. It would be great if app developers, advocates and health peak bodies combined their efforts to ensure that apps and other online pregnancy services meet certain quality standards, both in terms of quality of the information provided, privacy, and referrals to support services and the ability to extricate yourself in the case of loss.

The man

When I asked Associate Professor Mark Green whether there were any developments that he'd like to see in this space, he didn't miss a beat. 'I'd say at the moment, there's still probably too much emphasis on just the female side, very little emphasis on the male side; people need to wake up to it being 50 per cent of the equation.' Yep. The patriarchy strikes again.

He explains that we really haven't explored how we handle sperm very well. 'That's really been untouched since we started IVF forty years ago. Something I was looking at was different ways of processing sperm. We know a lot of male patients have DNA damage, they have problems with their sperm, yet we put them through these very archaic ways of processing the sperm that actually make it worse.'

Recent research showed that sperm fragmentation may be responsible for up to one third of miscarriages, and interventions such as sperm selection using hyaluronic acid before ICSI can improve live birth outcomes and reduce miscarriages.[306] Additionally, research from Wollongong-based IVF doctor, David Greening, released back in 2007, showed that ejaculating daily can decrease sperm fragmentation, a conclusion I'm sure will please many.

The good news is that if there is a sharpening of the focus on the contribution that men's physiology makes to miscarriage and other adverse pregnancy outcomes, it's sure to get more funding.

Right?

The Way I Are

I don't know why I had my septum pierced when I was forty-one. I think perhaps I'd finally made a decision to throw off the conservative shackles I'd felt bound by, working in large, formal newsrooms. My first and most enduring beat was business and finance and you weren't going to get far with the suited and booted crowd if you didn't fit in.

Either way, by the time I was forty-one, I'd shaved half my head, my body was covered in tattoos and I'd just had my septum pierced.

A couple of days after the piercing was done, I had an important interview. Apparently no one had told the kid who woke me up with a swift kick to the face. It was so hard I saw stars and my eyes took a good few minutes to relocate their focus. Good morning to you too, pumpkin.

The interview was with a highly regarded doctor who a few people had said was someone worth chatting to. She was extremely accomplished, super smart and had a special interest in miscarriage and pregnancy loss.

It was a 25-minute or so walk from our hotel down to her office. Masks weren't yet compulsory where I was visiting, unlike in Melbourne, so I walked along through the crisp May sunshine, enjoying the vitamin D being able to access my chin for the first time in a while. People stared at me as I walked down the street – probably because of my new piercing and my happy, laissez-faire air as I walked joyfully down that sunny street.

I found the building and I couldn't remember the last time I'd been to such a fancy place. They had lifts! I stepped inside and my own reflection greeted me, but as I stared back at myself, I blanched under the blood spatters covering the entire lower part of my face. It went from just above my nostrils all the way down to my chin. I looked like someone had punched me. Oh wait. The memory of a tiny little foot hurtling towards my face came roaring back to me, along with the whisper of a toddler's giggle.

I reached into my pocket and grabbed a mask, put it on, walked straight into reception, explained I was there for a meeting, but needed to use the ladies room. I spent a good ten minutes mopping up my face and came back into the reception area just as the good doctor had come out of her office to meet me.

With the most phenomenal sunshine-drenched cityscape acting as a backdrop to our conversation through her huge office windows, she told me her life story. She was accomplished, intelligent, professional and so impressive. She was sassy. And so funny. We talked about miscarriage and loss and IVF. We discussed my own history of loss and the lack of answers provided by any of the testing I underwent. But as I listened to her accent, I found my mind wandering, wondering when I'd be able to travel overseas again and show my kids the world.

Suddenly, I was jolted out of my reverie, by something she said.

'I think you have a problem in your quality control.'

My head snapped up from my notebook.

It wasn't the first time someone had suggested this as a possible reason for my multiple miscarriages. An 'overly receptive uterus' is how one doctor had phrased it. It means that while other uteruses decline to implant something not quite right, my uterus lets anything implant, leading to a pregnancy rate of 10/10 but a miscarriage rate of 7/9.

'I don't want to slut-shame your uterus. But I think you have a slutty uterus.'

I paused briefly and then I threw my head back and I laughed. I laughed so hard I felt tears forming in my eyes and my bloodied nose started to throb.

A slutty uterus.

Through my belly laughs I wheezed, 'How soon can I get it printed on a t-shirt?'

Hi, my name's Isy and I have a slutty uterus.

||||||||||||||||||||||||||||||||||||||||||||||||||||||||||||||||||||||||||||||||||||||||||||||||||||||||||||||||

16

Try Again

Shakespeare might not have written it this way, but whether to keep going or give up, that is the actual question.

Whether someone has one miscarriage or five, a subsequent pregnancy or just the prospect of it can be downright terrifying. How do I make it through each day when each day feels like a century? What are the chances I'll have another loss? What are the chances I won't? When do I start trying again? And the last and most confronting question of all: how do I know when it's time to stop?

Let's assume in the first instance that you have decided to try again. Many patients describe a 'yearning' or a 'desperation' for another child after experiencing early pregnancy loss. I remember acutely the feeling that every single person around me was pregnant, they were all gloating about their beautiful, big, round bellies and laughing at me through their pity. Such was my intense desire to be pregnant again and have another child. Loss is one thing, but a grief fuelled by hormones can be intense.

If you've seen the worst that pregnancy has to offer, it's entirely reasonable to fear it will happen again. This is why there is often a mission to 'do things differently' or 'try something new', even though, as we know, the results may be beyond our control. The loss of innocence in subsequent pregnancy, an inability to just enjoy the idea that 'everything will work out fine' can be incredibly painful and challenging, to say the least.

When to get going?

A miscarriage is similar to menstruation in the sense that its ultimate goal is to clear the contents of the uterus. The difference is that there are more contents to clear: the pregnancy tissue, as well as the thicker uterine lining. But the two ultimately have the same function, which is to clear the decks.

Barring any complicating factors such as, for instance, the identification of genetic abnormalities or clotting issues that would require additional medical interventions, physiologically the first and most important box you need to tick is that your miscarriage is complete and there are no signs of infection. That means either your hCG is at zero, your scans are clear or, in the case of a D&C, your treating doctor has given you clearance to try again. Once you have that, you can move onto the next stage, which is timing.

Two important studies show there may be an advantage to trying sooner, rather than later. The first was a literature review published in *Human Reproduction*, which showed that waiting less than six months after miscarriage to try again resulted in 'significantly reduced' risk of both further early pregnancy loss and preterm delivery.[307] This contradicted World Health Organization guidelines, which at the time the study was published in 2016 recommended waiting at least six months to try again after early pregnancy loss. When I contacted the WHO to ask for their more updated guidelines, a spokesman told me they haven't been updated since 2005. 'This recommendation and the underlying evidence is outdated and has not been used in more recent publications.' The spokesman was at pains to point out that the organisation is 'undertaking research into clinical management of miscarriage and their prevention, as well as impacts of Covid-19 infections on miscarriages'. It's seriously disappointing the guidelines haven't been updated, more than seventeen years after they were first published. Many clinicians, especially in developing countries, rely on this guidance for their medical practice.

Another study published in 2017 looked at 514 patients in North Carolina, Tennessee and Texas who had experienced miscarriage as their most recent pregnancy outcome. The research showed that, irrespective of race or previous pregnancies, an interval of less than three months after miscarriage was 'associated with the lowest risk of subsequent miscarriage'. They added that 'this implies counselling women to delay conception to reduce risk of miscarriage may not be warranted'.[308]

You might remember that I was recommended to delay conception for two menstrual cycles after my first loss. And this research begs the question why. The answer is simple: no pregnancy outcome is ever assured. Even if you've lived through one loss, it doesn't mean you're prepared for another. Before you try again, you have to be ready for whatever might happen. So no matter what the statistics say in terms of physical outcomes, there's no point rushing in unless you're mentally ready for another pregnancy and all that entails.

Time has to be taken to ensure you have the right supports around you; whether that is medical professionals, family or friends.

Likelihood of success

The data around the statistical likelihood of carrying a pregnancy to term after miscarriage is nothing like what you'd expect. It's actually exceptionally positive. It's baffling that medical professionals, including GPs, midwives and obstetricians, do not make this information more publicly available or understood. That's not to say that none do, of course. Just that it's not broadly understood or known among the general population. If this was to shift, it wouldn't just encourage patients to try again, but also help them emotionally prepare for a subsequent pregnancy, if they choose to try for one, with a more optimistic or hopeful lens through which to look.

So here is the data. After one miscarriage, there is absolutely no reason to think your next pregnancy will not be successful, and that's why doctors are so eager to encourage patients to 'just try again'. But surprisingly, even after multiple miscarriage, odds are likely that if you can conceive you will have a pregnancy resulting in a live birth, though it is important to note that these statistical likelihoods do decrease sharply with age.

For 'idiopathic' miscarriage, meaning losses with 'no apparent cause', at the age of twenty, even after two miscarriages, your likelihood of success in a subsequent pregnancy is 92 per cent. That comes down to 89 per cent at twenty-five, 84 per cent at thirty, 77 per cent at thirty-five, 69 per cent at forty and 60 per cent at forty-five.[309] Let me clarify: even at forty-five years of age and having had two miscarriages, there's a better than 2 in 1 chance that you will have a successful live birth.

Those stats decline, but stay higher than I think many would expect, even as the number of previous miscarriages and ages increase. At the other end of the spectrum, even after five idiopathic miscarriages, your likelihood of a successful pregnancy at twenty is still around 85 per cent. Again, it comes down with age, but remains surprisingly high; 79 per cent at twenty-five, 71 per cent at thirty, 62 per cent at thirty-five, 52 per cent at forty-two and 42 per cent at forty-five.[310]

And those odds, all things considered, really ain't bad.

Gettin' jiggy

Sex after loss can be incredibly challenging. Or it can be just what you need. There is no right answer. In terms of trying again, conception through sexual intercourse can be a very different ballgame when one or both partners are mourning a loss. One or both partners might not even have a sex drive, which can be dampened by fear, anxiety or depression. The birth partner can also be experiencing a degree of dissociation from or distrust in their body, due to a (misplaced) feeling that it may have 'failed them' in a previous pregnancy.

It's important, no matter how much you want another pregnancy, to take the time to prepare yourself physiologically and psychologically for two main reasons. The first is that you want to give yourself the best likelihood of success. Take the time to educate yourself about reproductive health, the way our reproductive systems work, as this can be invaluable. The second reason is that while statistics alone show that pregnancy after miscarriage is likely to be successful, you have to be prepared to weather another loss. Because no pregnancy comes with any sort of guarantee. Ever.

The sometimes overwhelming desire to be pregnant again can lead to a situation where sex becomes a duty or a transaction, rather than fun. Herein lies my first piece of solid advice: if you are planning to conceive a subsequent pregnancy with sex, make sure you have fun. Do whatever you need to do; invest in some sexy lingerie, buy some sex toys, suggest that position you've never done before that your partner has always wanted to (but maybe not anal, because that sort of defeats the purpose) and get busy.

If you're planning to conceive using IVF, IUI or a turkey baster, the same rules apply. Take a breath, practice self-care and make sure you're really ready before the process kicks off.

Try a little tenderness

Professor Lesley Regan is not just an exceptional clinician, she is probably one of the best health researchers in the world. Every aspect of her clinical approach is based on science and tangible evidence, as well as her years of experience in treating patients. She also has a great degree of compassion and empathy for those who live through loss. But I have to admit, I was somewhat surprised when I came to a chapter of her book entitled 'The Value of Tender Loving Care in Early Pregnancy'.

Back in 1984 a married Norwegian couple – Bahill and Sverre Stray-Pedersen, both doctors – published the results of a study that showed that among couples with no 'abnormal findings' after miscarriage, women receiving specific antenatal counselling and psychological support had a pregnancy success rate of 86 per cent, compared to 33 per cent in the remaining patients.[311]

A second study conducted in 1991 out of New Zealand showed very similar patterns. 'The formal programme of emotional support described in the paper appears to have contributed largely to the good outcome in the treatment group,' researchers noted. 'At the very least it is a far safer placebo than other medical and surgical therapies for this condition. Also the programme was a practical and greatly appreciated response to the very deep emotional distress that these women feel prior to and at the commencement of their pregnancies.'[312]

In 1997 Professor Regan published the results of her own study, along with two other researchers, into miscarriage outcomes among patients given additional supportive care. One hundred and twenty women (over 90 per cent of whom were Caucasian) who had experienced three or more consecutive miscarriages and were attending the early pregnancy clinic at St Mary's Hospital were encouraged to attend weekly ultrasound scans to confirm fetal viability and measurement of fetal growth. In the words of the researchers, 'attendance for supportive care conferred a significant beneficial effect on the outcome of pregnancy', independent of maternal age or the number of previous miscarriages. The miscarriage rate among patients who received supportive care was 26 per cent, while the remaining patients had a much higher rate of 51 per cent.

When I asked Professor Regan why TLC works, she was refreshingly honest. 'I don't know,' she said. But it's a remarkable and consistent pattern. She sums it up beautifully. 'If we're all a bit kinder to each other, the world would be a better place, wouldn't it?'

Professor Coomarasamy doesn't know why it works either. 'We know that pregnancy relies on you having a good immune balance and TLC might reduce the stress level, and that then has an impact on immunity. You can speculate.'

Estelle was a patient at her local recurrent miscarriage clinic after several losses and she was told that during her next pregnancy she could have more frequent scans. She and her partner decided to have fort-nightly scans. 'That was a huge help for us. We were absolute nervous wrecks every time we went for a scan, but it was really reassuring to have them and to know we would be having more regular checks. We felt like we could live our lives just a little bit more, not just be absolutely terrified.'

I would like to think that TLC is a little bit of inexplicable magic. If we treated all people with love and care, maybe there would be a little bit more magic – not just in medicine but in the world.

Is it time to stop?

I haven't met many patients who've had as many or more miscarriages than me. But I have met a lot of people who've had more than one. And often, they ask me two questions. The first is usually: 'How did you get through it?' And the advice I always give is in three parts: distraction, distraction, distraction.

Pregnancy after loss is overwhelming for so many reasons. And one of the worst aspects is the waiting. The sitting around, waiting to see if your scan will show a heartbeat, if your hCG is rising, if your NIPT will show anomalies. You cannot change any of these things. You just have to wait and see. The only way I stayed sane through this period was by focusing on other things. Taking myself out to shows, sewing, cooking, exercising, spending time with friends. I learned to ride a bicycle at thirty-eight. Giving my mind a rest and simply allowing myself to forget for an hour or two was the best strategy I could employ to get to the end of a day when each one felt like a millennium.

The second question I often get asked is, 'Why did you keep going?', which is just another way to ask me why I didn't stop. And that is usually followed up with a question that looks something like, 'How will I know when to stop?'

No one can tell you when it's time to stop. No one can tell you to keep going. I am one of the most stubborn, determined people you'll ever meet and I knew in my heart of hearts that I was meant to have another child and no one could ever convince me otherwise. I knew I had to keep going. I would have known it was time to stop, because I would have felt it in my heart. Obviously, there are financial considerations if you're using IVF and IUI, but in terms of your own inner strength, and the strength of your partner if there is one in the picture, only you know the answer to that question. Listen to your own heart and it will tell you what to do and how much you can handle.

Isn't She Lovely

Hey. I'm struggling mentally. I keep thinking the baby is not alive anymore.
I don't know if I can go another week without a scan. I've got an appointment
booked with you for next Thursday. Isy

||||||

The IVF specialist's office called me to book my follow-up appointment after my initial consultation with the baby-maker, but the two lines on a stick told me I didn't need one. Instead they started emailing me pathology slips for hCG and progesterone testing and prescriptions for progesterone supplements. I kept Dr Lovely up to date, with the intention of transferring back to her care the minute I felt the pregnancy was viable.

But I was in no rush. There was no reason to believe this pregnancy would be viable. I didn't hesitate to sign the contract for a new job, totally convinced that I would miscarry and then get on with life.

I knew as an absolute that this pregnancy would end before I was holding a baby. While husbo and I had agreed to keep trying for 2019, a plan to start IVF towards the end of the year was taking shape in my mind. I was turning forty that November and it felt like I was fast approaching the swinging doors of the last-chance saloon.

Annoyingly my hCG kept rising. And I knew that I was tipping into diabetes by my headaches and mood swings. Why couldn't my body just recognise another miscarriage and be done with it?

||||||

After five pregnancies together, Dr Lovely and I were like a well-oiled machine. But this time around I sensed a significant shift and I really did hope it wasn't sparked by pity. Looking back I think that Dr Lovely just knew what I didn't know yet: my biggest challenge through this pregnancy was going to be not totally falling apart mentally.

In a massive game-changer, her rooms now had an ultrasound machine. At the six-week mark, I was relieved to be transferred back to her care and weekly hCG tests were replaced with weekly scans. I was blessed to be distracted by a new job and a whole bunch of other dramas unfolding in my life. So I focused on those and, as always, I waited to bleed.

I had a scan at six weeks which showed a heartbeat, but I'd been here before, right?

|||||||

I looked at my friend, sitting across from me at my kitchen table. And my eyes widened. Suddenly, my pupils dilated and I went completely white. I whispered, 'I can't breathe.' He grabbed me, picked me up and carried me to my room. He lay me on the bed and sat on the carpeted floor next to me. And there he sat patiently, talking to me all the while, waiting for my first anxiety attack to pass.

The anxiety and fear gripping my body was just too much to handle. Sometimes even weekly scans weren't enough. I would turn up at the doctor's surgery convinced I was walking around with a dead baby inside me. I would wait for Dr Lovely to squeeze me in, knowing that unless I saw the flickering of a tiny heartbeat, it would only get worse. The nausea, the shaking, the nightmares. So many nightmares.

|||||||

'You know, you're ten weeks along now, Isy,' Dr Lovely said gently.
    'Yeah. So?'
    'I think it might be time to book you in for an NIPT test.'
    'Why the fuck would I waste the money on that?'
    'You never know.'

||||||

I shouldn't have taken a job in Collingwood, I chided myself, as I made the long, arduous, seemingly endless trek across the river, first thing on a Monday morning, no less. Most days I would arrive before the sun came up, just so I could sneak into an all-day parking spot and not worry about having to move my car every two hours through the day.

It was early, far too early, when I was at my desk and my phone rang. Dr Lovely's voice was shaky.

'Oh no. Just tell me. Just fucking say it,' I groaned, standing up and pacing in the space in front of my desk.

'Isy, it's clear,' she said gently.

I exhaled as I bent over in half, my hands supporting my shoulders by resting on my knees.

'There's something else,' Dr Lovely whispered. It was then that I realised she was trying not to cry.

'Oh gawd, what?' I started pacing again.

'It's a girl,' she said, her voice breaking a little.

My knees hit the ground hard as I started to sob.

'This is it, isn't it? I'm going to get my baby girl,' I gulped out, in what was less of a statement and more a prayer.

'I think so,' she whispered.

||||||

'I just can't do this anymore. I want it to be over,' I howled, sitting in the office of my brand spanking new psychologist. 'It's hell. Every single day is hell. And every day that I'm fucking miserable I feel like I'm being ungrateful. I just want it to be over and have this baby here safely.'

My GP and my psych offered me medication, but with a history of pregnancy loss, there was very little chance I was going to put anything into my body that didn't really need to be there. Even if every piece of irrefutable medical evidence showed it was safe.

Eventually the mental challenges of pregnancy caught up to me physically. My insulin doses ramped up. My hips started to give way. I was told I had to use crutches. When I didn't use the crutches I was warned in no uncertain terms that I was close to needing a wheelchair. I used the crutches.

||||||

I lay there. Staring at the ceiling. Silently, tears streamed down my face. Sheets rustled, instructions were barked. Because I was on my back, the tears rolled into my ears, pooling there, making the clanging of medical instruments sound dull and far away. Jack had his hand on my arm, squeezing intermittently. The anaesthetist had cancelled. The replacement was someone who didn't know me, didn't know my story, didn't understand what was happening.

'Hey,' he said quietly, when he saw my wet, pale face. 'Are you okay?'

'She's fine, please just leave her,' husbo said protectively. 'It's a lot.'

Marvin Gaye was playing in the operating theatre. I let myself indulge in a watery smile as Dr Lovely sang along. As she sliced me open.

Later, as I lay in recovery, she came to me. She looked me in the eye for what felt like the first time that day. And we just sat there. Looking at each other. I was the one who broke the silence.

'Thank you for never giving up on us.'

I spread one arm wide. She folded into me, in a hug. And we cried together, careful not to crush the little baby girl who was lying on my chest, her tiny, perfect mouth guzzling down her first feed.

||||||

Roxie-Rose Sophia Latimore was born in September 2019.

||||||||||||||||||||||||||||||||||||||||||||||||||||||||||||||||||||||||||||||||||||||||||||||||||||||

We're Going to Be Friends

This is an edited transcript of a conversation I had with Dr Lovely, over break-fast, just as I was in the final stages of writing this book. She had salmon on toast and I had avo and poached eggs (we're Jewish and catering is important). While Dr Lovely has become a close friend, we had never sat down and discussed the journey we went through together. This is the first time that conversation took place.

Q. *Have any of your other patients had more miscarriages than me?*
A. No, you're the most.

Q. *When you were treating me did you think it was gonna go on for as long as it did? What were you thinking? Like, say around the second or third miscarriage? Were you like, there's a problem here?*
A. So we look at patterns and you had . . . You had a beautiful, healthy, term baby. And to me, it seems more, rather than there being something inherently wrong with you, is that you were having a rubbish run of luck. And it just, like, it went too long. And I was sitting there thinking this has to stop at some stage, there is no reason for this to keep going.

Q. *Was there a point where you went, it's not going to happen for her?*
A. There was a point where I thought, you're at breaking point. I don't know how many more losses and how much more grief this woman has to take on board, and you genuinely every time surprised me at your resilience and your grit. I thought it would be a matter of just the sheer load of the grief stopped you before you got that baby that you so desperately wanted. I absolutely knew in my heart of hearts that that story had a happy ending. And I can't put my finger on it.

Q. *I was having lunch with someone yesterday. And I was telling her I was having lunch with you today. And she said to me (and I never knew this) that she and Jack actually had a conversation when it was all going down. And she asked him, 'Do you think it's going to happen?' And he actually said, 'She's going to keep going and she's gonna have a second baby.' Like it wasn't even a question in his mind. Because I was so determined.*

A. Yep, it was about whether you would have a breakdown, and I don't mean that lightly. But the stress and the trauma. I just in my gut knew that you'd get there. And for a lot of my patients, when they have two or three miscarriages in a row, they're going, 'Have you ever seen this before?' and 'Am I going to get there?' You're (de-identified, of course) a story of hope. And the question is just, how much more have you got in the tank? Because we will get there. It's a horrible numbers game. It's the worst lottery or casino roulette game in the world. But if you play it long enough, you'll hit it.

Q. *What do you think it was? If you had to guess? Do you think it was my slutty uterus?*

A. The more I read, the more I learn, I think it's exactly that. There are some women who don't implant, month after month after month, and they have a delayed time to conception, and they have some fertility or infertility. And then we have the opposite end of the spectrum where you've got this hyper-receptive endometrium, and everything sticks, whether it's healthy or unhealthy. And that's probably why you got pregnant so readily; every month, you'd be back in my inbox with another positive pregnancy test. And so there was maybe an element of that natural selection. That's the endometrium switch. I genuinely think that's the reason.

Q. *Were you shocked? I remember one time when I was pregnant you were like, 'How did you do that?'*

A. (Laughing hard.) Yeah, no, I don't think you've stopped shocking me. Typically, when I look after people with pregnancy losses, they get to a point where they just sit on the fence, or the sidelines rather, for a couple of days. So they just need to regroup, but your tenacity meant you had this attitude like, 'I'm going until I get it.'

Q. *The last pregnancy before Rox. The termination. How did you feel watching that play out?*

A. So that one really sticks very strongly in my mind because you hadn't had that bleeding and we'd gotten to six and a half weeks and then to ten before the wheels came off. And my heart just went through the floor for me. I was like, 'This is not fair.' And I remember calling you and you said, 'Dr Lovely, you have "that voice" on.' Around the time you'd started seeing me, it was before I was pregnant with my second. And in amongst all of that, you'd had so many losses, that I'd conceived and then was going to give birth to my second and I was heartbroken that it happened. I felt so guilty that I was lapping you. (Dr Lovely starts to cry and we pause for lots of cuddles.)

Q. *When you called me with the NIPT in the very last pregnancy with the clear result, I didn't understand your voice. It wasn't your sad voice or your pity voice (both laugh). But it wasn't your normal voice. And I realised you were trying not to cry.*

A. I'm always glued to my phone. And the results had come through on my phone. And I was in a stairwell and I just went, 'I have to call her right now, I can't even go to an office.'

Q. *So you never wanted me to give up?*

A. I genuinely hoped that you didn't stop and didn't give up. Because I just felt like you'd never be able to settle and that you deserved this baby and that you would get that happy ending, if we just stuck it out long enough.

Q. *I could see her. I knew she was there. I just had to grab her. It's like when you're at the start of a marathon, you end up falling over. But if you could just get to the finish line, I could see her waiting for me.*

A. I've never done a marathon but I've run 15 kilometres and there's that point of severe, severe pain. And if you can just get through it, you don't feel it anymore.

Q. *Why did you do my termination on a Saturday?*

A. Partly, I wanted to be emotionally available to you and physically available to you. And Saturday is a day that I don't have patients. I mean, yes, I have commitments with my family, but I have the support systems in place. And I can be at the hospital and stay until you're in recovery or do whatever I need to do without having to race out the door.

Q. *And how invested did you feel in those later pregnancies?*

A. I think by that stage I was holding my breath at every scan. Of course there's the doctor element. And I want good things for my patient. But this is now my friend who I care very deeply about and I don't want her to have more heartbreak. I remember praying, 'Just please be okay. Please be okay.'

Q. *What do you remember about the day Roxie was born?*

A. I was pretty emotional. I had tears in my eyes when I was operating. You couldn't see because it was on the other side of the drape. It was something that you had worked so very hard for, and Jack as well. I think I'd worked for it bloody hard as well (both laughing). You know I remember one of your first emails once we got over the low-risk NIPT result, detailing what monitoring you would like, and I was like, 'Babe, I've got it. I know you well enough by now.' (Both start laughing very hard and continue for quite some time.)

Q. *Yeah, I think a lot of doctors actually don't understand that those scans are psychological.*

A. It has really informed my practice moving forward. So when I first met you, I was probably in my second year of private practice, maybe even my first year. I knew how to follow the rules and follow protocols, but I was still evolving as a clinician. And I think that the degree of insight that I have, and after looking after you or working with you, whichever term you want to use, that I will ask women who've had pregnancy loss when they want to come in for their scans. I explain it's not going to change anything, but if it helps them among their anxiety, so they can tell themselves they only have seven days until they can see that heartbeat again, then that's what we do. I have this machine, this machine doesn't cost me any more whether I use it four times a day, or forty times a day, I might as well use the technology at my disposal, when it's completely safe to help.

Q. *(Starts to cry.) That makes me really emotional. Because the whole point of this whole thing is to help. The fact that someone else could benefit from me having explained my feelings to you . . . I was worried you wouldn't want to treat me anymore.*

A. I think I'm such a better practitioner for having been through all of that with you. I still think of you day to day in my practice, and going, 'Okay, what Isy needed isn't what everyone needs, but this is what I've learned.'

17

The Never-ending Story

Getting my happy ending didn't mean I was healed. My scar tissue is varied and I feel deeply that there are aspects of me that will never be whole. Severe and crippling anxiety is now a central part of my reality. Even two years after the arrival of my double-rainbow pot of gold baby, I check my underwear for blood every time I sit on a toilet. Sometimes when I see blood, I feel a jolt and the bile starts to rise; I'm panicking before my brain has even caught up to the fact that it's my period. I think about a beautiful line in a poem by Eleanor Jackson that describes a 'Rorschach on your underwear'.[313] During the pandemic, I cried watching the control line appear on my first rapid antigen test, as flashbacks of what felt like hundreds of pregnancy tests flew past my mind's eye. Abdominal ultrasounds fill me with dread and my breathing constricts from the moment they squeeze the cool gel onto my belly. But none of this compares to the people who don't get their happy ending.

When you are open about pregnancy loss, the floodgates open. All around you people want to tell you that you're not alone, that they too had a loss. Or their partner. Or their child. Or their sibling. Or their parent. Or their friend. Or their workmate. Because this is truly something that has touched everyone in some way. Everyone knows someone affected by miscarriage, even if they're not aware of it. Being someone whose life is built around storytelling, as I listened to story after story, I had a natural inclination to want to tell those stories, to effect change. Because within those stories there are commonalities both in kindness and in dereliction of care.

In writing *Hard to Bear*, I set out to forge a pathway for better care in early pregnancy loss. To use my understanding of the system as a patient and my research skills as a journalist to create visible, achievable ways to improve care and outcomes, reduce trauma and encourage empathy, kindness and understanding for the different journeys that patients make in this space. And make no mistake; there isn't just one journey. There are many, defined by the patient, the carers, the systems and so much more.

There are issues raised in this book that affect not just early pregnancy loss, but medical care in this country more broadly, especially as it relates to the marginalised among us. I hope that I have contributed to that discussion in a meaningful way, conscious of the lens of privilege through which I view those issues and the people they affect most.

The changes we have available to us as a society are far-reaching. Some are small and sit with individual practitioners. Some are structural and so deeply embedded they could take years to change. Others are financial and need the impetus of a government that understands how deeply our medical system is under-funded and strained.

For patients reading this book, I hope you walk away empowered, with a deeper sense of understanding about what's happened to you and the way forward, as well as the knowledge that you are far, far from alone. For those looking to support their close ones navigating this space, I hope you found insight into how they are feeling and the challenges they face, as well as tools to confidently offer support. For medical practitioners, I hope you can see how integral you are to every part of this process and your power to change someone's entire experience in this journey.

As a community I hope that we can see how all areas of care – social, medical and psychological – overlap to create the support network we all need. And this is where the next step in the *Hard to*

Bear journey comes in. The execution of a new strategy to make a real difference in people's lives. There is precedent that we can turn to for inspiration. I believe the two best examples are the endometriosis and domestic violence lobbies, because they represent various organisations in each space coming together to achieve aims that benefit the whole. If the various components that comprise miscarriage care – from hospitals to the people we love – formed a Venn diagram, there would be so many overlapping sections, we'd run out of shades of colour. The only way we're going to effect the change so badly needed is by working together on shared goals and targets as a powerful coalition of people who want to see change and are willing to make it happen.

To any medical or allied health practitioner who wants to see their industry do better. To parents who've experienced terrible care and don't want any parents to suffer like they have. To partners who feel unseen. To the nurses and midwives who don't know what to say but want to learn. We can do this. Together. Shall we?

18

Give Thanks and Praises

To every single person who agreed to be interviewed, to share their deepest pain and highest hopes, who did it with generosity and care: you are the backbone of this book and it is an absolute testament to your strength. Hear us roar.

Thank you to Roy and Roxie-Rose for being unapologetically you: totally and utterly perfect in every single way. Thank you to Jack for being my best friend, the love of my life and forever my partner in crime. Jack, I respect and cherish you beyond any words I could write down on a page and I'm so proud to be your wife.

To my mum, my dad, Jules and Loz, thank you for always being my greatest champions, I love all of you so much.

To my friends who saw me through the worst parts of this journey and the best, there are too many to name and you know who you are. I adore each and every one of you.

Dr Lovely, you are part of my family forever, thank you again for never ever giving up on us and for being my friend. And thank you to everyone at your clinic; a better team I have never known.

Sally Heath, your encouragement, kindness and generosity is probably the only reason this book exists. Thanks to my agent Melanie Ostell for believing in my work and being the firm, guiding, all-knowing handler (and friend!) that I need. Thanks also to Brigid

Mullane, Alisa Ahmed, Emily Cook and the whole team at Ultimo Press; I am so grateful that *Hard to Bear* found its way home to you. And my gratitude to Ang Savage and Karen Wyld for your early feedback and encouragement.

To John Spierings, I will never find the words. You're a guardian angel and without your faith and kindness, this book would never have happened. Well not this decade, anyway.

Mary Crooks and Janet Hailes Michelmore and the teams at The Victorian Women's Trust and Jean Hailes for Women's Health, what an amazing bunch of humans you are, who make real differences in people's lives. My grant from the VWT meant that I could take the time to write this book properly and truly do it justice. The auspicing of the grant by Jean Hailes came with a wealth of support and care, far beyond the task the team was engaged to execute.

Thank you to Cherisse Buzzacott for your collaboration, generosity, expertise, resilience, patience and for always being honest about the pain of your own journey. Sisters for life, I will always have your back.

Thank you to Dr Tess Ryan, Professor Bronwyn Fredericks, Professor Cath Chamberlain, Dr Lynore Geia and Professor Sandy O'Sullivan for your precious feedback, we truly cherish your guidance beyond words.

A special thank you to Kathy Kum-Sing who was the first to message my family when our daughter was born. We miss you always. Thank you to my Auntie Rhonda and my cousin Gulwanyang for giving me permission to use Gathang language in this book and for being the best family anyone could ask for; I love you.

Steph, Kate, Neela and Mariam, I don't even know where I would be without you. I love each of you individually and I love us as the weirdo little group that we are. Thank you for the love, laughs and your beautiful words. And yes, my spreadsheet will live forever. Let's never stop writing, hey?

Thank you to Dr Kyle Sheldrick for teaching me how to spot bullshit in a medical paper, to Dr Vijay Roach for always lending me an ear, to Brad Crammond for crunching my numbers over and over, to Dr Marilyn Clarke for being a champion among humans that I'm so grateful to know, Professor Craig Pennell for informing my early research, Professor Sarah Robertson and Professor Jeff Craig for always making time to point me in the right direction, and Quinn Guy for always helping me with my annoying data requests with patience and grace. Thank you to Laura Placella for doing a job that I just didn't have the strength to do; I know it was hard and I am grateful. Thank you to Katerina Weitkamp for holding my hand through my last pregnancy and never complaining about all the stupid jokes I made in an attempt to hide my abject terror. Thank you to Karen Percy for the training you gave me in trauma-informed reporting, both for my own welfare and that of my interviewees.

Gratitude also to Drs Jordan Walter and Devora Lieberman for stepping in to get my terminology and definitions right. Thank you to Associate Professor Mark Green and Dr Geoffrey Reid for your immense feedback and guidance. You make me seem far smarter than I am.

The stunningly beautiful cover of this book was a team effort. Thank you from the bottom of my heart to everyone who helped make it happen, including Pilgrim Hodgson, Amy Hiley and Alissa Dinallo.

Carly Findlay, thank you for your advice when I was just starting this journey. I am so lucky to have your counsel, but more importantly, your friendship. And thank you to my uncle Tony Latimore, the best word wrangler I know, for naming this book so beautifully.

Thank you to Rabbi Gersh Lazarow, who helped both in the research and healing aspects of this project, and to Jonathan Green, who as editor of *Meanjin* published my work and gave me permission to reprint one of those pieces in this book, in the vignette entitled The Way We Were.

To the best miscarriage brains trust anyone could ask for, two people whose work is helping change the way we view miscarriage and treat it; thank you Dr Jade Bilardi and Dr Melanie Keep.

Thank you to the immeasurable number of anonymous Twitter users who sent me medical papers because I couldn't afford access and sent me links to stories I'd missed or helped me brainstorm. The hell site can be pretty dang good on occasion. Also to all the friends who borrowed books from university libraries for me, thank you.

Thank you to every single doctor, scientist, academic, journalist and writer I interviewed. There are too many to name but whether you are named or whether you are not, your time, expertise and insight were invaluable and every single one of you gave it with limitless generosity.

To Jess Hill and Gabrielle Jackson, your books were the reason I wrote mine. Thank you for your support, guidance and, most of all, your crucial work in shining light on issues too long ignored.

And finally . . . To my seven angels. Not a day goes by that I don't think of you. Far from being forgotten, you are cherished and loved each day of our lives, and the work I do now, I do in your memory and with you as inspiration . . . until the day I see you again.

Additional Reading and Resources

Miscarriage Australia
https://miscarriageaustralia.com.au/

Red Nose Australia
https://rednose.org.au/

Tommy's National Centre for Miscarriage Research
https://www.tommys.org/

Miscarriage: What Every Woman Needs To Know by Professor
Dame Lesley Regan

*Not Broken: An Approachable Guide to Miscarriage and Recurrent Pregnancy
Loss* by Lora Shahine, MD

This work was made possible by the Victorian Women's Benevolent Trust through a grant to the Jean Hailes Foundation.

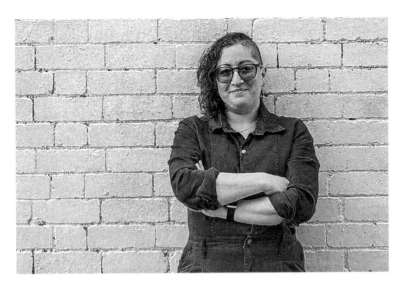

After growing up in Hong Kong, Isabelle Oderberg went to university in Melbourne. She has worked as a journalist for two decades in newsrooms across Europe, Asia and Australia, where she was the country's first social media editor for Melbourne's *Herald Sun*. Her work has appeared in *The Age/SMH*, *The Guardian*, *ABC*, *Meanjin* and elsewhere. She has also worked as a media and communications strategist across the not-for-profit sector. *Hard to Bear* is her first book.

Glossary

Abortion: Also known as termination, this is the intentional ending of a pregnancy using surgical or medical intervention.

Amish: Groups of traditionalist anabaptist Christians based mostly in America, with Swiss and German origins. Different groups follow different rules, but the strictest among them practice total isolation from modern society and eschewing of all modern technology.

Antiphospholipid syndrome: An auto-immune disease in which the immune system mistakenly creates antibodies to attack body tissue. It can cause blood clots in arteries, veins and the placenta.

ART: Assisted reproductive technology, such as in vitro fertilisation or intrauterine insemination.

Australian Bureau of Statistics (ABS): Australia's independent statutory body responsible for national data collection, collation and analysis.

Australian Institute of Health and Welfare (AIHW): The national agency responsible for information and statistics on the country's health and welfare.

Blastocyst: The stage that comes five days after fertilisation, a blastocyst is a rapidly dividing ball of cells, with two kinds of cells, an inner group and an outer shell. The inner group of cells will become an embryo, while the outer cells become the placenta. The blastocyst stage comes after the zygote stage.

Blighted ovum: An out-dated term that is still commonly used, this is the name of a pregnancy that has a gestational sac but no fetus. It can also be called an 'anembryonic pregnancy' because there's no embryo. It is confirmed by scan. This type of loss is thought to be caused by an embryo that doesn't develop properly being absorbed back into the body at a very early stage. Once this is confirmed, if the body does not naturally start to expel the pregnancy, the treatment options are the same as a missed miscarriage: a minor surgical procedure or medication.

BPA: Bisphenol A is an industrial chemical compound used commonly in plastics and resins since the 1950s.

Carbendazim: A widely used fungicide.

Cell-free DNA (cfDNA): Small fragments of 'unencapsulated' DNA, released from normal cells and circulating in our bloodstream.

Cerclage: A procedure in which the cervical opening is stitched shut to prevent preterm birth.

Cervix: The lower part of the uterus, shortened from cervix uteri, or 'neck of the uterus' in Latin.

Chemical pregnancy: A pregnancy that ends before reaching five weeks of gestation. It can show up on a high sensitivity pregnancy test or on a blood test, but it is too early to see in a scan. The patient may not even realise they're pregnant, they may just experience a 'very heavy period', then twig it is a miscarriage. A positive home pregnancy test or a trip to the doctor for a blood test can confirm the presence of hCG to indicate whether a miscarriage has occurred. Some patients will never realise (perhaps in some cases, mercifully) that a heavy period was in fact a pregnancy loss. Chemical pregnancies fuel a belief in the medical fraternity that miscarriage rates may be higher than the often-touted industry-standard of 20 to 25 per cent of all pregnancies.

Chromosomal abnormality: When added, missing, incomplete or altered chromosomes are present, which can lead to genetic disorders, or render an embryo or fetus incompatible with life.

Chromosome: A thread of DNA molecules responsible for carrying the genetic material of a living being. Humans should have

46 chromosomes, half from the biological mother and half from the biological father.

Complete miscarriage: This means the entire pregnancy has left your body. An incomplete miscarriage means that there may be some tissue left in the uterus and a small surgical procedure may be required to remove it all to prevent an infection from developing.

CRH (corticotrophin-releasing hormone): A hormone released in response to stress, also called the 'stress hormone'.

CVS (chorionic villus sampling): A test conducted to check the number of chromosomes of a fetus, by using a needle to penetrate the womb and extract a small number of cells from the placenta.

D&C (dilation and curettage): A procedure to remove pregnancy tissue or uterine lining. The cervix is dilated and, in most cases, suction is use to remove tissue. An instrument called a curette is used to ensure the uterus is empty. This procedure is commonly used for pregnancies under 14 weeks gestation.

D&E (dilation and evacuation): Similar to a D&C, but the tissue is removed using a suction device, as well as other instruments such forceps. This procedure is generally used at gestations over 14 weeks.

DES (diethylstilbesterol): A synthetic form of the hormone oestrogen, prescribed to women from around 1940 to around 1971 to prevent miscarriage and pre-term birth. It was found to be a carcinogen capable of crossing the placenta during pregnancy and causing cancer in both the biological parent and the child.

Diabetes: A chronic disease where the body cannot produce insulin or alternatively cannot effectively use the insulin it produces. Gestational diabetes is a form of diabetes present during pregnancy, whereby hormones produced by the placenta reduce the effectiveness of insulin, resulting in high blood sugar. It is usually diagnosed during pregnancy with a glucose tolerance test (GTT), though some patients only have elevated fasting levels (meaning overnight). It can sometimes be controlled with diet, but if not can be controlled with insulin until the baby is born. A follow up GTT test is done around six to 12 weeks after birth to ensure the diabetes is no longer present.

Dieldrin: A carcinogenic insecticide that is also an endocrine disruptor and a persistent organic pollutant, which means it's very difficult to break down both within humans and in the environment.

Dioxins: These are a group of chemicals that are part of the 'dirty dozen' persistent organic pollutants, not solely persistent in the environment, they are also persistent in the body, where they can cause endocrine disruption, immune system failure and a number of other negative effects.

DNA: DNA stands for deoxyribonucleic acid, which is a substance that stores our genetic material or genetic 'instructions'.

DNA fragmentation: This happens when strands of DNA break into pieces, which can cause chromosomal abnormalities.

DNA Methylation: Put in simple terms, DNA Methylation is when methyl groups are added to DNA molecules, affecting the way DNA behaves.

Down syndrome: Also known as Trisomy 21, Down syndrome is an intellectual and developmental disorder caused by extra material from, or copy of, chromosome 21.

Early pregnancy assessment service or centre (EPAS/EPAC): Outpatient clinics in hospital designed to support patients who have bleeding or other issues during the first 12 to 15 weeks of pregnancy.

Ectopic pregnancy: This occurs when an embryo implants outside of the uterus, often in a fallopian tube. There are a variety of possible treatments and outcomes for ectopic pregnancy, ranging from having to take medication to bring on a miscarriage all the way through to the condition being life threatening and requiring urgent surgery. In some cases when surgical removal of the pregnancy is necessary, it may result in the loss of a fallopian tube, if that is where the pregnancy has implanted, which can make conceiving naturally in future more difficult. About one or two in every hundred pregnancies are ectopic.[314] However, if you experience an ectopic pregnancy, the risk of another one is higher, at one in ten.[315]

Edwards syndrome: Also called Trisomy 18, Edwards syndrome causes severe disability and occurs when there is an extra copy of chromosome 18. It is usually fatal in utero or in the first year after birth.

Elective surgery: Any surgery that can be scheduled or pre-planned, meaning any surgery that is not an immediate emergency.

Endocrine disrupting chemicals: Chemicals that disrupt the hormone-producing and managing endocrine system. It controls growth, development, bodily function and the reproductive system.

Endometriosis: A condition in which cells similar to those in the inner lining of the uterus, grow outside the uterus. They can cover the ovaries, fallopian tubes and even the bowel and bladder.

Epigenetics: The study of how your environment, activity or behaviour affect the way your genes work.

Expectant management: This is the 'wait and see' strategy of miscarriage care, where you wait to see if the body will miscarry naturally.

Fecundity: This is the physiological ability of someone with a uterus to bear children. This is different to fertility rate, meaning the number of children a person bears.

Fetal monitoring unit: A FMU takes over the care of high-risk patients and babies who need monitoring after the cut-off for the EPAS (which is around 12 to 15 weeks).

Fetal personhood: The view of a fetus as a person or the personification of a fetus.

Fibroid: Benign growths in the uterus, usually made up of uterine muscle.

Genetic disorder: A disorder passed down through genes. These can be errors (such as too many copies of a single chromosome, like Down syndrome or Trisomy 21) or an inherited disease such as cystic fibrosis.

Gestation: The time between conception and birth, time spent in utero.

Hashimoto's disease: An auto-immune disorder in which antibodies attack thyroid cells.

hCG: Human chorionic gonadotrophin is a hormone produced by the placenta until about 10 to 12 weeks into a pregnancy.

Hutterite: Anabaptist agricultural communities based in America and Canada who share many similarities to the Amish.

Hyaluronic acid: A naturally occurring acid which can be used in sperm selection in IVF to exclude sperm affected by DNA fragmentation.

Hypothalamus: A part of the brain that links the endocrine system and pituitary gland.

ICSI: Intracytoplasmic sperm injection can be part of IVF treatment, when a single sperm is injected into an egg.

Idiopathic miscarriage: This is early pregnancy loss in which no cause has been identified.

Immunotherapy: Therapies designed to reduce a birth parent's immune response to a conception or to encourage conception, for instance immunosuppressant medication, or the injection of paternal cells. There is no convincing evidence that these therapies work.

Implantation: This is when a fertilised egg attaches to the uterine lining. In some cases it can cause a very small amount of bleeding.

IUI: Intrauterine insemination, a more sophisticated, medical form of turkey baster-style insemination, where a patient is given drugs to encourage ovulation and then washed sperm is injected into the vagina in a brief, outpatient appointment.

IVF: In vitro fertilisation is when eggs and sperm are extracted, fertilised in a lab to form an embryo, and then implanted into the uterus.

Karotype: An analysis of a person or fetus' full set of chromosomes, often to identify or check for chromosomal abnormalities or translocations (a rearrangement of chromosomes).

LGBTIQ+: An acronym standing for lesbian, gay, bisexual+, trans and gender diverse, intersex, Queer, and a range of other identities and experiences. Some communities also see the + as representing people who are HIV+.

Luteinising hormone: A hormone produced by the pituitary gland which controls menstruation and triggers ovulation (the release of eggs).

Medical management: The strategy of treating miscarriage where either misoprostol or a combination of misoprostol and mifepristone are given trigger to the miscarriage process and pass the pregnancy tissue.

Medicare codes: All medical services subsidised by the Australian government are given a unique code to identify them. These codes are subject to regular revision and expansion.

Meiosis: The process of cells dividing and multiplying.

Mennonite: Another Anabaptist denomination, similar to the Amish and Hutterite communities.

Methidathion: An insecticide for caterpillars, methidathion is banned in the European Union, America and China due to a range of health ill-effects and carcinogen concerns.

Microbiomes: These are communities of microorganisms that live both within and on our bodies, contributing to our health and wellness.

Microplastics: Tiny plastic particles that are damaging to both the environment and our health.

Mifepristone: A drug used in abortion and D&Cs, which blocks the production of progesterone and causes uterine contractions.

Misoprostol: A drug also used in abortion and D&Cs, misoprostol causes the cervix to dilate.

Missed or delayed miscarriage: This is when a pregnancy has stopped growing or an embryo has failed to develop and your body hasn't realised yet. That means that the body doesn't trigger the process of ending the pregnancy, i.e. bleeding. Missed miscarriages can come as a shock, because often there is no indication of miscarriage. Symptoms can persist because the body doesn't realise things aren't as they should be. Often the fetus has no heartbeat, although if you're being scanned as early as six weeks into the pregnancy you may be asked to wait a week or two to see if a heartbeat develops. In other cases the fetus has had heartbeat previously, but it that has since stopped. If you discover you've had a missed miscarriage at a scan, often the ultrasonologist can tell you approximately when the heartbeat or growth stopped.

Molar pregnancy (hydatidiform mole): A non-viable pregnancy that results in a placenta developing in an irregular way, with little sacs of fluid, a bit like a bunch of grapes. It is usually larger than it should be, resulting in higher production of hCG and stronger pregnancy symptoms. With a full molar pregnancy the fetus stops developing, in a partial molar pregnancy a fetus develops but rarely survives beyond 12 weeks. Around one in every 1200 pregnancies is a molar pregnancy.[316] Molar pregnancies are surgically removed. In some cases the placenta can become malignant and develop into a rare form of cancer called choriocarcinoma. It responds well to chemotherapy. Patients are monitored to ensure their hCG returns to zero, indicating all dangerous cells are gone from the body. Australia has several registries for Gestational Trophoblastic Disease, of which molar pregnancies are the most common form.

Monosomy: This is when there is only one chromosome present in cells instead of a pair. An example of a monosomy disorder is Turner syndrome, which only affects females and occurs when one of the X sex chromosomes is missing, causing a range of medical and developmental issues.

MTHFR gene: Methylenetetrahydrofolatereductase is the gene that helps your body process folate.

Nitrogen dioxide: A chemical compound that can cause swelling of the throat and respiratory system, inflammation, reduced oxygenation of body tissues and a range of other adverse health effects. In very high doses it can cause death.

Non-binary: People who identify as living outside the prescribed gender binaries of male and female.

Non-Invasive Prenatal Testing (NIPT): A screening tool used usually in the first trimester of a pregnancy. It works by analysing a blood sample from the birth parent, locating the fetal blood cells and testing them for anomalies. And yes, a baby's DNA flows through its mother's veins, in some cases for decades after they are born. The test is staggeringly accurate, boasting accuracy rates of at least 99.5 per cent.

Oestrogen: Known as the 'female hormone', oestrogen is the sex hormone which assists in the development of the female reproductive system.

Particle matter: Tiny, microscopic solid particles or liquid drops that are carried in the air, small enough that they can be inhaled.

Per and polyfluoroalkyl substances (PFASs): These are man-made chemicals used to create water resistance in a range of products. They are persistent organic pollutants (POPs), also known as forever chemicals, because they take so long to break down.

Perchlorate: A by-product of pharmaceutical production and other manufacturing, also used in food packaging. It is an endocrine disruptor and is toxic to the thyroid.

Persistent Organic Pollutants (POPs): POPs, also called 'forever chemicals', are known for their longevity in breaking down, leading to deeply concerning build-ups in the environment, and organisms, like humans. They cause significant health and environmental issues.

Personification: See fetal personhood.

PGT-A: Used in IVF, PGT-A is preimplantation genetic testing on embryos, checking for aneuploidy or an irregular number of chromosomes.

Phthalates: Industrial chemicals commonly used in plastics production, as well as cosmetics. They can cause damage to the liver, lungs and kidneys, and as endocrine disruptors can cause significant damage to reproductive system.

Pituitary gland: A pea-sized part of the brain, weighing in at around half a gram, located off the hypothalamus. It is an essential part of the endocrine system, which has a central role in regulating sexual reproduction.

Polycystic ovary syndrome: A hormonal disorder that can cause over-sized ovaries with small cysts.

Pregnancy tissue: Tissue that develops as part of pregnancy, including but not limited to fetal tissue and the placenta.

Products of conception: The 'formal' medical terminology for pregnancy tissue, which is now becoming more widely used as a more compassionate and delicate alternative.

Progesterone: A hormone produced by the ovaries, it has many roles in the body, such as regulation of menstruation. During pregnancy, progesterone is responsible for preparing the body for implantation, reducing the immune response so the body doesn't reject the pregnancy and preventing preterm labour. When progesterone production falls after a pregnancy, this is thought to be the trigger for lactation to begin. Progesterone is produced by the ovaries and the adrenal gland. Around week seven of pregnancy, the placenta takes over progesterone production.

Recurrent miscarriage: Either two or three consecutive miscarriages, depending on who you're asking. The Royal Women's Hospital in Melbourne defines it as three losses,[317] but the Australian Journal of General Practice defines it as two.[318] It can be any combination of the types of miscarriages I've described, and many women's hospitals have recurrent miscarriage clinics that address and treat this issue. Less than five per cent of couples experience recurrent miscarriage,[319] or one in 200 women.[320] Unfortunately it is often only when you're classified as a recurrent miscarriage patient that you are offered any medical investigation.

Reproductive immunology: The study of the relationship between the immune system and sexual reproduction.

Septate uterus: This is a uterus divided into two parts either partially or completely, by a band of uterine tissue called a septum running downwards inside the cavity.

Spontaneous abortion: The formal medical terminology for a miscarriage or early pregnancy loss. Its usage was formally abandoned in the UK, but it is still used the Australian context and many others.

Stillbirth: The death of a baby after 20 weeks of gestation either before or during labour.

Surgical management: One of the three options for miscarriage management, surgical management of a miscarriage is a procedure to end the pregnancy, usually a D&C or a D&E (see above).

Termination for medical reasons (TFMR): An abortion due to a fetal abnormality or because a pregnancy threatens the life of the birth parent.

Thalidomide: A drug given to birth parents from the late 1950s to early 1960s to treat, among other things, morning sickness. It caused significant birth defects in affected babies, the most well-known of which was malformation of the upper limbs.

Threatened miscarriage: A threatened miscarriage usually occurs in the context of vaginal bleeding in a confirmed pregnancy before 20 weeks gestation, where the cervix is closed. Threatened miscarriages require ongoing monitoring (such as blood tests and scans), as they may progress into a miscarriage, or continue as a viable pregnancy. It is important to note that early pregnancy bleeding is common and does not always mean a miscarriage is inevitable.

Transmasculine: Someone who was assigned the female gender at birth, but does not identify as female. For instance they may identify as male, masculine or non-binary.

Trisomy: The name given when someone has three copies of a chromosome instead of two. An example of trisomy is Down syndrome, also known as Trisomy 21, in which someone has a third copy of chromosome 21.

Uterus: Also known as a womb, this is the hollow organ in which a fetus or baby gestates and grows.

World Health Organization: The arm of the United Nations responsible for messaging and information provision to support international public health.

Zygote: A fertilised egg. The zygote stage comes before that of a blastocyst.

Endnotes

Foreword: It's Only the Beginning

1 Stirrat, Gordon. 'Recurrent Miscarriage II: Clinical Associations, Causes, and Management,' *The Lancet* 336, no. 8717 (September 1990): 728-733.

Introduction: Hello

2 Nanda, Kavita, Laureen M Lopez, David A Grimes, Alessandra Peloggia, Geeta Nanda and Cochrane Pregnancy and Childbirth Group (ed.). 'Expectant Care versus Surgical Treatment for Miscarriage.' *Cochrane Database of Systematic Reviews*, March 2012.

3 Moscrop, Andrew. '"Miscarriage or abortion?" Understanding the medical language of pregnancy loss in Britain; a historical perspective.' *Medical humanities* 39, no. 2 (December 2013): 98-104.

4 Hutchon, David and Sandra Cooper. 'Terminology for early pregnancy loss must be changed,' *BMJ* 317, no. 7165 (October 1998): 1081.

1: Don't Speak

5 Bardos, Jonah, Daniel Hercz, Jenna Friedenthal, Stacey Missmer and Zev Williams, 'A national survey on public perceptions of miscarriage,' *Obstetrics & Gynecololgy* 125, no. 6 (June 2015): 1313-1320.

6 Exodus 23:26. The Holy Bible, English Standard Version: revised 2016. biblia.com, accessed 2022.

7 Hosea 9:14. The Holy Bible, English Standard Version: revised 2016. biblia.com, accessed 2022.

8 Freidenfelds, Lara. *The Myth of the Perfect Pregnancy: A History of Miscarriage in America*. New York: Oxford University Press, 2019. p.23.

9 Firth, John (trans.) 'Book 8, To Fabatus,' Letters to Pliny, 1900. http://www.attalus.org/old/pliny8.html#10

10 Stivala, Joan. 'Malaria and Miscarriage in Ancient Rome.' *Canadian Bulletin of Medical History* 32, no. 1 (Spring 2015): 143–161.

11 Leroy, Margaret. *Miscarriage.* London: Macmillian Optima, 1988.

12 Ibid. p.96.

13 Withycombe, Shannon. *Lost: Miscarriage in Nineteenth-Century America.* New Brunswick: Rutgers University Press, 2018, p.4.

14 Ibid. p.28.

15 Freidenfelds, Lara. *The Myth of the Perfect Pregnancy: A History of Miscarriage in America.* New York: Oxford University Press, 2019. p.43.

16 Withycombe, Shannon. *Lost: Miscarriage in Nineteenth-Century America.* New Brunswick: Rutgers University Press, 2018, p.5.

17 Ibid. p.72.

18 Cox, Rebecca. 'The ancient taboo of miscarriage.' *InnovAiT* 13, no. 1 (2019): 61–62.

19 Blei, Daniela. 'The History of Talking About Miscarriage.' The Cut, 2018. https://www.thecut.com/2018/04/the-history-of-talking-about-miscarriage.html

20 Cecil, Rosanne. *The anthropology of pregnancy loss: Comparative studies in miscarriage, stillbirth, and neonatal death.* Washington, DC: Berg Publishers, 1996.

21 Ibid. p.9.

22 Elisa Sobo, 'Cultural Explanations for Pregnancy Loss In Rural Jamaica.' In Rosanne Cecil (ed.), *The Anthropology Of Pregnancy Loss*, Berg, Oxford, 1996, p.43.

23 Kilshaw, Susie. 'How Culture Shapes Perceptions of Miscarriage.' SAPIENS, July 2017. https://www.sapiens.org/biology/miscarriage-united-kingdom-qatar/

24 World Health Organization, 'Larai's Story.' who.int, 2018. https://www.who.int/news-room/spotlight/why-we-need-to-talk-about-losing-a-baby/larai's-story

25 Pickering, Karen and Bennett, Jane. *About Bloody Time.* Melbourne: Victorian Women's Trust, 2019. p.97.

26 Oderberg, Isabelle. 'Talking about grief is something we need to get better at.' *The Age*, 2022. https://www.theage.com.au/lifestyle/life-and-relationships/talking-about-grief-is-something-we-need-to-get-better-at-20221025-p5bsm1.html

27 Oderberg, Isabelle. 'The "ugly" side of pregnancy loss is the part we most need to see.' *Sydney Morning Herald*, 2020. https://www.smh.com.au/lifestyle/life-and-relationships/the-ugly-side-of-pregnancy-loss-is-the-part-we-most-need-to-see-20201002-p561di.html

2: The Fame

28 *Party of Five.* 1996. Season 2, episode 18, 'Before and After.' Directed by Steven Robman. Aired on February 21 1996, on Fox.

29 *Beverly Hills 90210*. 1996. Season 7, episode 30, 'Senior Week.' Directed by Jefferson Kibbee. Aired on 14 May 1997, on Fox.

30 *Girls*. 2012. Season 1, episode 2, 'Vagina Panic.' Directed by Lena Dunham. Aired on 22 April 2012, on HBO.

31 *Criminal Minds*. 2014. Season 9, episode 14, '200.' Directed by Larry Teng. Aired on 7 April 2014, on CBS.

32 *Chicago P.D.* 2020. Season 7, episode 13, 'I Was Here.' Directed by Charles Carroll. Aired on 5 February 2020, on NBC.

33 *Dallas*. 1978. Season 1, episode 5, 'Bar-B-Que.' Directed by Robert Day. Aired on 29 September 1978, on CBS.

34 Grey's Anatomy Universe Wiki. 'Katie Kent.' greysanatomy.fandom.com, revised 2019.

35 *Grey's Anatomy*. 2020. Season 16, episode 10, 'Help Me Through the Night.' Directed by Allison Liddi-Brown. Aired on 6 May 2020, on ABC.

36 *Grey's Anatomy*. 2010. Season 6, episode 24, 'Suicide Is Painless.' Directed by Jeannot Szwarc. Aired on 25 March 2010, on ABC.

37 Stafford, Andrew. '"I dreaded that interview coming out": Ben Folds on Brick, William Shatner and hitting rock bottom.' *The Guardian*, 2019. https://www.theguardian.com/books/2019/aug/29/ben-folds-william-shatner-brick-melbourne-writers-festival

38 Durham, Judith, 'I Celebrate Your Life My Baby,' recorded 1998. Track 6 on *Epiphany*, Musicoast, 2011, compact disc.

39 Art Gallery of New South Wales. 'The Miscarriage.' artgallery.nsw.gov.au. https://www.artgallery.nsw.gov.au/artboards/frida-kahlo-diego-rivera/lines-of-connection/item/3ymo6k/

40 Espinoza, Javier. 'Frida Kahlo's last secret finally revealed.' *The Guardian*, 2007. https://www.theguardian.com/world/2007/aug/12/artnews.art

41 Maslen, Kylie. *Show Me Where it Hurts*. Melbourne: Text Publishing, 2020. p.91.

42 *The Bold Type*. 2020. Season 4, episode 13, 'Lost.' Directed by Erin Ehrlich. Aired on 25 June 2020, on Freeform.

43 Oderberg, Isabelle. 'From undercooked statistics to over-simplification: what The Bold Type got wrong about pregnancy loss.' *The Guardian*, 2020. https://www.theguardian.com/tv-and-radio/2020/jul/22/from-undercooked-statistics-to-over-simplification-what-the-bold-type-got-wrong-about-pregnancy-loss

44 *Bluey*. 2020. Season 2, episode 19, 'The Show.' Directed by Richard Jeffery. Aired on 4 April 2020, on Disney.

3: Count on Me

45 Quenby, Sibohan, Ioannis Gallos, Rima Dhillon-Smith, Marcelina Podesek; Mary Stephenson, Joanne Fisher, Jan Brosens, et al. 'Miscarriage matters: the epidemiological, physical, psychological, and economic costs of early pregnancy loss.' *The Lancet* 397, no. 10285 (May 2021): 1658–1667.

46 Jakab, Zsuzsanna. 'Health information – backbone of public health.' *Public Health Panorama* 5, no. 1 (March 2019): 4–6.

47 The Stillbirth Foundation and PWC. 'The economic impacts of stillbirth in Australia.' stillbirthfoundation.org, 2016. https://stillbirthfoundation.org.au/wp-content/uploads/2020/08/Economic-Impacts-of-Stillbirth-2016-PwC.pdf

48 Rice, William R. 'The High Abortion Cost of Human Reproduction.' Preprint, July 2018, https://doi.org/10.1101/372193

49 Cleveland Clinic. 'Female Reproductive System.' my.clevelandclinic.org, reviewed 2022. https://my.clevelandclinic.org/health/articles/9118-female-reproductive-system

50 The British Broadcasting Corporation. 'Nine things that shape your identity before birth.' BBC, accessed 2022. https://www.bbc.co.uk/teach/nine-things-that-shape-your-identity-before-birth/zdwbhbk

51 Linnakaari, Reeta, Nea Helle, Maarit Mentula, Aini Bloigu, Mika Gissler, Oskari Heikinheimo and Maarit Niinimäki. 'Trends in the incidence, rate and treatment of miscarriage – nationwide register-study in Finland, 1998–2016.' *Human Reproduction* 134, no. 11 (November 2019): 2120–2128.

52 Wilcox, Allen, Clarice Weinberg, John O'Connor, Donna Baird, John Schlatterer, Robert Canfield, Glenn Armstrong and Bruce Nisula. 'Incidence of Early Pregnancy Loss.' *The New England Journal of Medicine* 319, no. 4 (July 1988): 189–194.

53 Quenby, Sibohan, Ioannis Gallos, Rima Dhillon-Smith, Marcelina Podesek, Mary Stephenson, Joanne Fisher, Jan Brosens, et al. 'Miscarriage matters: the epidemiological, physical, psychological, and economic costs of early pregnancy loss.' *The Lancet* 397, no. 10285 (May 2021): 1658–1667.

54 Hure, Alexis, Jennifer Powers, Gita Mishra, Danielle Herbert, Julie Byles and Deborah Loxton. 'Miscarriage, Preterm Delivery, and Stillbirth: Large Variations in Rates within a Cohort of Australian Women.' *PLoS One* 7, no. 5 (2012): e37109. https://doi.org/10.1371/journal.pone.0037109

55 Wilcox, Allen, Clarice Weinberg, John O'Connor, Donna Baird, John Schlatterer, Robert Canfield, Glenn Armstrong and Bruce Nisula. 'Incidence of Early Pregnancy Loss.' *The New England Journal of Medicine* 319, no. 4 (July 1988): 189–194.

56 Office of the DiPHR Director. 'Longitudinal Investigation of Fertility and the Environment (LIFE) Study.' National Institute of Child Health and Human Developed, reviewed 2021. https://www.nichd.nih.gov/about/org/diphr/od/research/longitudinal

57 Watkins, Adam. 'How men's damaged sperm could play significant role in recurrent miscarriage.' The Conversation, 2019. https://theconversation.com/how-mens-damaged-sperm-could-play-significant-role-in-recurrent-miscarriage-109683

58 Rossen, Lauren M., Katherine A. Ahrens and Amy M. Branum. 'Trends in Risk of Pregnancy Loss Among US Women, 1990–2011.' *Paediatric and Perinatal Epidemiology* 32, no. 1 (January 2018): 19–29.

59 Nonaka, Koichi, Teiji Miura and Karl Peter. 'Recent Fertility Decline in Dariusleut Hutterites: An Extension of Eaton and Mayer's Hutterite Fertility Study.' *Human Biology* 66, no. 3 (1994): 411–420.

60 Newman, Jade, Repon Paul, and Georgina Chambers. 'Assisted reproductive technology in Australia and New Zealand 2019.' Sydney: National Perinatal Epidemiology and Statistics Unit, the University of New South Wales, 2021.

61 Australian Institute of Health and Welfare. 'Separation statistics by principal diagnosis (ICD-10-AM 10th edition), Australia, 2018–19.' aihw.gov.au, 2019. https://www.aihw.gov.au/reports/hospitals/principal-diagnosis-data-cubes/contents/data-cubes

62 Homer, Hayden Anthony. 'Modern Management of Recurrent Miscarriage.' *Australian and New Zealand Journal of Obstetrics and Gynaecology* 59, no. 1 (February 2019): 36–44.

63 Andersen, Anne-Marie Nybo, Jan Wohlfahrt, Peter Christens, Jørn Olsen and Mads Melbye. 'Maternal age and fetal loss: population based register linkage study.' *British Medical Journal* 320, no. 7251 (June 2000): 1708–1712.

4: Bad Medicine

64 Green, Lawrence W. 'Closing the Chasm between Research and Practice: Evidence of and for Change: L. W. Green.' *Health Promotion Journal of Australia* 25, no. 1 (April 2014): 25–29.

65 Australia Institute of Health and Welfare. 'More patients, longer waiting times for both elective surgery and emergency department care.' aihw.gov.au, 2019. https://www.aihw.gov.au/news-media/media-releases/2019/december/more-patients-longer-waiting-times-for-both-electi

66 The Royal Australian College of General Practitioners. 'General Practice: Health of the Nation 2019.' East Melbourne, VIC: RACGP, 2019. p.53.

67 Jackson, Gabrielle. *Pain and Prejudice.* Sydney: Allen & Unwin, 2019.

68 Ibid. p.319.

69 Merone, Lea. 'The unattractive truth about misogyny in medicine and medical research.' Croakey Health Media, 2019. https://www.croakey.org/the-unattractive-truth-about-misogyny-in-medicine-and-medical-research/

70 Angstmann, Melanie, Cindy Woods and Caroline M. De Costa. 'Gender Equity in Obstetrics and Gynaecology – Where Are We Heading?' *Australian and New Zealand Journal of Obstetrics and Gynaecology* 59, no. 2 (April 2019): 177–180.

71 Mackee, Nicole. 'A new generation.' *The Medical Journal of Australia* 197, no. 5 (September 2015). https://www.mja.com.au/journal/2012/197/5/new-generation

72 Australian Government Department of Health. 'Obstetrics & Gynaecology: 2016 Factsheet.' hwd.health.gov.au, 2016. https://hwd.health.gov.au/resources/publications/factsheet-mdcl-obstetrics-gynaecology-2016.pdf

73 Farren, Jessica, Maria Jalmbrant, Lieveke Ameye, Karen Joash, Nicola Mitchell-Jones, Sophie Tapp, Dirk Timmerman and Tom Bourne. 'Post-Traumatic Stress, Anxiety and Depression Following Miscarriage or Ectopic Pregnancy: A Prospective Cohort Study.' *BMJ Open* 6, no. 11 (November 2016): e011864.

74 Quenby, Siobhan, Ioannis Gallos, Rima Dhillon-Smith, Marcelina Podesek, Mary Stephenson, Joanne Fisher, Jan Brosens, et al. 'Miscarriage Matters: The Epidemiological, Physical, Psychological, and Economic Costs of Early Pregnancy Loss.' *The Lancet* 397, no. 10285 (May 2021): 1658–1667.

75 Blackmore, Emma Robertson, Denise Côté-Arsenault, Wan Tang, Vivette Glover, Jonathan Evans, Jean Golding and Thomas G. O'Connor. 'Previous Prenatal Loss as a Predictor of Perinatal Depression and Anxiety.' *British Journal of Psychiatry* 198, no. 5 (May 2011): 373–378.

76 'Miscarriage: Worldwide Reform of Care Is Needed.' *The Lancet* 397, no. 10285 (May 2021): 1597.

77 Quenby, Sibohan; Ioannis Gallos; Rima Dhillon-Smith; Marcelina Podesek; Mary Stephenson; Joanne Fisher; Jan Brosens et al. 'Miscarriage matters: the epidemiological, physical, psychological, and economic costs of early pregnancy loss.' *The Lancet* 397, no. 10285 (May 2021): 1658–1667.

78 Coomarasamy, Arri, Rima K Dhillon-Smith, Argyro Papadopoulou, Maya Al-Memar, Jane Brewin, Vikki M Abrahams, Abha Maheshwari, et al. 'Recurrent Miscarriage: Evidence to Accelerate Action.' *The Lancet* 397, no. 10285 (May 2021): 1675–1682.

79 Better Health Channel. 'Patient-centred care explained.' betterhealth.vic.gov. au, reviewed 2015. https://www.betterhealth.vic.gov.au/health/servicesandsupport/patient-centred-care-explained

80 Lloyd, Bradley, Mark Elkins and Lesley Innes. 'Barriers and Enablers of Patient and Family Centred Care in an Australian Acute Care Hospital: Perspectives of Health Managers.' *Patient Experience Journal* 5, no. 3 (November 2018): 55–64.

81 McCormack, Brendan, Jan Dewing and Tanya McCance. 'Developing person–centred care: addressing contextual challenges through practice development.' *Online Journal of Issues in Nursing* 16(2), no. 3.

82 Luxford, Karen, Dana Gelb Safran and Tom Delbanco. 'Promoting patient-centered care: a qualitative study of facilitators and barriers in healthcare organizations with a reputation for improving the patient experience.' *International Journal for Quality in Health Care* 23, no. 5 (October 2011): 510–515.

83 Engel, Joyce and Lynn Rempel. 'Health Professionals' Practices and Attitudes About Miscarriage.' *MCN: The American Journal of Maternal/Child Nursing* 41, no. 1 (January 2016): 51–57.

84 Diamond, David J. and Martha O. Diamond. 'Parenthood after reproductive loss: How psychotherapy can help with postpartum adjustment and parent-infant attachment.' *Psychotherapy* 54, no. 4 (December 2017): 373–379.

85 Cheng, Connie Yu Heng. 'Effects Of Race, Socioeconomic Factors On Emergency Management Of Threatened And Early Pregnancy Loss.' *Yale Medicine Thesis Digital Library* (2016).

86 Oderberg, Isabelle. '"Just a miscarriage": has anything improved in NSW since Jana Horska's shocking experience in 2007?' *The Guardian*, 2021. https://www.theguardian.com/society/2021/sep/26/just-a-miscarriage-has-anything-improved-in-nsw-since-jana-horskas-shocking-experience-in-2007

87 Oderberg, Isabelle. 'Miscarriage is the most common pregnancy complication. So why are we so bad at treating it?' *The Guardian*, 2021. https://www.theguardian.com/commentisfree/2021/oct/13/miscarriage-is-the-most-common-pregnancy-complication-so-why-are-we-so-bad-at-treating-it

5: Fast Car

88 Duckett, Stephen. 'Young people dropping private health hurts insurers most, not public hospitals.' The Conversation, 2020. https://theconversation.com/young-people-dropping-private-health-hurts-insurers-most-not-public-hospitals-132004

89 Australian Prudential Regulation Authority. 'Quarterly private health statistics.' apra.gov.au, 2022. https://www.apra.gov.au/quarterly-private-health-insurance-statistics

90 Australian Institute of Health and Welfare, *Australia's mothers and babies*. (Canberra, ACT, 2022), https://www.aihw.gov.au/reports/mothers-babies/australias-mothers-babies/contents/labour-and-birth/place-of-birth

91 Australian Institute of Health and Welfare, *Australia's mothers and babies*. (Canberra, ACT, 2022), https://www.aihw.gov.au/reports/mothers-babies/australias-mothers-babies/contents/labour-and-birth/place-of-birth

92 Department of Health. 'Australia's Future Health Workforce – Obstetrics and Gynaecology.' health.gov.au, 2018. https://www.health.gov.au/sites/default/files/documents/2021/03/obstetrics-and-gynaecology-australia-s-future-health-workforce-report.pdf

93 Hutchens, Gareth. 'Want to know how much a job pays? Here's the income for hundreds of Australian occupations.' ABC News, 2021. https://www.abc.net.au/news/2021–06–13/income-averages-for-different-occupations-jobs/100209972

94 Women's Ultrasound Melbourne. 'Screening for Chromosomal Abornormalities in Pregnancy.' womensultrasound.com.au. https://womensultrasound.com.au/services/screening/

95 Ross, Loretta and Rickie Solinger. *Reproductive Justice: An Introduction*, 1st edition. Berkeley: University of California Press, 2017, p.47.

96 Quann, Jack. 'Man says trying to console his wife through text as she miscarried was "barbaric".' Newstalk, 2021. https://www.newstalk.com/news/man-says-trying-to-console-his-wife-through-text-as-she-miscarried-was-barbaric-1212904

6: Rolling in the Deep

97   Wheeler, Sara Rich. 'After Perinatal Loss.' *Journal of Obstetric, Gynecologic & Neonatal Nursing* 21, no. 2 (March 1992): 140.

98   Riggs, Damien W., Ruth Pearce, Carla A. Pfeffer, Sally Hines, Francis Ray White and Elisabetta Ruspini. 'Men, Trans/Masculine, and Non-Binary People's Experiences of Pregnancy Loss: An International Qualitative Study.' *BMC Pregnancy and Childbirth* 20, no. 1 (December 2020): 482.

99   Zucker, Jessica. *I Had a Miscarriage: A Memoir, a Movement.* New York: Feminist Press, 2021, p.13.

100 Côté-Arsenault, Denise and Mary-T. B. Dombeck. 'Maternal Assignment of Fetal Personhood To a Previous Pregnancy Loss: Relationship to Anxiety in The Current Pregnancy.' *Health Care for Women International* 22, no. 7 (October 2001): 649–665.

101 Deegan, Mary Jo and Michael R. Hill. *Women and Symbolic Interaction.* London: Allen & Unwin, 1987, p.232.

102 Jansen, Charlotte. 'Foetus 18 Weeks: the greatest photograph on the 20th century?' *The Guardian*, 2019. https://www.theguardian.com/artanddesign/2019/nov/18/foetus-images-lennart-nilsson-photojournalist

103 Withycombe, Shannon. *Lost: Miscarriage in Nineteenth-Century America.* New Brunswick: Rutgers University Press, 2018, p.168.

104 Freidenfelds, Lara. *The Myth of the Perfect Pregnancy: A History of Miscarriage in America.* New York: Oxford University Press, 2019. p.84.

105 Ibid. p.84.

106 Layne, Linda L. *Motherhood Lost: A Feminist Account of Pregnancy Loss in America.* New York: Routledge, 2003, p.118.

107 Freidenfelds, Lara. *The Myth of the Perfect Pregnancy: A History of Miscarriage in America.* New York: Oxford University Press, 2019. p.109.

108 Woodburn, Woody. 'Woodburn: Faithful vow to remember thee.' VC Star, 2021. https://www.vcstar.com/story/opinion/columnists/2021/07/09/woodburn-faithful-vow-remember-thee/7906000002/

109 Beutel, Manfred, Hans Willner, Rainer Deckardt, Michael Von Rad and Herbert Weiner. 'Similarities and Differences in Couples' Grief Reactions Following a Miscarriage: Results from a Longitudinal Study.' *Journal of Psychosomatic Research* 40, no. 3 (March 1996): 245–253.

110 Wheeler, Sara Rich. 'Psychosocial Needs of Women During Miscarriage or Ectopic Pregnancy.' *AORN Journal* 60, no. 2 (August 1994): 221–231.

111 Engel, Joyce and Lynn Rempel. 'Health Professionals' Practices and Attitudes About Miscarriage.' *MCN: The American Journal of Maternal/Child Nursing* 41, no. 1 (January 2016): 51–57.

112 Côté-Arsenault, Denise and Mary-T. B. Dombeck. 'Maternal Assignment of Fetal Personhood To a Previous Pregnancy Loss: Relationship to Anxiety in The Current Pregnancy.' *Health Care for Women International* 22, no. 7 (October 2001): 649–665.

113 Taft, Angela J and Lyndsey F Watson. 'Depression and Termination of Pregnancy (Induced Abortion) in a National Cohort of Young Australian Women: The Confounding Effect of Women's Experience of Violence.' *BMC Public Health* 8, no. 1 (December 2008): 75.

7: We're All in This Together

114 Miller, Ellena J., Meredith J. Temple-Smith and Jade E. Bilardi. '"There Was Just No-One There to Acknowledge That It Happened to Me as Well": A Qualitative Study of Male Partner's Experience of Miscarriage.' Edited by Virginia Zweigenthal. *PLOS ONE* 14, no. 5 (May 2019): e0217395.

115 Nguyen, Van, Meredith Temple-Smith and Jade Bilardi. 'Men's Lived Experiences of Perinatal Loss: A Review of the Literature.' *Australian and New Zealand Journal of Obstetrics and Gynaecology* 59, no. 6 (December 2019): 757–766. https://doi.org/10.1111/ajo.13041.

116 Voss, Pauline, Maren Schick, Laila Langer, Asrin Ainsworth, Beate Ditzen, Thomas Strowitzki, Tewes Wischmann and Ruben J. Kuon. 'Recurrent Pregnancy Loss: A Shared Stressor – Couple-Orientated Psychological Research Findings.' *Fertility and Sterility* 114, no. 6 (December 2020): 1288–1296.

117 Creagh, Sunanda. 'Pregnancy loss linked to depression in young men.' The Conversation, 2011. https://theconversation.com/pregnancy-loss-linked-to-depression-in-young-men-2683

118 Puddifoot, John E., and Martin P. Johnson. 'Active Grief, Despair and Difficulty Coping: Some Measured Characteristics of Male Response Following Their Partner's Miscarriage.' *Journal of Reproductive and Infant Psychology* 17, no. 1 (February 1999): 89–93.

119 Cohen, Jon. *Coming To Term: Uncovering The Truth About Miscarriage.* New Jersey: Rutgers University Press, 2005, p.217.

120 Beutel, Manfred, Hans Willner, Rainer Deckardt, Michael Von Rad and Herbert Weiner. 'Similarities and Differences in Grief Reactions Following a Miscarriage: Results from a Longitudinal Study.' *Journal of Psychosomatic Research* 40, no. 3 (March 1996): 245–253.

121 Obst, Kate Louise, Clemence Due, Melissa Oxlad and Philippa Middleton. 'Men's Grief Following Pregnancy Loss and Neonatal Loss: A Systematic Review and Emerging Theoretical Model.' *BMC Pregnancy and Childbirth* 20, no. 1 (December 2020): 11.

122 Beutel, Manfred, Hans Willner, Rainer Deckardt, Michael Von Rad and Herbert Weiner. 'Similarities and Differences in Couples' Grief Reactions Following a Miscarriage: Results from a Longitudinal Study.' *Journal of Psychosomatic Research* 40, no. 3 (March 1996): 245–253.

123 Gouveia, Aaron and MJ Gouveia. *Men and Miscarriage: A Dad's Guide to Grief, Relationships and Healing After Loss.* New York: Skyhorse Publishing, 2021, p.11.

124 Ibid. p.13.

125 Swanson, Kristen M., Zahra A. Karmali, Suzanne H. Powell and Faina Pulvermakher. 'Miscarriage Effects on Couples' Interpersonal and Sexual Relationships During the First Year After Loss: Women's Perceptions.' *Psychosomatic Medicine* 65, no. 5 (September 2003): 902–910.

126 Ibid.

127 Van Kan, Frankie. 'Shouting Through The Silence.' *Archer*, Issue 15, 2021, p.94.

128 Gouveia, Aaron and MJ Gouveia. *Men and Miscarriage: A Dad's Guide to Grief, Relationships and Healing After Loss*. New York: Skyhorse Publishing, 2021, p.24.

129 hooks, bell. *The Will to Change: Men, Masculinity, and Love*. New York: Atria Books, 2004, p.66.

130 Earle, Sarah, Carol Komaromy and Linda Layne. *Understanding Reproductive Loss: Perspectives on Life, Death and Fertility*. 1st ed. London: Routledge, 2012, p.88.

131 Reilly, Kate. 'Emotional trauma of miscarriage on men is often overlooked.' The Washington Post, 2021. https://www.washingtonpost.com/health/miscarriage-men-grief/2021/07/02/f7d7f388-ceed-11eb-8014-2f3926ca24d9_story.html

132 Lockton, Jane, Clemence Due and Melissa Oxlad. 'Love, Listen and Learn: Grandmothers' Experiences of Grief Following Their Child's Pregnancy Loss.' *Women and Birth* 33, no. 4 (July 2020): 401–407.

133 Lorch, Danna. 'When Losing a Pregnancy Leads to Losing Friends.' The Atlantic, 2022. https://www.theatlantic.com/family/archive/2022/01/pregnant-friend-ghost-after-miscarriage/621297/

134 Keep, Melanie, Samantha Payne and Jane Ellen Carland. 'Experiences of Australian Women on Returning to Work after Miscarriage.' *Community, Work & Family* (October 2021): 1–10.

135 Ibid.

8: I Wanna Be Sedated

136 Layne, Linda L. *Motherhood Lost: A Feminist Account of Pregnancy Loss in America*. New York: Routledge, 2003, p.69.

137 Van Kan, Frankie. 'Shouting Through The Silence.' *Archer*, Issue 15, 2021, p.91.

138 Quenby, Sibohan, Ioannis Gallos, Rima Dhillon-Smith, Marcelina Podesek; Mary Stephenson, Joanne Fisher, Jan Brosens, et al. 'Miscarriage matters: the epidemiological, physical, psychological, and economic costs of early pregnancy loss.' *The Lancet* 397, no. 10285 (May 2021): 1658–1667.

139 Layne, Linda L. *Motherhood Lost: A Feminist Account of Pregnancy Loss in America*. New York: Routledge, 2003, p.109.

140 Riggs, Damien W., Ruth Pearce, Carla A. Pfeffer, Sally Hines, Francis Ray White and Elisabetta Ruspini. 'Men, Trans/Masculine, and Non-Binary People's Experiences of Pregnancy Loss: An International Qualitative Study.' *BMC Pregnancy and Childbirth* 20, no. 1 (December 2020): 482.

141 Lind, Emily R. M. and Angie Deveau. *Interrogating Pregnancy Loss: Feminist Writings on Abortion, Miscarriage, and Stillbirth.* Bradford: Demeter Press, 2017. p. 132.

142 Ibid. p.152.

143 Prior, Matthew, Carmel Bagness, Jane Brewin, Arri Coomarasamy, Lucy Easthope, Barbara Hepworth-Jones, Kim Hinshaw, et al. 'Priorities for Research in Miscarriage: A Priority Setting Partnership between People Affected by Miscarriage and Professionals Following the James Lind Alliance Methodology.' *BMJ Open* 7, no. 8 (August 2017): e016571.

144 Nishmat's Women's Health and Halacha. 'Pregnancy Loss & Neonatal Loss.' yoatzot.org, reviewed 2020. https://www.yoatzot.org/miscarriage/627/

145 Van der Kolk, Bessel. *The Body Keeps the Score: Brain, Mind, and Body in the Healing of Trauma.* New York: Penguin Books, 2015, p.190.

146 Ibid. p.190.

147 Ibid. p.176.

148 Teigen, Chrissy. 'Hi.' Medium, 2020. https://chrissyteigen.medium.com/hi-2e45e6faf764

149 Kint, Esther Lea. 'Women's Experiences of Pregnancy Loss: An Interpretative Phenomenological Analysis.' PhD thesis, Edith Cowan University, 2015, p.343.

150 Brin, Deborah J. 'The Use of Rituals in Grieving for a Miscarriage or Stillbirth.' *Women & Therapy* 27, no. 3–4 (March 2004): 123–132.

151 Limbo, Rana, Kathie Kobler and Elizabeth Levang. 'Respectful Disposition in Early Pregnancy Loss.' *MCN: The American Journal of Maternal/Child Nursing* 35, no. 5 (September 2010): 271–277.

152 Ibid.

153 Regan, Lesley. *Miscarriage: What Every Woman Needs To Know.* 2nd ed. London: Orion Books, 2001, p.231.

154 Australian Human Rights Commission. 'Supporting Working Parents website and online resources.' humanrights.gov.au, 2016. https://humanrights.gov.au/our-work/sex-discrimination/projects/supporting-working-parents-pregnancy-and-return-work-national

155 Ibid.

156 Ibid.

157 Cheryl, 'Disability Discrimination in the Workplace.' Women With Disabilities, 2021. https://wwda.org.au/blog/disability-discrimination-in-the-workplace/

158 Keep, Melanie, Samantha Payne and Jane Ellen Carland. 'Experiences of Australian Women on Returning to Work after Miscarriage.' *Community, Work & Family* (October 2021): 1–10.

159 The British Broadcasting Corporation. 'Now other women won't be haunted by the labour ward.' bbc.com, 2021. https://www.bbc.com/news/uk-scotland-glasgow-west-58348827

160 Dux, Monica. *Things I Didn't Expect (When I Was Expecting).* 1st ed. Melbourne: Melbourne University Press, 2013, p.119.

161 Oderberg, Isabelle. 'When it comes to delivering would-be parents the worst news in the world, we can and must do better.' *The Guardian*, 2022. https://www.theguardian.com/commentisfree/2022/mar/15/when-it-comes-to-delivering-would-be-parents-the-worst-news-in-the-world-we-can-and-must-do-better

9: More Than Words

162 Cohen, Jon. *Coming To Term: Uncovering The Truth About Miscarriage*. New Jersey: Rutgers University Press, 2007, p.102.

163 Layne, Linda L. *Motherhood Lost: A Feminist Account of Pregnancy Loss in America*. New York: Routledge, 2003, p.69.

10: Papa Don't Preach

164 Hughes, Kelly and Eugene Boisvert. 'Coronavirus border restrictions led to an outback ordeal for this Adelaide couple.' ABC News, 2021. https://www.abc.net.au/news/2021–01–05/sa-woman-endures-miscarriage-after-nsw-coronavirus-border-ban/13030750

165 Layne, Linda L. *Motherhood Lost: A Feminist Account of Pregnancy Loss in America*. New York: Routledge, 2003, p.239.

166 Chu, Justin J, Adam J Devall, Leanne E Beeson, Pollyanna Hardy, Versha Cheed, Yongzhong Sun, Tracy E Roberts, et al. 'Mifepristone and Misoprostol versus Misoprostol Alone for the Management of Missed Miscarriage (MifeMiso): A Randomised, Double-Blind, Placebo-Controlled Trial.' *The Lancet* 396, no. 10253 (September 2020): 770–778.

167 Mazza, Danielle; Gwendoline Burton; Simon Wilson; Emma Boulton; Janet Fairweather and Kirsten I Black. 'Medical abortion.' *Australian Journal of General Practice* 49, no. 6 (June 2020): https://doi.org/10.31128/ajgp-02-20-5223

168 Levinson-King, Robin. 'US women are being jailed for having miscarriages.' The BBC, 2021. https://www.bbc.com/news/world-us-canada-59214544

169 Glenza, Jessica. 'Ohio bill orders doctors to "reimplant ectopic pregnancy" or face "abortion murder" charges.' *The Guardian*, 2019. https://www.theguardian.com/us-news/2019/nov/29/ohio-extreme-abortion-bill-reimplant-ectopic-pregnancy

170 Ross, Loretta and Rickie Solinger. *Reproductive Justice: An Introduction*. 1st ed. Berkeley: University of California Press, 2017, p.55.

171 Allen, Amanda and Cari Sietstra. 'Miscarriages Are awful, and Abortion Politics Make Them Worse.' The New York Times, 2021. https://www.nytimes.com/2021/06/22/opinion/miscarriage-abortion.html

172 Reagan, Leslie. 'From Hazard to Blessing to Tragedy: Representations of Miscarriage in Twentieth-Century America.' *Feminist Studies* 29, no. 2 (June 2003): 357–378.

173 Parsons, Kate. 'Feminist Reflections on Miscarriage, in Light of Abortion.' *IJFAB: International Journal of Feminist Approaches to Bioethics* 3, no. 1 (March 2010): 1–22.

174 Huggins, Jackie. *Sister Girl: Reflections on Tidaism, Identity and Reconciliation.* 2nd ed, St Lucia: University of Queensland Press, 2022, p.2.

175 Huggins, Jackie. 'Black Women and Women's Liberation.' *Hecate* 13 (1987): 77.

176 Australian Institute of Health and Welfare. 'Mothers are older, smoking less and having healthy babies.' aihw.gov.au, 2021. https://www.aihw.gov.au/news-media/media-releases/2021–1/august/mothers-are-older-smoking-less-and-having-healthy

177 Decker, Megan. '30 Celebrity Moms Who Had Kids After 40.' Harper's Bazaar, 2019. https://www.harpersbazaar.com/celebrity/latest/g18196402/celebrities-children-after-40-infertility/

178 Bucklow, Andrew. 'Michelle Bridges admits her pregnancy comment was "naive".' News, 2021. https://www.news.com.au/entertainment/celebrity-life/celebrity-kids/michelle-bridges-admits-her-pregnancy-comment-was-naive/news-story/e6f5555387f9b5f51c19669a5a7a1f02

179 Khalil, Shireen. 'IVF and egg freezing: Sonia Kruger opens about the simple procedure that helped her fall pregnant.' News, 2020. https://www.news.com.au/lifestyle/parenting/pregnancy/ivf-and-egg-freezing-sonia-kruger-opens-about-the-simple-procedure-that-helped-her-fall-pregnant/news-story/2afafe62bfe548f08526f7bc85ed34c2

180 Lu, Donna. '"Very pragmatic": 42% of Australian women are open to egg freezing as a work perk.' *The Guardian*, 2021. https://www.theguardian.com/science/2021/jul/13/a-very-pragmatic-decision-42-of-australian-women-are-open-to-egg-freezing-as-a-work-perk

181 Lai, Krista, Erin Garvey, Cristine Velazco, Manrit Gill, Erica Weidler, Kathleen van Leeuwen, Eugene Kim, Erika Rangel and Gwen Grimsby. 'High Fertility Rates and Pregnancy Complications in Female Physicians Indicate a Need for Culture Change.' *Annals of Surgery* online (October 2022): https://doi.org/10.1097/sla.0000000000005724

182 Lu, Donna. '"Very pragmatic": 42% of Australian women are open to egg freezing as a work perk.' *The Guardian*, 2021. https://www.theguardian.com/science/2021/jul/13/a-very-pragmatic-decision-42-of-australian-women-are-open-to-egg-freezing-as-a-work-perk

183 Henriques-Gomes, Luke. 'Australia's jobless benefits will be among worst in OECD after Covid supplement cut.' *The Guardian*, 2020. https://www.theguardian.com/business/2020/sep/08/australias-jobless-benefits-will-be-among-worst-in-oecd-after-covid-supplement-cut

184 Williams, Zoe. 'Unspeakable grief: breaking the silence around terminations for medical reasons.' *The Guardian*, 2021. https://www.theguardian.com/lifeandstyle/2021/aug/09/unspeakable-grief-breaking-the-silence-around-terminations-for-medical-reasons

11: Who Are You?

185 Ross, Loretta and Rickie Solinger. *Reproductive Justice: An Introduction.*
Berkeley: University of California Press, 2017, p.9.

186 Crenshaw, Kimberlé. *Demarginalizing the Intersection of Race and Sex: A Black
Feminist Critique of Antidiscrimination Doctrine, Feminist Theory and Antiracist
Politics.* University of Chicago Legal Forum 140, no. 1 (1989): 139–167.

187 Best, Odette (ed.) and Bronwyn Fredericks (ed.). *Yatdjuligin: Aboriginal And
Torres Strait Islander Nursing and Midwifery Care.* 3rd ed. Cambridge:
University of Cambridge Press, 2021, p.112.

188 Tudor Hart, Julian. 'The Inverse Care Law.' *The Lancet* 297, no. 7696
(February 1971): 405–412.

189 '50 Years of the Inverse Care Law'. *The Lancet* 397, no. 10276 (February 2021): 767.

190 Ross, Loretta and Rickie Solinger. *Reproductive Justice: An Introduction.*
Berkeley: University of California Press, 2017, p.102.

191 Mukherjee, Sudeshna, Digna R. Velez Edwards, Donna D. Bird, David A.
Savitz and Katherine E. Hartmann. 'Risk of Miscarriage Among Black
Women and White Women in a US Prospective Cohort Study.' *American
Journal of Epidemiology* 177, no. 11 (June 2013): 1271–1278.

192 Norsker, Filippa Nyboe, Laura Espenhain, Sofie á Rogvi, Camilla Schmidt
Morgen, Per Kragh Andersen and Anne-Marie Nybo Andersen.
'Socioeconomic Position and the Risk of Spontaneous Abortion: A Study
within the Danish National Birth Cohort.' *BMJ Open* 2, no. 3 (2012): e001077.

193 Zoila, Miriam. 'A Tale of Two Movements.' Color Lines, 2015. https://
www.colorlines.com/articles/tale-two-movements

194 Ayoola, Adejoke B., Krista Sneller, Tega D. Ebeye, Megan Jongekrijg Dykstra,
Victoria L. Ellens, HaEun Grace Lee, and Gail L. Zandee. 'Preconception
Health Behaviors of Low-Income Women'. *MCN: The American Journal of
Maternal/Child Nursing* 41, no. 5 (September 2016): 293–298.

195 Cheng, Connie Yu Heng. 'Effects Of Race, Socioeconomic Factors On
Emergency Management Of Threatened And Early Pregnancy Loss.' *Yale
Medicine Thesis Digital Library* (2016): 2043.

196 Edwards, Susan; Melanie Birks; Ysanne Chapman and Karen Yates.
'Miscarriage in Australia: The Geographical Inequity of Healthcare Services.'
Australasian Emergency Nursing Journal 19, no. 2 (May 2016): 106–111.

197 Australian Human Rights Commission. 'Indigenous Deaths in Custody:
Chapter 3 Comparison: Indigenous and Non-Indigenous Deaths.' humanrights.
gov.au, 1996. https://humanrights.gov.au/our-work/indigenous-deaths-
custody-chapter-3-comparison-indigenous-and-non-indigenous-deaths

198 Watego, Chelsea, David Singh and Alissa Macoun. *Partnership for Justice in
Health: Scoping Paper on Race, Racism and the Australian Health System.*
Discussion paper. Melbourne: The Lowitja Institute, 2021.

199 Australia Institute of Health and Welfare. 'Access to health services by
Australians with disability.' aihw.gov.au, 2017. https://www.aihw.gov.au/
reports/disability/access-health-services-disability/contents/content

200 Buzwell, Simone. 'Gender Dysphora.' *O&G Magazine* vol. 20, no. 04, p.22.

201 Zucker, Jessica. *I Had A Miscarriage*, 1st ed. New York: The Feminist Press, 2021, p.105.

202 Ross, Loretta and Rickie Solinger. *Reproductive Justice: An Introduction*. Berkeley: University of California Press, 2017, p.197.

203 Riggs, Damien W., Ruth Pearce, Carla A. Pfeffer, Sally Hines, Francis Ray White and Elisabetta Ruspini. 'Men, Trans/Masculine, and Non-Binary People's Experiences of Pregnancy Loss: An International Qualitative Study.' *BMC Pregnancy and Childbirth* 20, no. 1 (December 2020): 482.

204 Lens, Jill Weiber. 'Miscarriage, Stillbirth, & Reproductive Justice.' *Washington University Law Review* 98, no. 2 (2021): 1059–1115.

205 Australian Bureau of Statistics, *COVID-19 Mortality in Australia, Deaths registered to 31 January 2022* (Canberra, ACT, 2022), https://www.abs.gov.au/articles/covid-19-mortality-australia#death-due-to-covid-19-country-of-birth

206 Australian Bureau of Statistics, *COVID-19 Mortality in Australia, Deaths registered to 31 January 2022*. 'Country of Birth' (Canberra, ACT, 2022), https://www.abs.gov.au/articles/covid-19-mortality-australia#deaths-due-to-covid-19-socio-economic-status-seifa-

207 Australian Human Rights Comission. The Involuntary or Coerced Sterilisation of People with Disabilities in Australia. Sydney, NSW: Australian Government, 2012.

208 Fredericks, Bronwyn, Karen Adams, Angus, The Australian Women's Health Network Talking Circle and Judy Gregory (ed.). *National Aboriginal and Torres Strait Islander Women's Health Strategy*. Melbourne, VIC: Australian Women's Health Network, 2010. p.10.

209 Dudgeon, Pat and Abigail Bray. 'Reproductive Justice and Culturally Safe Approaches to Sexual and Reproductive Health for Indigenous Women and Girls.' In *Routledge International Handbook of Women's Sexual and Reproductive Health*, edited by Jane M. Ussher, Joan C. Chrisler and Janette Perz 1st ed. London: Routledge, 2019, 542–555.

12: *Gagil Marrung*

210 Buzzacott, Cherisse. 'I supported other women to have babies but faced my own battle alone.' IndigenousX, 2021. https://indigenousx.com.au/i-supported-other-women-to-have-babies-but-faced-my-own-battle-alone/

211 Australian Bureau of Statistics, *Housing Statistics for Aboriginal and Torres Strait Islanders Peoples*, Cat. no. 4744.0 (Canberra: ACT, 2021), https://www.abs.gov.au/statistics/people/aboriginal-and-torres-strait-islander-peoples/housing-statistics-aboriginal-and-torres-strait-islander-peoples/2021

212 Nelson, Doreen (ed.), Rhonda Marriot (ed.) and Tracy Reibel (ed.). *Ngangk Waangening: Mothers' Stories*. 1st ed. Fremantle: Fremantle Press, 2021, p.55.

213 Ibid. p.52.

214 Best, Odette (ed.) and Bronwyn Fredericks (ed.). *Yatdjuligin: Aboriginal And Torres Strait Islander Nursing and Midwifery Care*. 3rd ed. Cambridge: University of Cambridge Press, 2021, p.52.

215 Dudgeon, Pat and Abigail Bray. 'Reproductive Justice and Culturally Safe Approaches to Sexual and Reproductive Health for Indigenous Women and Girls'. In *Routledge International Handbook of Women's Sexual and Reproductive Health*, edited by Jane M. Ussher, Joan C. Chrisler and Janette Perz, 542–555. Melbourne: Routledge, 2019.

216 Bell, Ann V. '"It's Way out of My League": Low-Income Women's Experiences of Medicalized Infertility.' *Gender & Society* 23, no. 5 (October 2009): 688–709.

217 Griffiths, Emma, Julia V. Marley and David Atkinson. 'Preconception Care in a Remote Aboriginal Community Context: What, When and by Whom?', *International Journal of Environmental Research and Public Health* 17, no. 10 (May 2020): 3702.

218 Ibid.

219 Moreton-Robinson, Aileen. *Talkin' Up to the White Woman: Indigenous Women and Feminism (10th Anniversary Edition)*. Queensland: University of Queensland Press, 2020, p.171.

220 Brady, Susan and Sonia Grover. 'The Sterilisation of Girls and Young Women in Australia.' Australian Human Rights Commission, 1997. https://humanrights.gov.au/our-work/disability-rights/projects/sterilisation-girls-and-young-women-australia-1997-report

221 Ross, Loretta and Rickie Solinger. *Reproductive Justice: An Introduction*. Berkeley: University of California Press, 2017, p.167.

222 Family Matters. 'The Family Matters Report 2020.' familymatters.org.au, 2020. https://www.familymatters.org.au/the-family-matters-report-2020/

223 Hunter, Sue-Anne. 'Family Matters Report 2020 reveals Aboriginal and Torres Strait Islander children continue to be separated from families and culture at an alarming rate.' snaicc.org.au, 2020. https://www.snaicc.org.au/family-matters-report-2020-reveals-aboriginal-and-torres-strait-islander-children-continue-to-be-separated-from-families-and-culture-at-an-alarming-rate/

224 Ross, Loretta and Rickie Solinger. *Reproductive Justice: An Introduction*. Berkeley: University of California Press, 2017, p.96.

225 Best, Odette (ed.) and Bronwyn Fredericks (ed.). *Yatdjuligin: Aboriginal And Torres Strait Islander Nursing and Midwifery Care*. 3rd ed. Cambridge: University of Cambridge Press, 2021, p.65.

13: The Key, The Secret

226 Burrowes, Kelly. 'Gender bias in medicine and medical research is still putting women's health at risk.' The Conversation, 2021. https://theconversation.com/gender-bias-in-medicine-and-medical-research-is-still-putting-womens-health-at-risk-156495

227 Mirin Arthur. 'Gender Disparity in the Funding of Diseases by the U.S. National Institutes of Health.' *J Womens Health* 30, no. 7 (July 2021): 956–963.

228 Jayasena, Channa N, Utsav K Radia, Monica Figueiredo, Larissa Franklin Revill, Anastasia Dimakopoulou, Maria Osagie, Wayne Vessey, Lesley Regan, Rajendra Rai and Waljit S Dhillo. 'Reduced Testicular Steroidogenesis and Increased Semen Oxidative Stress in Male Partners as Novel Markers of Recurrent Miscarriage.' *Clinical Chemistry* 65, no. 1 (January 2019): 161–169.

229 Science Mueseum. 'Thalidomide.' sciencemueseum.org.uk, 2019. https://www.sciencemuseum.org.uk/objects-and-stories/medicine/thalidomide

230 Cancer Australia. 'Cervical Cancer.' canceraustralia.gov.au, accessed 2022. https://www.canceraustralia.gov.au/node/4003

231 Dux, Monica. *Things I Didn't Expect (When I Was Expecting)*, 1st ed. Melbourne: Melbourne University Press, 2013, p.122.

232 Jauniaux, Eric; Roy G. Farquharson; Ole B. Christiansen and Niek Exalto. 'Evidence-Based Guidelines for the Investigation and Medical Treatment of Recurrent Miscarriage.' *Human Reproduction* 21, no. 9 (June 2006): 2216–2222.

233 Dorothy Warburton. 'Cytogenetics of Reproductive Wastage: From Conception to Birth,' in *Medical Cytogenetics*, ed. Hong Fong L. Mark (Florida, CRC Press, 2000), p.224.

234 Ibid. p. 232.

235 Cohen, Jon. *Coming To Term: Uncovering The Truth About Miscarriage*. New Jersey: Rutgers University Press, 2007, p.44.

236 Ibid. p.45.

237 Robinson, Lynee, Ioaniss Gallos, Sarah Conner, Madhurima Rajkhowa, David Miller, Sheena Lewis, Jackson Kirkman-Brown and Arri Coomarasamy. 'The Effect of Sperm DNA Fragmentation on Miscarriage Rates: A Systematic Review and Meta-Analysis.' *Human Reproduction* 27, no. 10 (October 2012): 2908–2917.

238 Dorothy Warburton. 'Cytogenetics of Reproductive Wastage: From Conception to Birth,' in *Medical Cytogenetics*, ed. Hong Fong L. Mark (Florida, CRC Press, 2000), p.237.

239 Komine-Aizawa, Shihoko, Sohichi Aizawa and Satoshi Hayakawa. 'Periodontal Diseases and Adverse Pregnancy Outcomes.' *Journal of Obstetrics and Gynaecology Research* 45, no. 1 (January 2019): 5–12.

240 Layne, Linda L. *Miscarriage: What Every Woman Needs To Know*. London: Hachette, 2001, p.180.

241 Ibid. p.181.

242 Lashen, Hany. 'Obesity Is Associated with Increased Risk of First Trimester and Recurrent Miscarriage: Matched Case-Control Study.' *Human Reproduction* 19, no. 7 (July 2004): 1644–1646.

243 Coomarasamy, Ari. 'Giving some pregnant women progesterone could prevent 8,450 miscarriages a year, say experts.' Tommy's, 2020. https://www.tommys.org/about-us/charity-news/giving-some-pregnant-women-progesterone-could-prevent-8450-miscarriages-year-say-experts

244 Duncan, Colin. 'Did the NICE Guideline for Progesterone Treatment of Threatened Miscarriage Get It Right?' *Reproduction and Fertility* 3, no. 2 (April 2022): C4–C6. https://doi.org/10.1530/RAF-21–0122

245 Kamalanathan, Sadishkumar; Jaya Prakash Sahoo and Thozhukat Sathyapalan. 'Pregnancy in polycystic ovary syndrome.' *Indian J Endocrinol Metab* 17, no. 1 (2019): 37–43.

246 Min, Yu; Xing Wang; Hang Chen and Guobing Ying. 'The exploration of Hashimoto's Thyroiditis related miscarriage for better treatment modalities.' *Int J Med Sci.* 17, no 16 (2020): 2402–2415.

247 Gaysina, Darya. 'Folic acid in pregnancy – MTHFR gene explains why the benefits may differ.' The Conversation, 2018. https://theconversation.com/folic-acid-in-pregnancy-mthfr-gene-explains-why-the-benefits-may-differ-95302

248 Tamblyn, Jennifer A., Nicole S.P. Pilarski, Alexandra D. Markland, Ella J. Marson, Adam Devall, Martin Hewison, Rachel K. Morris and Arri Coomarasamy. 'Vitamin D and Miscarriage: A Systematic Review and Meta-Analysis.' *Fertility and Sterility* 118, no. 1 (July 2022): 111–122.

249 Zhou, Ang and Elina Hyppönen. 'Vitamin D Deficiency and C-Reactive Protein: A Bidirectional Mendelian Randomization Study.' International Journal of Epidemiology (May 2022) https://doi.org/10.1093/ije/dyac087

250 Gallagher, James. 'Endometriosis "risks miscarriage".' bbc.com, 2015. https://www.bbc.com/news/health-33115478

14: Toxic

251 Layne, Linda L. *Motherhood Lost: A Feminist Account of Pregnancy Loss in America.* New York: Routledge, 2003, p.73.

252 Negro-Vilar, Andres. 'Stress and Other Environmental Factors Affecting Fertility in Men and Women: Overview.' *Environmental Health Perspective* 101, no. 2 (July 1993): 59–64.

253 Cohen, Jon. *Coming To Term: Uncovering The Truth About Miscarriage.* New Jersey: Rutgers University Press, 2007, p.155.

254 Ibid.

255 Short, Kate in *The Sydney Morning Herald*, March 17, 1991, p.18.

256 The British Broadcasting Corporation. 'Pesticide made us sterile, banana workers say.' bbc.com, 2022. https://www.bbc.co.uk/news/world-latin-america-62120058

257 Greenwood, Michael. 'Commonly used chemicals associated with miscarriage, Yale School of Public Health study finds.' Yale School of Medicine, 2020. https://medicine.yale.edu/news-article/commonly-used-chemicals-associated-with-miscarriage-yale-school-of-public-health-study-finds/

258 National Institute of Environmental Health Sciences. 'Endocrine Disruptors.' niehs.nih.gov, 2022. https://www.niehs.nih.gov/health/topics/agents/endocrine/

259 Carrington, Damian. 'Microplastics found in human blood for first time.' *The Guardian*, 2022. https://www.theguardian.com/environment/2022/mar/24/microplastics-found-in-human-blood-for-first-time

260 Environment Protection and Heritage Council. *NChEM: A National Framework for Chemicals Management in Australia: Discussion Paper*. Adelaide, S. Aust.: Environment Protection and Heritage Council, 2005, p.6.

261 Bray, Karina. 'What you need to know about endocrine-disrupting chemicals.' Choice, 2019. https://www.choice.com.au/health-and-body/beauty-and-personal-care/skin-care-and-cosmetics/articles/endocrine-disrupting-chemicals

262 Zanolli, Lauren and Mark Oliver. 'Explained: the toxic threat in everyday products, from toys to plastic.' *The Guardian*, 2019. https://www.theguardian.com/us-news/2019/may/22/toxic-chemicals-everyday-items-us-pesticides-bpa

263 Office of the DiPHR Director Research. 'Reproductive Endocrinology.' nichd.nih.gov, 2021. https://www.nichd.nih.gov/about/org/dir/dph/od/research/longitudinal

264 Rossen, Lauren M., Katherine A. Ahrens and Amy M. Branum. 'Trends in Risk of Pregnancy Loss Among US Women, 1990–2011.' *Paediatric and Perinatal Epidemiology* 32, no. 1 (January 2018): 19–29.

265 Noosa Council. 'The Noosa River Plan: Whole of catchment management.' noosa.qld.gov.au, 2019. https://www.noosa.qld.gov.au/downloads/file/2726/draft-noosa-river-plan-2019-ver-2 (page 23)

266 Oderberg, Isabelle. 'Air grievances: silence swirls around the toll of bushfire smoke during pregnancy.' *The Guardian*, 2021. https://www.theguardian.com/lifeandstyle/2021/jan/11/air-grievances-silence-swirls-around-the-toll-of-bushfire-smoke-during-pregnancy

267 Zhang, Liqiang, Weiwei Liu, Kun Hou, Jintai Lin, Chenghu Zhou, Xiaohua Tong, Ziye Wang, et al. 'Air Pollution-Induced Missed Abortion Risk for Pregnancies.' *Nature Sustainability* 2, no. 11 (November 2019): 1011–1017.

268 Leiser, Claire L., Heidi A. Hanson, Kara Sawyer, Jacob Steenblik, Ragheed Al-Dulaimi, Troy Madsen, Karen Gibbins, et al. 'Acute Effects of Air Pollutants on Spontaneous Pregnancy Loss: A Case-Crossover Study.' *Fertility and Sterility* 111, no. 2 (February 2019): 341–347.

269 Zhou, Wenzheng, Xin Ming, Qing Chen, Xiaoli Liu, and Ping Yin. 'The Acute Effect and Lag Effect Analysis between Exposures to Ambient Air Pollutants and Spontaneous Abortion: A Case-Crossover Study in China, 2017–2019.' *Environmental Science and Pollution Research* 29, no. 44 (September 2022): 67380–67389.

270 Abdo, Mona, Isabella Ward, Katelyn O'Dell, Bonne Ford, Jeffrey Pierce, Emily Fischer and James Crooks. 'Impact of Wildfire Smoke on Adverse Pregnancy Outcomes in Colorado, 2007–2015.' *International Journal of Environmental Research and Public Health* 16, no. 19 (October 2019): 3720.

271 Oderberg, Isabelle. 'Air grievances: silence swirls around the toll of bushfire smoke during pregnancy.' *The Guardian*, 2021. https://www.theguardian.com/lifeandstyle/2021/jan/11/air-grievances-silence-swirls-around-the-toll-of-bushfire-smoke-during-pregnancy

272 Ibid.

273 Ibid.

274 Oderberg, Isabelle. 'Doctors issue official guidance on effects of air pollution and bushfire smoke on pregnant people.' *The Guardian*, 2021. https://www.theguardian.com/environment/2021/jul/19/doctors-issue-official-guidance-on-effects-of-air-pollution-and-bushfire-smoke-on-pregnant-people

275 Australian Medical Association. 'Climate change is a health emergency.' ama.com.au, 2019. https://www.ama.com.au/media/climate-change-health-emergency

276 Barreca, Alan, Olivier Deschenes and Melanie Guldi. 'Maybe Next Month? Temperature Shocks and Dynamic Adjustments in Birth Rates.' *Demography* 55, no. 4 (August 2018): 1269–1293.

277 Simonis, Magdalena and Kimberly Humphrey. 'Climate change impacts women more than men.' InSight, 2021. https://insightplus.mja.com.au/2021/33/climate-change-impacts-women-more-than-men/

278 Giakoumelou, Sevi, Nick Wheelhouse, Kate Cuschieri, Gary Entrican, Sarah E.M. Howie and Andrew W. Horne. 'The Role of Infection in Miscarriage.' *Human Reproduction* Update 22, no. 1 (January 2016): 116–133.

279 Megli, Christina J. and Carolyn B. Coyne. 'Infections at the Maternal–Fetal Interface: An Overview of Pathogenesis and Defence.' *Nature Reviews Microbiology* 20, no. 2 (February 2022): 67–82.

280 Johri, Mira, Rosa E Morales, Jean-François Boivin, Blanca E Samayoa, Jeffrey S Hoch, Carlos F Grazioso, Ingrid J Barrios Matta, et al. 'Increased Risk of Miscarriage among Women Experiencing Physical or Sexual Intimate Partner Violence during Pregnancy in Guatemala City, Guatemala: Cross-Sectional Study.' *BMC Pregnancy and Childbirth* 11, no. 1 (December 2011): 49.

281 Maconochie, Noreen, Pat Doyle and Rebecca Kate Simmons. 'Risk Factors for First Trimester Miscarriage-Results from a UK-Population-Based Case-Control Study.' *BJOG: An International Journal of Obstetrics & Gynaecology* 114, no. 2 (February 2007): 170–186.

282 Arck, Petra C, Mirjam Rücke, Matthias Rose, Julia Szekeres-Bartho, Alison J Douglas, Maria Pritsch, Sandra M Blois, et al. 'Early Risk Factors for Miscarriage: A Prospective Cohort Study in Pregnant Women.' *Reproductive BioMedicine Online* 17, no. 1 (January 2008): 101–113.

283 INTRuST Clinical Consortium, VA Mid-Atlantic MIRECC Workgroup, PGC PTSD Epigenetics Workgroup, Alicia K. Smith, Andrew Ratanatharathorn, Adam X. Maihofer, Robert K. Naviaux, et al. 'Epigenome-Wide Meta-Analysis of PTSD across 10 Military and Civilian Cohorts Identifies Methylation Changes in AHRR.' *Nature Communications* 11, no. 1 (December 2020): 5965.

284 Eisenberg, Michael L., Zhen Chen, Aijun Ye and Germaine M. Buck Louis. 'Relationship between Physical Occupational Exposures and Health on Semen Quality: Data from the Longitudinal Investigation of Fertility and the Environment (LIFE) Study.' *Fertility and Sterility* 103, no. 5 (May 2015): 1271–1277.

285 Levine, Hagai, Niels Jørgensen, Anderson Martino-Andrade, Jaime Mendiola, Dan Weksler-Derri, Irina Mindlis, Rachel Pinotti and Shanna H

Swan. 'Temporal Trends in Sperm Count: A Systematic Review and Meta-Regression Analysis.' *Human Reproduction Update* 23, no. 6 (November 2017): 646–659.

286 The Observer. 'Shanna Swan: "Most couples may have to use assisted reproduction by 2045".' *The Guardian*, 2021. https://www.theguardian.com/society/2021/mar/28/shanna-swan-fertility-reproduction-count-down

287 Cook, Katsi. 'Cook: Women are the First Environment.' ictnews.org, 2018. https://indiancountrytoday.com/archive/cook-women-are-the-first-environment

288 Your Fertility. 'Chemicals in our environment.' yourfertility.org.au, update 2023. https://www.yourfertility.org.au/everyone/lifestyle/chemicals-our-environment

15: *Video Killed the Radio Star*

289 Australian Broadcast Corporation. 'VIDEO: The Baby Business.' abc.net.au, 2016. https://www.abc.net.au/4corners/the-baby-business-promo/7449646

290 Victorian Assisted Reproductive Treatment Authority. 'One in six women fall pregnant spontaneously after IVF.' varta.org.au, 2019. https://www.varta.org.au/resources/news-and-blogs/one-six-women-fall-pregnant-spontaneously-after-ivf

291 Tommy's. 'Why miscarriage happens.' tommys.org, accessed 2022. https://www.tommys.org/baby-loss-support/miscarriage-information-and-support/miscarriage-statistics#ivf

292 Hogan, Jen. 'Prof Robert Winston: "The Publicity around IVF is very misleading".' *The Irish Times*, 2021. https://www.irishtimes.com/life-and-style/health-family/parenting/prof-robert-winston-the-publicity-around-ivf-is-very-misleading-1.4590525

293 Human Fertilisation & Embryology Authority. 'Press release: Age is the key factor for egg freezing success says new HFEA report, as overall treatment numbers remain low.' hfea.gov.au, 2018. https://www.hfea.gov.uk/about-us/news-and-press-releases/2018-news-and-press-releases/press-release-age-is-the-key-factor-for-egg-freezing-success-says-new-hfea-report-as-overall-treatment-numbers-remain-low/

294 Taylor, Natasha. 'Slater and Gordon investigating class action into IVF add-ons.' Lawyers Weekly, 2021. https://www.lawyersweekly.com.au/biglaw/31303-slater-and-gordon-investigating-class-action-into-ivf-add-ons

295 Manning, Sanchez. 'Couple who spent £20,000 on IVF treatment before shelling out another £7,000 on "add-ons to boost their chances of a baby" become first in the UK to sue over the "worthless and unproven" extras.' Daily Mail UK, 2018. https://www.dailymail.co.uk/news/article-6375673/Couple-spent-20-000-IVF-treatment-7-000-add-ons-UK-sue.html

296 Lensen, Sarah, Karin Hammarberg, Alex Polyakov, Jack Wilkinson, Stephen Whyte, Michelle Peate and Martha Hickey. 'How Common Is Add-on Use

and How Do Patients Decide Whether to Use Them? A National Survey of IVF Patients.' *Human Reproduction* 36, no. 7 (June 2021): 1854–1861.

297 Lensen, Sarah, Sheng Chen, Lucy Goodman, Luk Rombauts, Cindy Farquhar and Karin Hammarberg. 'IVF Add-ons in Australia and New Zealand: A Systematic Assessment of IVF Clinic Websites.' *Australian and New Zealand Journal of Obstetrics and Gynaecology* 61, no. 3 (June 2021): 430–438.

298 Regan, Lesley. *Miscarriage: What Every Woman Needs To Know.* 3rd ed., London: Hachette, 2018, p.93.

299 Kucherov, Alexander, Jessica Atrio and Zev Williams. 'Patient-Controlled Tissue Collection for Genetic Testing after Early Pregnancy Loss: A Pilot Study.' *Prenatal Diagnosis* 38, no. 3 (February 2018): 204–209.

300 Colley, Emily, Adam J. Devall, Helen Williams, Susan Hamilton, Paul Smith, Neil V. Morgan, Siobhan Quenby, Arri Coomarasamy and Stephanie Allen. 'Cell-Free DNA in the Investigation of Miscarriage.' *Journal of Clinical Medicine* 9, no. 11 (October 2020): 3428.

301 Mor, Amir, Mursal Gardezi, Karen Jubanyik, Burcin Simsek, David B. Seifer, Pasquale Patrizio, Ecem Esencan, et al. 'Miscarriage Determination in First Trimester Based on Alpha-Fetoprotein Extracted from Sanitary Pads.' *Fertility and Sterility* 116, no. 2 (August 2021): 462–469.

302 Hayman, Melanie J, Kristie-Lee Alfrey, Kim Waters, Summer Cannon, Gregore I Mielke, Shelley E Keating, Gabriela P Mena, et al. 'Evaluating Evidence-Based Content, Features of Exercise Instruction, and Expert Involvement in Physical Activity Apps for Pregnant Women: Systematic Search and Content Analysis.' *JMIR MHealth and UHealth* 10, no. 1 (January 2022): e31607.

303 Lupton, Deborah and Sarah Pedersen. 'An Australian Survey of Women's Use of Pregnancy and Parenting Apps.' *Women and Birth* 29, no. 4 (August 2016): 368–375.

304 Freidenfelds, Lara. *The Myth of the Perfect Pregnancy: A History of Miscarriage in America.* New York: Oxford University Press, 2019.

305 Buchanan, Limin, Emi Anderson, Huilan Xu MBiostat, Philayrath Phongsavan, Chris Rissel, and Li Ming Wen. 'Sources of Information and the Use of Mobile Applications for Health and Parenting Information during Pregnancy: Implications for Health Promotion.' *Health Informatics Journal* 27, no. 3 (July 2021): https://doi.org/10.1177/14604582211043146

306 West, Robert, Arri Coomarasamy, Lorraine Frew, Rachel Hutton, Jackson Kirkman-Brown, Martin Lawlor, Sheena Lewis, et al. 'Sperm Selection with Hyaluronic Acid Improved Live Birth Outcomes among Older Couples and Was Connected to Sperm DNA Quality, Potentially Affecting All Treatment Outcomes.' *Human Reproduction* 37, no. 6 (May 2022): 1106–1125.

16: Try Again

307 Kangatharan, Chrishny, Saffi Labram and Sohinee Bhattacharya. 'Interpregnancy Interval Following Miscarriage and Adverse Pregnancy

Outcomes: Systematic Review and Meta-Analysis.' *Human Reproduction Update* 23, no. 1 (March 2017): 221–231.

308 Sundermann, Alexandra C., Katherine E. Hartmann, Sarah H. Jones, Eric S. Torstenson and Digna R. Velez Edwards. 'Interpregnancy Interval After Pregnancy Loss and Risk of Repeat Miscarriage.' *Obstetrics & Gynecology* 130, no. 6 (December 2017): 1312–1318.

309 Brigham, Sara, Cathryn Conlon, and Roy Gibb Farquharson. 'A Longitudinal Study of Pregnancy Outcome Following Idiopathic Recurrent Miscarriage'. *Human Reproduction* 14, no. 11 (November 1999): 2868–2871.

310 Ibid.

311 Stray-Pedersen, Babill and Sverre Stray-Pedersen. 'Etiologic Factors and Subsequent Reproductive Performance in 195 Couples with a Prior History of Habitual Abortion.' *American Journal of Obstetrics and Gynecology* 148, no. 2 (January 1984): 140–146.

312 Liddell, Hilary, Neil Pattison and Angi Zanderigo. 'Recurrent Miscarriage - Outcome After Supportive Care in Early Pregnancy.' *The Australian and New Zealand Journal of Obstetrics and Gynaecology* 31, no. 4 (November 1991): 320–322.

16: *The Never-ending Story*

313 Jackson, Eleanor. *Gravidity and Parity*. Melbourne: Vagabond Press, 2021, p.26.

Glossary

314 'Ectopic pregnancy.' The Women's, https://www.thewomens.org.au/health-information/pregnancy-and-birth/pregnancy-problems/early-pregnancy-problems/ectopic-pregnancy

315 'Ectopic pregnancy.' NHS, 2022. https://www.nhs.uk/conditions/ectopic-pregnancy/

316 'Pregnancy & birth.' The Women's, https://www.thewomens.org.au/health-information/pregnancy-and-birth/pregnancy-problems/early-pregnancy-problems/hydatidiform-mole

317 'Hydatidiform mole.' The Women's, https://www.thewomens.org.au/patients-visitors/clinics-and-services/pregnancy-birth/pregnancy-care-options/recurrent-miscarriage-clinic

318 Hong Li, Ying and Anthony Marren. 'Recurrent pregnancy loss: A summary of international evidence-based guidelines and practice.' *Australian Journal of General Practice* 47, no. 7 (July 2018): 432–436.

319 Ibid.

320 'Recurrent miscarriage.' Tommy's, 2020, https://www.tommys.org/pregnancy-information/pregnancy-complications/baby-loss/miscarriage/recurrent-miscarriage